Natural Labor and Birth

An Evidence-Based Guide to the Natural Birth Plan

An Evidence-Based Guide to the Natural Birth Plan

MICHELLE ARISTIZABAL, MD, FACOG

President, Owner, and Principal Physician in ObGyn
Wombkeepers Obstetrics and Gynecology and Maternity Wellness Center
Attending Physician, St. Barnabas Medical Center and Hackensack Meridian Health
Mountainside Medical Center
Montclair, New Jersey

Mc
Graw
Hill
Education

New York Chicago San Francisco Athens London Madrid
Mexico City Milan New Delhi Singapore Sydney Toronto

Natural Labor and Birth: An Evidence-Based Guide to the Natural Birth Plan

1 2 3 4 5 6 7 8 9   DSS   23 22 21 20 19 18

ISBN 978-1-259-86287-8
MHID 1-259-86287-9

This book was set in WarnockPro-Light by MPS Limited
The editors were Andrew Moyer and Christie Naglieri
The production supervisor was Richard Ruzycka
Project management was provided by MPS Limited
Photographs were provided by Holland Logan, Violet's Bloom Photography.
The cover designer was Randommatrix.
This book is printed on acid-free paper.

Library of Congress Cataloging-in-Publication Data

Names: Aristizabal, Michelle, author.
Title: Natural labor and birth: an evidence-based guide to the natural birth
    plan / editors, Michelle Aristizabal, MD, FACOG, President, Owner,
    and Principle Physician in ObGyn, Wombkeepers Obstetrics and Gynecology
    and Maternity Wellness Center, Montclair, New Jersey, Attending Physician,
    St. Barnabas Medical Center and Hackensack Meridian Health, Mountainside
    Medical Center, Montclair, New Jersey.
Description: New York : McGraw-Hill, [2019]
Identifiers: LCCN 2018013861 | ISBN 9781259862878 (paperback)
Subjects: LCSH: Pregnancy—Popular works. | Natural childbirth—Popular works. |
    Midwives—Popular works. | Obstetricians—Popular works. | BISAC: MEDICAL /
    Gynecology & Obstetrics.
Classification: LCC RG525 .A75 2018 | DDC 618.4—dc23
LC record available at https://na01.safelinks.protection.outlook.
    com/?url=https%3A%2F%2Flccn.loc.gov%2F2018013861&data=01%7C01%7Cleah.
    carton%40mheducation.com%7Cd0b5a46050484e1d19c708d5903093ba%7Cf919b1ef
    c0c347358fca0928ec39d8d5%7C0&sdata=nC3ajDNklzJEmIzNQ%2BeaRMw%2FfiFX
    HkdkI5QMT6Kpt4c%3D&reserved=0

This book is dedicated to the many mothers who constantly challenge us to find better, safer, and kinder options for childbirth.

ABOUT THE AUTHOR

Michelle Aristizabal, MD, FACOG, is a board-certified General Obstetrician and Gynecologist in Montclair, New Jersey. She runs a busy, private practice with a special focus on supporting women who desire low-intervention, unmedicated births. Dr. Aristizabal earned her medical degree from the University of Arizona and completed her obstetrics residency training at Saint Barnabas Medical Center in Livingston, New Jersey. As an attending physician, she has worked tirelessly to expand the acceptance of natural birth practices within her local medical community and 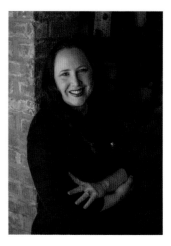 educates medical students and resident physicians in alternative labor management techniques. When she's not delivering babies, she and her husband of fourteen years are busy with their own two incredible children, who fill their lives with much hilarity and love. Dr. A, as she's known to her patients, also enjoys hiking, archery, and various creative pursuits, including painting and writing poetry and fiction.

CONTENTS

My journey into natural birth began late in my training as an obstetrician. My residency occurred within a classic, heavy-intervention obstetrics program, although I had attended a very open and liberal medical school which informed many of my core beliefs regarding patient autonomy and the role of medical intervention and alternative medicine. In my last year of residency, I found myself in the uncomfortable role of the patient, pregnant with my second child. I had given birth to my first child via cesarean section and was determined to avoid a second surgery. I quickly realized how few options I had for a vaginal delivery, even within my own hospital, where I was a senior resident. I began researching both medical and lay literature in an effort to identify any strategies that might increase my chances of a successful VBAC. In doing so, I discovered an entirely different philosophy toward childbirth and the very loud outcry from women who were unhappy having babies in the manner in which I had been taught. Although I had delivered over a thousand babies by this point in my career, I was completely ignorant about natural birth practices and the large movement away from medically managed birth. I also discovered that the medical evidence in support of the standard labor management I performed on any given day was lacking. I learned natural birth techniques, many of which made perfect sense from my knowledge of anatomy and labor physiology and applied them to my own birth. My son was born vaginally 2 months prior to my graduation.

As a new attending, I found myself eager to support women who wanted to have babies in a different way. I continued reading as many books and journal articles that I could find regarding alternative approaches to labor management and attended workshops and conferences given by midwives, childbirth educators, doulas, and other "birthworkers" in order to learn better techniques for supporting naturally laboring mothers. My own mother also completed training in doula support, childbirth education, and lactation support and helped to expand my knowledge base as she worked with patients and began to support my practice. She also helped me to understand how much resistance naturally laboring women faced when the doctor left the room.

Word of the young obstetrician supporting natural birth and VBAC quickly spread throughout my community and within a year of graduating residency, I found myself with a very busy, primarily natural birthing practice. Within 2 years, I had opened a solo medical practice, dedicated to helping women achieve unmedicated deliveries and VBACs, which included childbirth education, doula support, prenatal yoga, and lactation counseling and support groups. However, as I attempted to help my patients reach their goals, I frequently found myself in conflict with the institution that had trained me, mainly the nurses and other doctors who were uncomfortable with my patients ambulating, eating, and spending more time in labor. The goal of my literature searches rapidly transitioned from self-education to defense of my management and my patients' labor plans. I spent many hours in the hospital library pulling articles in order to support how I was caring for a woman laboring upstairs. I began to wish for a better resource that I could draw upon when these challenges arose. This recognition of the need for a single, evidence-based resource for natural birth practices was furthered over the years by the increasing number of colleagues who began to reach out to me for information and article links to help them care for their own patients.

The aim of this book is to make the case for natural labor as a reasonable, evidence-based, alternative to aggressive labor management in a way that is valuable to both women exploring their birth options and the doctors, midwives, nurses, doulas, and other individuals caring for them. It does this through a thorough, scientific examination of each of the points of a typical natural birth plan. It also offers alternative, nonmedical strategies for common labor challenges and a framework for care providers and patients to work together toward satisfying birth processes and outcomes. At times, this goal was frustrated by a lack of evidence regarding common natural birthing requests; however, in these situations I made a strong effort to also demonstrate, if applicable, the lack of evidence for denying a certain birth request. I approached this project from the ethical viewpoint that, as most natural birth requests constitute the avoidance of intervention and maintenance of normalcy in the birth process, the burden of proof should fall to the intervention, not the other way around.

I am extremely grateful to McGraw-Hill Education for taking on this unusual project and considering it an important addition to the body of educational resources regarding childbirth. I am especially appreciative of my editor Andrew Moyer, who believed in this lofty idea of mine and helped it become a reality, patiently guiding a novice author and busy doctor through the writing process. I would also like to acknowledge the teachers and mentors throughout my medical training who have encouraged me to continue striving to learn more and be better for my patients. To the staff of Saint Barnabas Medical Center and Mountainside Medical Center, despite our moments of conflict, I know without your willingness to be open to new ideas, as well as challenge them, this book would not exist and I will always be appreciative for your support of both me and our shared patients. Finally, I would like to express my love and gratitude for my husband and children, who have unconditionally loved and supported me even when they have had to share me far too often with this calling, and my mother, Catherine Galle, who has always nurtured my every dream and built the vision that truly enabled us all to become wombkeepers.

MICHELLE ARISTIZABAL, MD, FACOG

The Battle for Natural Birth in the American Maternity System

Change, before you have to.

—Jack Welch

Understanding the Motives for the Natural Birth Movement and Why the Medical Community Needs to Embrace It

REMEMBERING SOPHIA

That summer was in the year of the seventeen year cicada. First, we saw only their shells haunting the trees and bushes and occasionally the children would find one of the strange moths on the driveway, breathing out its last bit of life after waiting under the ground for so many years. An entire existence in the dark for this one moment in the sunshine, this one moment's claim on immortality.

With the warming days, swarms seemed to appear over night. As I peeled a sticky child from my chest with one hand, reaching with my other to silence the beeping phone that was causing him to stir, I heard their machinery-like love song over the hum of the window air conditioner. I tiptoed around the house, feeling the heat of the day beginning to sink in even at the early hour and, as I stepped outside, the full chorus of the cicada greeted me. For a moment, it sounded like an alarm sounding all around me. The heaviness of the air clung to me and every other living thing. The overgrown grass in our unkempt yard seemed to sweat. I placed my bags in the car and forced myself in, turning on the air-conditioning as quickly as I could. I took a long slow breath and felt a day's worth of fatigue already overwhelming me. It was a bad day to be covering the labor floor.

My drive to the hospital was a quick one. We had bought our house several years before with the single goal of a very quick commute. When you spend as many continuous hours locked inside a brick building as I did, the thought of spending any significant amount of time getting there and back is unconscionable. Though, as far as hospitals go, it was a nice one. Set in the green suburban hills a short distance from New York City, it had a more serene ambiance than most. The grounds were always perfectly manicured with new seasonal flowers appearing each month. There were even beautiful gardens, ponds, and walking paths designed for the emotional well-being of patients, staff, and other guests, though I know very few staff who had ever seen them. The hallways in the main entrance were marble and friendly women greeted you upon entering. Each day, one of the local florists brought a fresh arrangement of flowers for the entry. It all made for a nice picture on the pamphlets and billboards advertising maternity services to the community. Only the creaking and stalling of the elevators revealed the building's age and the administration's reluctance to address bare bones issues. Compared to some of the more urban hospitals I had visited while exploring residency options, it was a paradise.

The morning started off quiet enough. After getting the morning report, I went to see a few patients who had delivered their babies with other physicians in my coverage group in the days before. The list was typical, fairly evenly split between women who had vaginal deliveries and the less fortunate women who had their babies in an operating room. Our labor and delivery unit was a busy one, where close to six thousand babies entered the world each year. The high risk care and neonatology unit were some of the most highly regarded in the country and most patients came for access to that level of care, should they need it.

The close to even split in mode of delivery had earned our hospital a place on the national naughty list of "bad" "high intervention" hospitals with unnecessarily high cesarean section rates. Occasionally, demonstrators would gather outside the hospital and hold a little protest to warn the public about all the supposed inappropriate things that went on inside. There was even a book that used our hospital as a central illustration of the many broken things about the obstetrical system in America.[1] However, as I went from woman to woman that day and read the reasons for their cesarean, I did not find glaring examples of cesareans that should not have been performed. Most of the indications fell into the "shrug" category. Maybe if the patient had not received an epidural so early, maybe if they had not broken her water, maybe if they did not start this medicine, something could have gone differently, but who could know for sure? It was a big baby. The baby was in a bad position and the fetal heart rate tracing did not look good. Maybe no matter what the woman, the residents, her nurses, or her doctor had done, she would have ended up in the same place, with her baby born the same way just under a different set of circumstances. For myself, I could not think of a single cesarean I had performed as an attending obstetrician where, at the time I headed into the operating room, I did not feel I had exhausted every other option. It was a subject that frequently occupied my mind as I tried to keep my own cesarean rate low and as the hospital pushed for more and more reforms to improve their overall rate. Where did this very normal activity of having babies really all fall apart?

As the day wore on, the rooms on labor and delivery quickly began to fill. The heat brought them out in droves. Tired doctor after tired doctor entered the unit, sweat still dripping from their foreheads from the walk through the parking lot. Just as one room emptied, another belly, either in labor or simply wanting to be, occupied it again. Baby after baby rolled down the hallway. However, even by the afternoon, no patient had arrived for me to care for. I was the service doctor, there to provide care for any patient who showed up without a private physician to care for them, and I was feeling the nervous charm of my good fortune at having no work before me.

Every few hours, I emerged from my call room to inspect "The Board," a listing of all the patients in labor that was hung in the center of the labor and delivery nursing station. Each patient was indicated by room number, doctor, number of previous babies they had borne, cervical exam, whether their water was broken, and what medications they were receiving. On most days, the entire patient list would have a "P" in the medication column, which indicated that they were receiving pitocin, a synthetic variant of the natural hormone oxytocin that brings about contractions. Nearly half the patients on any given day would have also been induced and had their membranes artificially ruptured. There was not a question of whether a patient was going to receive an epidural for pain management during labor, it was simply a matter of when the check appeared in the box to indicate that it was done.

My good luck came crashing to a halt twenty minutes after five, just as I was sitting down to my recently delivered nochi bolognese. One of the junior residents called, her voice urgent with concern on the other end of the phone.

"We just brought a patient to room nine. She is fully dilated but the baby's heart rate is down."

Unimpressed, assuming the patient was going to rapidly deliver, I reluctantly pushed back from my meal and asked, "Who is her doctor?"

"She doesn't have one. She got her care with some midwife."

Now I was interested. I briskly walked from my call room to the Labor and Delivery unit and entered the frantic room nine, where two residents were yelling at the woman to push while the patient was screaming and flailing out of control. Several nurses were slamming cabinet doors, quickly assembling delivery equipment, and preparing the infant warmer for a resuscitation. Multiple alarms were sounding over the methodical thudding of the fetal heart rate monitor, it's slow sound obvious enough to make an actual observation of the heart rate unwarranted. As is my typical response to a crisis situation, I became very calm and quiet. I walked to the cabinet and retrieved a pair of gloves, while simultaneously questioning the residents.

"What number baby is this for her?"

"Second, previous baby was section."

"She's a VBAC?" I demanded incredulously. The situation now much more dire. The resident nervously nodded in assent.

"I am going to examine you," I informed the patient. The patient's labia were purple and swollen. I felt for the baby's head. It was low in her pelvis, but molded and swollen. The realization of what was going on washed over me. I tried to get the patient to look in my eyes.

"How long have you been pushing?"

No response. I now noticed her companions for the first time. A middle aged woman in street clothes stood attentively at the patient's side, along with the panicked father. I mentally went through the woman's list of possible identities: mother, aunt, sister, friend, doula, or midwife. I decided it was one of the latter and now met her gaze.

"How long has she been pushing?"

She quickly looked back and forth at the patient and then her husband, the conflict raging on her face. Finally the patient's husband responded reluctantly, "Two hours."

I did the quick mental calculation to determine the quickest way to get the baby out, running through all the possibilities that got them here and the consequences of each decision I had before me. I decided in under five seconds.

"Vacuum," I demanded and promptly applied the suction cup to the baby's head, not bothering to instruct the residents and feeling my own pulse begin to rise. I took a moment to settle myself and then did what I had been trained to do.

The infant emerged pale and purple in color, not crying, with four little limbs hanging limply at it's side. The cord that had been tight around the child's neck had been quickly cut and the baby was handed off to the awaiting neonatologist. Once I gave it up, I felt my hands begin to shake, as the adrenalin finally had its effect, and heard the mother weakly ask as they were busy forcing air into the baby's lungs,

"What is it?"

"A girl," one of the nurses replied.

"Sophia," the mother smiled to her husband, not grasping what our quiet, serious glances implied.

The woman at her side encouraged her with a forced smile, "You did it!"

"I did it, I'm so happy."

Baby Sophia spent many weeks in the Neonatal Intensive Care Unit before being discharged home with a presumed anoxic brain injury. After the delivery, I saw the woman from Sophia's birth in the hall outside labor and delivery. Initially, I meant to simply pass her by, but I could not hold back the question that had been plaguing my mind.

"Why did she try to have her baby at home? She was high risk."

The woman shrugged and then replied unapologetically, "She wanted a natural birth. She wanted a vaginal delivery. No one would even let her try."

The urge to blame someone for Sophia's birth is strong in most people who hear her birth story. It is easy to blame Sophia's mother. That blame is the natural conclusion that arises from the presumption that a pregnant mother's first and foremost duty is to make decisions that prioritize the safety of the infant she carries, even if that is to her personal detriment.

That presumption is so ingrained in our society that it is rendered incontrovertible and any perceived deviation from that norm draws criticism from even the strongest proponents of personal autonomy. The woman sacrificing herself on the altar of motherhood is female glorification in its highest form. The lines of sacrifice are repeated in movie after movie, television show after show, often spoken between couples clutching hands with emotional music playing in the background, "If you have to make a choice, to save me or save the baby, you save the baby! Save the baby!" The decision made by Sophia's mother to pursue a "high-risk" vaginal delivery, in a way that may have put her child at increased danger, is deemed an inherently selfish act according to our collective moral consciousness, so conditioned by a subjective valuing of child over mother. Selfishness is the most damning judgment we can place on a mother and the gravest of insults.

It is easy to blame the midwife. Again, according to our modern viewpoint, by choosing to attend Sophia's birth within the home, she presumably prioritized mode of delivery and her patient's birth experience over Sophia. She failed to recognize fetal distress and arrange transfer to the hospital in a timely fashion. She was also clearly practicing outside of her scope of care and, according to some state laws, outside of the legal limitations of her midwifery license. Home birth, in and of itself, is not supported by the American College of Obstetricians and Gynecologists and a history of previous cesarean delivery is considered an absolute contraindication to delivery within the home.[2] In 4 out of 28 states where Certified Professional Midwives, midwives without a formal nursing background, are licensed to practice, a midwife who attends an out-of-hospital VBAC can actually be arrested and imprisoned for providing this care.[3]

However, it is exceedingly more difficult for those within the medical community to consider that they may share in the blame for Sophia's birth and examine the ways in which their own system creates the sequence of decisions that culminate in births like Sophia's. In this case, the labeling of VBAC as "high risk" immediately restricted the options for Sophia's delivery and created risk by offering only extremes of care. It is particularly interesting to note that in this circumstance, it was not the "high-risk" vaginal delivery after a previous cesarean delivery that resulted in Sophia's compromise. It was simply a routine challenge that impeded Sophia's blood supply, a tight umbilical cord around the neck, a complication which could have occurred in any "low-risk" delivery. The reason this problem was not detected and acted upon before it caused harm was because Sophia's mother was not in a hospital. The reason Sophia's mother was not in a hospital was because she could not find a doctor who would be willing to "let" her have a vaginal delivery after her previous cesarean section. The question I should have been asking was not why Sophia's mother tried to have her baby at home, but why she felt she did not have the option of a hospital birth.

Women throughout the country are finding themselves with limited options when it comes to the delivery of their children. The cesarean section rate has remained steady at 32% for the last 2 years.[4] While overall induction rates have decreased, one in five women still have their labors induced artificially and the list of medical indications for induction has expanded to include advanced maternal age, maternal obesity, and an ever-declining definition of postdates pregnancies. In a survey of over 2000 women, 14.8% of respondents felt pressured into an induction and 13.3% felt pressured into a cesarean delivery.[5,6] In the same survey, 76% of women indicated that they were unable to walk in labor and 92% delivered lying on their backs. Nearly all the women who were surveyed, four out of five, had continuous fetal heart rate monitoring, received IV fluids, and had food and drink restricted.[7] Of those women like Sophia's mother, who had a history of a previous cesarean delivery, 90% had another cesarean delivery.[8]

The hospital, once a harbor of safety through an unpredictable labor process, has become an institutional representation of the battle being waged over women's bodies and reproductive rights and the stage upon which women feel horrific atrocities are committed, not prevented. Obstetricians and nurses, rather than being viewed as guardians of women and infants through a tumultuous birth process, have been cast as central villains in a performance of unwanted cesarean sections, unnecessary medical interventions, and disrespect toward laboring women that plays itself out in countless labor and delivery units across the country and is recounted in tale after tale featured in various films, news articles, and mommy blogs. Births are managed in a machinery fashion under the guise of ensuring safety. Labor and delivery protocols, one of the last vestiges of a patriarchal medical system, tell women what they are and are not allowed to do with their own bodies and babies. Women are "not allowed" to walk, eat, or take off their blood pressure cuff or fetal monitor. They must labor in bed, deliver on their back, and often receive medications and episiotomies without appropriate explanations or even specific consent being obtained, beyond that of an all-inclusive consent they sign upon admission to the hospital but rarely read. Women are "not allowed" to remain pregnant past a certain gestational age and must present at the hospital for their induction. Many hospitals and physicians "do not do" VBACs.

In response to this over-medicalization of the birth process and the lack of autonomy experienced in many maternity wards, an ever-growing percentage of women have begun to speak with their feet and reject part or all of standard prenatal care and seek options for their labor and delivery along the fringes of the traditional medical establishment or outside it. It is not only women who want a VBAC who are fleeing obstetricians and hospitals, but also women who simply want to give birth without technological interventions, without epidurals, and without an increased risk of surgery. According to data released by the CDC, in the short time period from 2004 to 2012, there has been a 56% increase in out-of-hospital births and the percentage of births attended by midwives both in and out of hospital has more than doubled to represent 7.9% of all births in the United States.[9,10]

Multiple advocacy groups have arisen out of the current climate, working to combat the injustices and inappropriate care that are felt to be pervasive within the maternity health care system. The Coalition for Improving Maternity Services, the Maternity Center Association, Childbirth Connection, Choices in Childbirth, the International Cesarean Awareness Network (ICAN), ImprovingBirth Network, and VBAC Facts are some of the more prominent examples of these groups. An entire natural birth industry has formed as well, offering various products and services, including childbirth educators, doulas, and lactation counselors, that are meeting the needs of women that are being unmet by the medical community and with varying levels of expertise. DONA INTERNATIONAL, the leading doula certification program, has seen its membership grow from 750 in 1994 to over 6000 in 2012. Over half of women in the United States attend some form of natural childbirth education, with a wide range of options including Lamaze, the Bradley Method, BirthWorks, HypnoBirthing, or one of the many hospital-sponsored classes taught at nearly every maternity center in the country. Multiple natural birth promoting online communities, such as BabyCenter, TheBump, Mothering.com, have grown and flourished, where women offer support, share information, and discuss birth experiences. Countless books have been written describing the problems with US maternity system and offering natural alternatives to its norm.

Those that go by the term "birthworkers," the midwives, doulas, childbirth educators, and lactation counselors in the natural birth community, advocate for a physiological birth model, defined as labor and birth powered by the innate human capacity of the woman and the fetus without medical intervention. Specifically, this model calls for the spontaneous onset and progression of labor, appropriate biological and psychological conditions to enable labor to progress in an unhindered fashion, a vaginal delivery of the infant and placenta, and skin-to-skin contact of the mother and newborn infant with no separation in the postpartum period and early initiation of breastfeeding. Proponents of a physiological birth model are often highly critical of obstetricians and hospitals alike and strongly call into question much of what has become standard in both prenatal and labor and delivery care, including ultrasound, antibiotics for prevention of group beta Streptococcus—related sepsis and meningitis, intrapartum fetal monitoring, vitamin K administration in the newborn for prevention of hemorrhagic disease of the newborn, antibiotic eye ointment for prevention of birth-related conjunctivitis, and cesarean birth for breech presentation or multiple gestations. They routinely raise the question of whether low-risk women should even be receiving care from obstetricians, who they view as surgeons first and foremost, who are without the knowledge or philosophy of care to be able to properly support a physiologic birth process. Most believe birth is safer in the home or in a midwife-run birth center because medical interventions, rather than the birth process itself, result in the greatest number of bad outcomes and what bad outcomes that do occur in homebirth or a birth center could not be prevented in a hospital birth to any large degree.

Most people within the medical community consider these positions to be dangerous anti-medical extremism that will ultimately result in the loss of more women and babies during the birth process. Some of the more vocal critics of the natural birth movement, such as Dr. Amy Tuteur, accuse these organizations of promoting an idealized vision of birth and shepherding women toward unmedicated deliveries in order to sell a product, in this case: midwives, doulas, childbirth education, lactation counseling, natural birth books, and birth supplies. Rather than answering a need, they are creating it by convincing women there is a perfect birth that they need to obtain, similar to the way the wedding industry sells the idea of the perfect wedding.[11] From the medical perspective, the complaints of natural birth proponents and the women they support represent "high-class problems" in a world where real neonatal and maternal mortality still exist to a startling degree in underdeveloped countries and underserved populations. They argue that American obstetricians and the modern maternity system are merely victims of their own success; women only lament unpleasant birth experiences because they have no knowledge of or experience with the very real horrors that can occur in birth and are prevented by medical intervention. Any birth process that results in a healthy mother and a healthy baby is, by a medical definition, a success and any process that exposes mothers and babies to an increased real or perceived risk is rigidly avoided.

There is, however, a growing voice within the medical community that is questioning the priorities of current obstetrical practices because, even from a purely medical standpoint, the case for change is strong. In the short period of time from 1991 to 2014, the number of cesareans performed in the United States increased by 33%, while the perinatal mortality rate, defined as the percentage of babies 28 weeks gestation or greater at delivery who died prior to or within 7 days of delivery, decreased only from 13.12 in 1000 births to 9.98 in 1000 births. This decrease in perinatal mortality is statistically significant yet it represents only a small difference when the actual number of overall births are taken into account. In addition, the decrease is a result of a number of factors, not simply that more cesareans mean more babies saved. However, the association of cesarean delivery with an increased rate of severe maternal complications of delivery and maternal mortality has been well documented in the medical literature and impacts a large number of births. Intraoperative surgical complications of cesarean include damage to adjacent organs, such as the bowel, bladder, or other urinary tract structures and unintentional injury to the uterus, vagina, or cervix via extension of the uterine surgical extension. Other complications include significant blood loss, the need for blood transfusion, and hysterectomy. When the results of the multitude of studies that have detailed the risks of cesarean are averaged, approximately 12% of women undergoing a cesarean delivery experience one or more of these surgical complications, with 1 in 200 cesareans requiring a concurrent hysterectomy, which is associated with significantly higher rates of all other intraoperative complications than that observed with cesarean delivery alone and has an associated maternal mortality rate of 1.6%. The risks of all complications and maternal mortality increase with each subsequent cesarean delivery a women undergoes.[12,13] Given that 9 out of 10 women who have one cesarean will have a repeat cesarean in their subsequent births, the percentage of all pregnant women delivering in a higher risk repeat cesarean section rises in direct proportion to the overall primary cesarean section rate.

The reasons for the increasing cesarean section rate are numerous and debated at length. Some blame increasing levels of technology that needlessly raise alarms or a changing patient population that is older, heavier, and with a greater number of indications for cesarean. Others believe doctors are the main source of the problem, performing greater numbers of cesareans for convenience or to minimize their chances of being sued in an ever more litigious environment. While undoubtedly each of these factors are, at least to some degree, influencing the cesarean rate, the causes most commonly cited by medical professionals themselves center around ensuring a safe and healthy delivery for the baby. In terms of the actual indications for cesarean provided at the time of delivery, failure of labor progression (34%) and non-reassuring fetal heart rate pattern (23%) are most common, followed by fetal malpresentation (17%), multiple gestations, maternal–fetal indications, preeclampsia, and maternal request.[14] However, given the known risks of cesarean delivery, even if the improvement in perinatal mortality could be exclusively attributed to greater numbers of cesareans and the practices that lead to them, the question begs to asked whether benefit is worth the cost. Maternal mortality is thankfully a rare event, but in the same time frame in which the cesarean section rate has rapidly increased, there has been a 27% increase in the maternal mortality rate in the United States.[15] Are we losing more mothers, at least in part, due to an intolerance of any risk for babies?

There is also a growing concern that current obstetrics practices are not just increasing women's risk of physical harm, but mental and emotional harm also. Women report feeling victimized by the way they were treated during their labor and delivery, that they were not given the right to make their own medical decisions during labor, and that they were met with extreme resistance if they desired anything outside of the standard, intervention heavy, medical birth model. In fact, one in four women would describe their labor and delivery experience as traumatic.[16] A significant number of women actually meet criteria for post-traumatic stress disorder (PTSD) in the postpartum period as a result of their delivery experience, with a mean prevalence of 4% in multiple studies, and the number of women who demonstrate at least some post-traumatic symptoms in relation to their birth has been shown to be as high as 30%.[17] Birth-related factors that increase a woman's likelihood of experiencing PTSD or PTSD-related symptoms include negative subjective birth experiences, having an operative delivery, and lack of support during the labor process.[18] Clearly, there is a maternal need that is being unmet by our system and traditional obstetrics care is failing a significant number of women to some degree. Those who provide that care must begin to ask themselves if they have been judging their success by the same ruler as their patients. Perhaps a healthy mom goes beyond the immediate physical outcome.

A written birth plan is the manifestation of the conflict between maternal needs and the overly simplistic medical goal of healthy mom, healthy baby. Often several pages long and detailing preferences for as many contingencies as she can imagine, a woman's birth plan is her attempt to regain personal autonomy over an unpredictable process that medicine has so overzealously tried to control that one out of three births ends in an operating room. Physicians and medical staff, however, most often view the birth plan with hostility, taking it as a personal affront that questions both their expertise and their motives. Birth plans are frequently passed around by nurses, residents, and doctors and openly mocked or, with seeming less malice, simply tucked into the chart and ignored. Few regard them as opportunity for dialogue about the care their patient desires and a legitimate expression of what that woman does and does not consent to in labor.

The American College of Obstetrics and Gynecology has recognized this and has issued several recommendations to decrease the cesarean section rate and broaden the approach toward labor management to include low-intervention models of care. In their obstetrics consensus, Safe Prevention of the Primary Cesarean Section, recommendations mainly center around relaxing the definitions on what constitutes a failure of labor progression and allowing women more time to deliver their babies in all stages of labor. In their 2017 Committee Opinion, they also acknowledged the importance of women's preferences for their birth experience, especially for low-risk women, and offered a set of guidelines for providers to more confidently care for women using a low-intervention approach.[19] These efforts represent a large step forward in expanding women's childbirth options, but recommendations alone do not necessarily bring about a rapid change in the culture and practices across the country.

In order for change to occur, medical providers must first accept that they should change. This seems simple, given the growing and varied number of voices making the case for that change. However, due to the very technical way physicians and nurses are trained in decision making, it is more challenging than one might think. "Good medicine," evidence-based medicine, involves examining the way in which a specific treatment brings about a specific measurable outcome that can be compared to that produced by a separate specific treatment. The studies that are performed are most often initiated from a place of bias which assumes the superiority of the medical model and it is only the implementation of that medical model that is examined. Natural birth practices, which are largely void of any treatment or even the strict avoidance of a treatment, are more challenging to quantify and compare. Subjective things, such as experience, are nearly impossible to study in randomized control trials, the gold standard of medical evidence. In order to motivate members of the medical community to change, one must look for reasons outside of the strict scientific framework. The initial question providers should ask is not whether a particular medical or natural approach is "better" statistically, but rather does the patient have the right to choose nonintervention or a natural technique whether or not it is technically better by scientific standards or is the medical intervention so superior to nonintervention that it should be considered the only viable option.

This question is one of medical ethics, specifically the principle of respect for patient autonomy. Again, in theory, it seems simple. The United States was founded on the principle of personal autonomy and most of us hold deep respect for the "moral right of every competent individual to choose and follow his or her own plan of life and actions" (p. 49).[20] It would follow that undoubtedly a woman should be able to decline an epidural, an IV, or whatever other medical intervention she did not desire. But should she be able to refuse an induction or a cesarean, even if it is necessary to save the life of the baby she carries? What rights does the baby have, while encased within its mother's body, at what gestational age does it obtain them, and what happens when what is deemed best for the baby is in direct conflict with what is best for the mother, either medically or by her own subjective judgment? It is this inherent contradiction in the right of the mother to bodily autonomy and the intradependent right of the unborn baby to bodily well-being that fills the pages of ethics textbooks and has created endless hours of political and legal contention. Connections to the abortion debate are also hard to deny and the same emotions that complicate that ethical debate complicate debates concerning the obligations of women to the infants they carry. While the conservative and liberal viewpoint differ greatly in terms of whether the fetus should be granted full moral status, entitled to the same protections of more fully developed human beings, most ethicists agree that if a woman has the intention to carry her fetus to term, she has some moral responsibility to minimize the likelihood that her child will be born unhealthy. It is the degree to which that responsibility obligates her to submit to lifestyle modifications and medical treatments that is so heavily debated.[20,21]

To make the debate even more complicated is the fact that it is rare for conflicts in maternal–fetal interests to reach life or death extremes. It is hard to find a woman who would not readily consent to and seek out a medical intervention in order to truly save the life of her unborn child. However, in obstetrics, the majority of interventions performed are done preventatively, without a black or white outcome to choose between. The disagreements that arise between medical providers and their patients, particularly in respect to birth plans and labor management, are concerning interpretations of risk, usually only as it applies to the unborn child, and the level to which medical intervention should be utilized to mitigate that risk.

For example, a woman's water may break before labor has started and her doctor recommend an induction. This purpose of the induction would be to decrease the chance of infection, as the greater the time interval from membrane rupture to infant delivery, the greater the likelihood of infection. A woman desiring a natural, low-intervention approach may prefer to wait and see if labor will occur spontaneously, as she worries an induction will increase her chance of needing an epidural and other medical interventions. She may also worry about that the induction itself may expose her baby to more stress and possible harm. At the time the induction is being discussed, neither the woman nor her baby is in any danger. Any outcome is possible. Labor may begin on its own. An infection may occur with or without the induction. The induction may prevent an infection. This is where evidenced-based medicine attempts to solve the dilemma and compare induction to expectant management, waiting for labor to begin spontaneously, and recommend a clear course of action. However, studies frequently conflict one another and they only inform providers and women about the most likely outcome given one particular course of action, not what will happen in any one individual's case. Furthermore, even if a course of action is only marginally more beneficial, it can be statistically significant enough to become the standard of care.

The "evidence," the way one was trained, and personal experience often result in strong opinions on the part of medical providers about what is the "right" thing to do and frequently that opinion is presented to the patient as the only safe option. This tendency has resulted in many women calling foul on the medical community, claiming that providers are playing "the dead baby card" in order to convince patients to agree to interventions they do not feel comfortable with. Canadian researchers explored and substantiated this claim, finding that providers themselves reported using extreme language in their conversations with patients regarding management decisions, saying things like, "Well, you don't want your baby to die do you?" even in situations that were not life or death.[22] Certainly a woman's ability to make an autonomous decision to forgo a recommended medical intervention is limited when the choice is presented in such dire terms, when it is made to seem that refusal will endanger the life of her child.

Even when less frightening language is used, it can be coercive. For example, if a woman is told she is at an increased risk for stillbirth if her pregnancy extends beyond a certain gestational age, though the information may be technically true, without providing her with the details about how much of an increased risk and compared to what, she is unable to make a truly independent and informed decision. Our medical culture has become so risk-adverse that any course of action that has an "increased risk" has become equated with bad care, without a clear definition of how much of an increased risk is too much risk, and it is most often "risk" that is cited as the reason for denying part or all of a woman's natural birth plan.

One way we might begin to better define how much risk is too much risk, is by considering one of the extremes in obstetrical managment, one with a well-documented neonatal morbitiy and mortality. Breech presentation, which occurs in 4% of singleton pregnancies at term, is when the baby enters the pelvis in a bottom or feet down position, as opposed to the normal head down position. Cesarean delivery is routinely recommended if a breech presentation has persisted past 39 weeks gestation because multiple, reliable studies demonstrate that for every 100 vaginal breech deliveries, approximately 1 baby will die or suffer significant injury during delivery that would have been born healthy had a cesarean been performed.[23] While most women feel a 1 in a 100 chance of losing their baby during delivery is a too heavily weighted game of Russian Roulette, if viewed from an alternative perspective, 99% of women undergoing cesareans for breech could have a safe vaginal breech delivery. Consequently, the American College of Obstetrics and Gynecology still firmly states that a well-informed patient should be allowed to choose a vaginal delivery in the setting of a breech baby. Medical ethicists concur that a woman should not be coerced into a surgical procedure, even a potentially lifesaving one for her infant, when 99% of the time her baby can be safely delivered without surgery. A vaginal delivery, while not a recommended course of action given the significantly lower risk alternative, is still a reasonable alternative.

Yet, the purpose of this discussion is not to make the case for or against vaginal breech deliveries. The purpose is to demonstrate that if a vaginal breech delivery, with a 1 in 100 risk of neonatal mortality or significant morbidity, is still considered a reasonable alternative, then when considering whether a woman has the right to choose a low-intervention approach or decide against a particular medical intervention, any perceived risk should be considered against that extreme. For example, a "high-risk" VBAC carries a risk of neonatal mortality of 1.24 per 1000 births.[24] The risk of stillbirth with expectant management at 41 weeks gestation, the most commonly cited cutoff for when a patient "must be" induced, is 17.6 per 10,000 compared to 14.9 per 10,000 at 40 weeks gestation, when it is still considered "safe" to be expectantly managed.[25] How can a woman be pressured into an induction with a 0.027% difference in the risk to her baby from one week to the next?

The risks associated with the more tedious points of natural birth plans are even lower. For example, the ability to ambulate in labor is one of the most common requests made by women wishing to labor naturally. Often they are told this is not safe because there is a risk the umbilical cord could prolapse, or escape ahead of the baby's head into the vagina, causing constriction and decreased blood flow to the baby. Interestingly, there is no medical evidence whatsoever indicating that ambulation in labor, at term, with the baby in a cephalic, head down, position is associated with umbilical cord prolapse. However, suppose ambulation were a risk for this complication, umbilical cord prolapse is a very rare event, only occurring in between 1.4 and 6.2 per 1000 births and the risk of perinatal mortality in the setting of a prolapse is less than 10%, particularly when it occurs in the hospital setting with the ability to perform an immediate cesarean.[26,27] Yet, even with risks in these ranges, patients are not often not "allowed" to choose VBAC, expectant management past a certain gestational age, ambulation, or countless other "noninterventions" in a similar or lower risk category. This practice certainly is not ethical, does not respect a woman's autonomy, and is a misrepresentation of the risk involved. There is not one aspect of the typical natural birth plan that will be discussed in the coming chapters that carries so much risk to a woman's baby that she should not be free to choose it without being unduly frightened that she is endangering her unborn child. Discussions of risk are a necessary part of obstetrics care. Doctors and midwives are obligated to discuss risk in order to provide informed consent, but that risk must be discussed in context and not exaggerated in order to obtain compliance. There is no risk-free option to get a child out of a woman's body. It is the provider's role to work with their patient to help identify the options that make the most sense for her.

If obstetricians fail to do this and continue to resist the natural birth trend, there will be multiple negative impacts. The most damaging to the profession as a whole and patients themselves will be a loss of women's confidence in obstetricians, the most highly trained providers of obstetrical care, to provide that very care for which they are so well trained. Long gone are the days when patients simply accepted everything their doctors said without question. Today, any patient, with the aid of a simple Google search, can access relevant journal articles, committee opinions, and practice guidelines. They can also access any number of websites and news articles discussing and frequently criticizing obstetrics practices. If obstetricians are misrepresenting risk when discussing care and restricting women's options without due cause, their patients are quite capable of finding out and, when they do, they will no longer trust their doctor and their trust of the profession in general will be diminished. Like Sophia's mother, this will lead patients to reject potentially life saving medical care in the future and open the door for them to deliver their babies in situations that are significantly less safe than the original situation their doctor was trying to protect them and their babies from. If obstetricians want to continue to be seen as leaders in the field, with the moral authority to make recommendations that mid-level providers and patients will trust and follow, they must begin to discuss risk in a more honest, relevant way that respects a woman's ability to make an intelligent, informed choice. They must work to help their patients reach their goals instead of working against them.

It behooves obstetricians to do so also from a purely economic standpoint. Doctors are notoriously bad at business, but it does not take a brilliant business mind to recognize that the tide of patients and their associated revenue is turning away from doctors and hospitals to midwives, birthing centers, and homebirths. Whether or not this is a good change is a topic for further discussion, but in terms of obstetrician's self-interest, it undoubtedly is a bad prognostic sign in a climate of rising costs and decreasing reimbursements where medical practices depend on large volume to stay afloat. Any other business that was losing market share in a similar fashion would perform a root cause analysis and initiate promotional and product changes to meet the changing demands of their customers.

Obstetricians certainly have a marketing problem. Midwives are strongly making the case that they should be the primary providers of obstetrical care for low-risk women and much of the evidence supports their cause, with midwives demonstrating lower cesarean rates and higher patient satisfaction with their care. The media has jumped on the bandwagon, with multiple articles, news reports, and documentaries encouraging women to choose midwives for a lower risk of unnecessary medical interventions. While the American College of Obstetrics and Gynecology took a first step in their Committee Opinion, providing support for a low-intervention approach, they have yet to publically campaign that obstetricians are as equally qualified as midwives to care for low-risk women and offer them a low-intervention option, with the reassurance of having a physician able to readily recognize and respond should a low-risk situation suddenly become high risk. Perhaps this is because there are too few obstetrician actually providing this option in practice. They cannot market a product they are not able to produce.

Brookwood Medical Center, a hospital in Birmingham, Alabama, learned this the hard way. In 2016, a jury awarded a Caroline Malatesta, a prior obstetrics patient, $16 million dollars in return for the medical negligence and reckless fraud committed by the hospital where she delivered her fourth child. The case centered around the hospital's failure to honor the promises made in their extensive natural birth advertising campaign, which offered women water birth, freedom of movement, and individualized birth plans. The plaintiff successfully argued that she was misled by the hospital and injured by their implementation of medical interventions that she did not consent to.[28] While many have criticized the judgment as excessive and out of proportion to the injuries received, the jury sent a strong message that a patient's birth experience matters, women have the right to have their wishes respected in labor, and hospitals and doctors cannot offer something they are unwilling to deliver.

The medical community may not agree with its negative portrayal by natural birth community, but, without a doubt, women are feeling repressed by the implementation of maternity care within the current medical model. History has shown us time and time again that individuals who feel oppressed will rise up and demand a change and go to extremes to obtain it. Whether it is deciding to have a high-risk birth within the home, suing hospitals and doctors who take away their autonomy, or abandoning physicians as care providers, women are making it known that they want something else than they are being offered. They want the ability to have the best of both worlds. They want qualified care providers who can respond to a bad situation but who judiciously utilize medical interventions and can be trusted to recommend a change in a woman's birth plan only if it is truly warranted. They want the resources of the hospital available, but they do not want to sacrifice their desire for a natural birth in order to have that reassurance. Obstetricians and the rest of the medical community can continue to stick their collective head in the sand or they can reclaim a leadership role in this debate and begin to dialogue with patients, midwives, doulas, and lactation consultants about what women need. By discontinuing both their blatant opposition toward and willful ignorance of natural birth practices, obstetricians can calm the anti-medical sentiment within the natural birth community and more effectively develop ways to safely provide natural birth options without sacrificing good medicine. Change will happen regardless. It would be better for everyone if the medical community and especially obstetricians were part of the process.

REFERENCES

1. Block J. *Pushed: The Painful Truth about Childbirth and Modern Maternity Care.* Cambridge, MA: Da Capo Press; 2008.
2. American College of Obstetricians and Gynecologists. *ACOG Committee Opinion 669.* Washington, DC: American College of Obstetricians and Gynecologists; 2016.
3. Kamel J. "No one can force you to have a cesarean" is false. VBAC Facts. January 2016.
4. Martin JA, Hamilton BE, Osterman MJ. Births in the United States, 2015. NCHS Data Brief No. 258. Hyattsville, MD: National Center for Health Statistics; 2016.
5. Osterman MJ, Martin JA. Recent declines in induction of labor by gestational age. NCHS Data Brief No. 155. Hyattsville, MD: National Center for Health Statistics; 2014.
6. Jou J, Kozhimann KB, Johnson PJ, Sakala C. Patient-perceived pressure from clinicians for labor induction and cesarean delivery: a population-based survey of US women. *Health Serv Res.* 2015;50(4):961-981.
7. Declercq ER, Sakala C, Corry MP, et al. Listening to mothers II: report of the second national U.S. survey of women's childbearing experiences. *J Perinat Educ.* 2007; 16:9-14.
8. Martin JA, Hamilton BE, Sutton PD, et al. Births: final data for 2006. National Vital Statistics Reports, vol 57, no. 7. Hyattsville, MD: National Center for Health Statistics; 2009.
9. MacDorman MF, Mathews TJ, Declercq E. Trends in out-of-hospital births in the United states 1990-2012. NCHS Data Brief No. 144. Hyattsville, MD: National Center for Health Statistics; 2014.
10. Declercq E. Midwife-Attended Births in the United States, 1990–2012: Results from Revised Birth Certificate Data *J Midwifery Women's Health.* 2015;60(1):10-15.
11. Tuteur A. *Push Back: Guilt in the Age of Natural Parenting.* New York, NY: Harper-Collins Publishers; 2016.
12. Grivell RM, Dodd JM. Short- and long-term outcomes after cesarean section. *Expert Rev Obstet Gynecol.* 2011;6(2):205-215.
13. Shellhass CS, Gilbert S, Landon MB, et al. The frequency and complication rates of hysterectomy accompanying cesarean deliveries. *Obstet Gynecol.* 2009;114(2 pt 1): 224-229.
14. American College of Obstetrics and Gynecology; Society for Maternal-Fetal Medicine. Obstetrics care consensus no. 1: safe prevention of the primary cesarean section. *Obstet Gynecol.* 2014;123(3);693-711.

15. MacDorman MF, Declercq E, Cabral H, et al. Recent increases in the US maternal mortality rate: disentangling trends from measurement issues. *Obstet Gynecol.* 2016;128(3):447-455.

16. Declercq E, Sakala C, Corry M, Applebaum S. *New Mothers Speak Out: National Survey Results Highlight Women's Postpartum Experiences.* New York, NY: Childbirth Connection; 2008.

17. Yildiz PD, Ayers S, Phillips L. The prevalence of posttraumatic stress disorder in pregnancy and after birth: A systematic review and meta-analysis. *J Affect Disord.* 2017;208(1):634-645.

18. Furuta M, Sandall J, Cooper D, Bick D. Predictors of birth-related post-traumatic stress symptoms: secondary analysis of a cohort study. *Arch Womens Ment Health.* 2016;19(3):521-528.

19. American College of Obstetricians and Gynecologists. *ACOG Committee Opinion 687.* Washington, DC: American College of Obstetricians and Gynecologists; 2017.

20. Jonsen A, Siegler M, Winslade W. *Clinical Ethics.* New York, NY: McGraw Hill; 2015.

21. Mappes T, Degrazia D. *Biomedical Ethics.* New York, NY: McGraw Hill; 2001.

22. Hall WA, Tomkinson J, Tomkinson MCK. Canadian care providers' and pregnant women's approaches to managing birth: minimizing risk while maximizing integrity qualitative health research. 2011. doi:10.1177/1049732311424292. Published online September 22, 2011.

23. Kotaska A, Menticoglou S, Gagnon R, et al. Vaginal delivery of breech presentation. Society of Obstetricians and Gynaecologists. Clinical Practice Guideline No. 226. *J Obstet Gynaecol Can.* 2009;31:557-566.

24. Menacker F, MacDorman MF, Declercq E. Neonatal mortality risk for repeat cesarean compared to vaginal birth after cesarean (VBAC) deliveries in the United States, 1998–2002 birth cohorts. *Matern Child Health J.* 2010;14(2):147-154.

25. Rosenstein MG, Cheng YW, Snowden JM, Nicholson JM, Caughey AB. Risk of stillbirth and infant death stratified by gestational age. *Obstet Gynecol.* 2012;120(1): 76-82.

26. Kahana B, Sheiner E, Levy A, et al. Umbilical cord prolapse and perinatal outcomes. *Int J Gynaecol Obstet.* 2004;84:127-132.

27. Boyle JJ, Katz VL. Umbilical cord prolapse in current obstetrics practice. *J Reprod Med.* 2005;50:303-306.

28. Nathman AN. Caroline Malatesta was just awarded $16 million in a lawsuit against the hospital where she delivered her fourth child. *Cosmopolitan.* Available at http://www.cosmopolitan.com/lifestyle/news/a62592/caroline-malatesta-brookwood-childbirth-lawsuit/. Accessed August 2016.

CHAPTER 2

Current Barriers to Natural Birth

The obstacles preventing natural birth practices from becoming part of the routine options presented to women are numerous and complex, but they are important to understand, both for medical providers working with patients who desire a natural birth and for women themselves who may be meeting resistance toward their natural birth plan. One of the harder to define barriers is the general culture of labor and delivery units that often stands in opposition to the natural birth plan. That culture can be a product of the stressful, dynamic, and fast-paced working environment nurses and doctors find themselves within, but it is also a result of the way in which nurses and resident doctors are trained and their own life experiences. An obstetrical residency is one of the most challenging and often demoralizing residencies a physician may undergo and this impacts both their relationship with patients and their approach to labor management. Obstetrical residencies also rarely include formal training in low-intervention techniques. This is because most training tends to occur within busy, high-risk centers which provide the opportunity for residents to be exposed to a large volume of delivery and surgical experiences, as well as a wide range of complications and unusual pathology, but little time for the actual one-on-one work with laboring women that really promotes understanding of the labor process.

Much of the other impediments to the natural birth approach are, unattractively, all business. Birthing babies takes considerable time and our medical system is based mainly on procedural reimbursements, meaning obstetricians earn the same amount of money for a procedure, or delivery, that takes 10 minutes as one that takes 10 hours. The risk of litigation for performing that procedure also continues to rise, with physicians assuming large costs for malpractice and living under the constant threat of a lawsuit that would increase those costs further or even threaten their personal property and their ability to continue to practice medicine in their specialty. It is a complicated set of challenges that often pit the interests of physicians against the interests of their own patients.

RESIDENCY: THE BARRIER OF THE MACHINE

An Obstetrics and Gynecology residency is an intense four year training program that competes only with surgical residencies in terms of its reputation of suffering among the residents completing it. While all residents work hard, it is only in OB/GYN that a resident can go an entire twenty-four hour shift without sitting down or eating. In my hospital, there was always a patient in need and it was always urgent. We divided our time between delivering babies and triaging pregnant patients on labor and delivery, learning to perform gynecologic surgery with up to fourteen hour stints in the operating room, managing all the postpartum and postoperative patients recovering on the hospital floors, caring for patients with gynecologic issues in the emergency room, and seeing patients in the hospital's outpatient clinic. A normal week consisted of eighty hours of physically, mentally, and emotionally draining work. In recent years, more attention has been given to the plight of doctors in training and the dangers of sleep deprived physicians delivering care. Several new regulations have been implemented which have improved residency hours, however when I started my residency several of those regulations were not in place and the ones that were in place were often intentionally ignored. Residents frequently lied about their hours under the threat of their program being put on probation or because they were convinced their life would actually be worse with some different system.

I began my residency with a q3 call schedule. This meant I worked two back-to-back twelve to fourteen hour days followed by a third day and night, over twenty-four consecutive hours, in the hospital, where I literally never saw my call room bed. I only had four consecutive twenty-four hour periods off each month and that could include a post-call day, where a large part of the time was spent in bed recovering from the day and night before. As we moved up in the hierarchy, we transitioned into a night float system, which was significantly better and meant we only had to work overnight every other weekend. Still, that equated to working two weeks straight, with one twenty-four hour stint in the middle, to get two days off. In exchange for this "better" working schedule, we gave up two months of our lives to work the vampire shift of fifteen hours, overnight, five days in a row, trying to fit in a few hours of sleep during the day. Our weekends were free until Sunday night, but again much of that free time was spent in bed recovering. The demands of the night float shift were so intense that most people were physically sick for a large portion of it. The level of exhaustion I experienced literally made me nauseous to the point that I would often vomit if I tried to eat after long shifts.

Beyond the physical and mental demands of this level of training, residency also took a tremendous toll on all our personal relationships. Of the residents I trained with, four marriages dissolved during residency and three nearly did. One of the most common complaints from all of our partners was that no matter how bad their day had been, ours was always worse. They could never be the one that needed taken care of. They could never be tired. They could never be sick. In the battle of who had it worst, we always won and that can be very difficult to live with, especially if there are kids involved. There was also the problem that the further into the medical world we got, the farther away from the real world we went and the journey back into everyday life was often difficult if not impossible to make. Slowly, people began to feel closer to the people in the medical world than their own spouses. Infidelity was and remains common in our program.

I started my residency with an eleven month old baby girl. She had been born during my fourth year of medical school, which had granted much flexibility in terms of her care, as the last year of medical school tends to be filled with elective rotations and light schedules. She was a happy, chubby little baby with a mess of dark curls and deep black eyes that would search my soul in the quiet nighttime hours when we would walk the halls alone. I was as in love with her as I was naive in my belief that my training would not take me from her for too much. I had not even weaned her before I started. Somehow that thought did not even occur to me. I assumed I would find time to pump at the hospital, that somehow doctors in training to deliver children and care for women would be sympathetic to my situation and supportive. I was mistaken.

Twenty hours into my first shift, I had not eaten or emptied my bladder and my swollen breasts were leaking through my last set of breast pads. I quickly realized that having a child was not a strength in the eyes of those who were training me. It was a weakness. It also, above all, was not a permitted excuse. Others could use personal situations as cause for needing some special request met, but whether it was scheduling calls and holidays or getting out of the hospital on time, having a child was unmentionable. It could never be the reason. It was a liability. There was no empathy because for someone to have empathy meant they had to do more work. By the time my residency was done, I realized I could not even remember what my daughter was like between the ages of one and three. At least my husband took a lot of videos.

For whatever reason, the intolerance was worse between women in the department. All too often, as one of my male senior residents with a thick Southern accent so memorably put it, it was "girl on girl action," and girls are not just mean, they are ruthless. Whether it was the nurses or female attendings relating to the female residents or interactions between the female residents themselves, there was little kindness. My first morning presenting "The Board," complete exhaustion won out and my mind became a blank slate. I was simply unable to remember the details of the patients who I was supposed to be passing off to the next team. Instead of coming to my aid, the upper year residents who had worked with me overnight, who were in charge of teaching me and guiding me, smelled the blood in the water and began circling for the kill. Each bit of information I forgot, they were there, nipping, until the point that I had lost all composure and any chance of performing my job. After the sign out was done, the resident who had been doing most of the shaming, came to me laughing, saying she had "been there too" and that some day it would be funny for me as well. It never was and, to this day, I feel humiliated when I recount the experience. However, it was by no means the last time such a thing happened to me during my training. Each mistake made in residency opened the door for someone to yell at you, belittle you, or, the most dreaded consequence of all, pile on even more work when all you wanted in the entire world was to just go home. When my classmates reached the top of the totem pole, they even tried to implement a demerit system which would force people to work in the triage unit after their shift was complete if they stepped out of line.

This process hardens most people and they usually end up repeating the cycle. Upper year residents and attending doctors would recount their stories of residency abuse with certain pride. Most considered it a necessary part of the training of young obstetricians. Unfortunately, that hardness often carried over into their relationships with their patients. Poor bedside manner is a one of the most frequent criticisms of doctors in a field where one should expect nothing but patience and sensitivity. However, it is difficult to have sympathy for uncomfortable pregnant women when you have been emotionally battered and sleep deprived for years, especially if you spent any of that time pregnant yourself.

One evening call, I was paged to evaluate a patient in the triage unit. She was contracting frequently but was not dilating and was not yet even term. This was the fourth or fifth time she had come to the hospital with these complaints and was very tired and frustrated. I was thirty five weeks pregnant with my second child at the time and had just spent ten hours on my feet in the operating room before heading up to labor and delivery to take over the night call. As I explained to her that she was to go home, a terrible rant ensued. How was she supposed to go on like this? Did I just expect her to live with these contractions? Her other baby had been born early and been fine. She insisted that this baby be delivered early or, at the very least, that I would take her out of work, though I had no power to do that as a resident. As she carried on and on, the annoyance boiled up within me and my own belly tightened into one of the many contractions I had been having since twenty-eight weeks. I simply walked out of the room. Poor bedside manner indeed.

The principle of soldiering on is ingrained in us from the very beginning of our training. The first day of our orientation, we sat in a nice conference room and were informed of how many sick days we had in our contract. We were then informed that, while it did not say so in the contract, the only sick day you were permitted was when you were either in the ER or dead. I spent many days vomiting or having diarrhea between my surgical cases. When it became really bad, we would have an IV placed by one of the nurses, get some fluids and anti-nausea medication, and go see the next patient. A cold did not even get you sympathy. Pregnant residents kept the same schedule as everyone else, often working more calls to make up for the call they would miss during their four weeks of maternity leave, which was taken out of their vacation time. Pregnant residents literally worked until their water broke or they were dilated enough to be admitted themselves. I wrote up my own history and physical on the day I delivered my son and would have put in my own orders if my water had not have been broken.

While the necessity of this method of training could and should be debated, its effectiveness cannot. Our training program had amazingly consistent results in terms of clinical knowledge and surgical expertise. Residency makes you into a machine. You develop a sequence of movements to complete each task before you as quickly and efficiently as possible, while simultaneously being distracted by the next page, the next patient. You become fast. You become good. In the operating room, your hands begin to move with a fluid, dance-like motion and by the end of your third year, you walk with a swagger of purpose and confidence. When the emergency presents itself, your muscle memory kicks in and you tackle the situation with complete calm because you know you can handle it, just as you have done it or seen it done so many times before. When the bad, scary moments come, the machine is reliable. The machine is consistent. The machine saves a life. The machine gets it done. And if you are a patient, finding yourself on the receiving end of that emergency, you want the machine.

But somewhere the people get lost. You get lost. Most people do not even know it has happened. I was fortunate enough to have a cabinet door fall on my head and let me know it had happened to me. Our labor and delivery unit was in desperate need of a makeover. Lovely pink and teal adorned the walls and the cheap cabinets hung loosely from their hinges and creaked each time they were opened and closed. One evening, at the start of a night shift, I was called to check "Room 9." I had yet to meet her but my focus was absolute.

Task: Check patient
Step 1: Get glove
Step 2: Check fetal heart rate monitor
Step 3: Inform patient you are going to check her while putting glove on. Do not ask.
Step 4: Check patient
Step 5: Update labor board
Step 6: Write note
Step 7: Call attending.

Somewhere between step one and two, I felt a very sharp thud land on my skull, as the cabinet door I had just opened to retrieve my glove came crashing to the floor. I immediately felt tears come to my eyes and a gash in my head. The surprise of the patient took my attention to her for the first time since I had come in and, as I looked into her eyes, I realized I had entered the room not knowing her name, not informing her of who I was, and had not even looked at her. I could not believe that I had become "that doctor"; I could not believe I had become that person.

The first time I thought I might want to be an obstetrician, I was actually still in high school. I participated in an amazing program where, at age fifteen, I was able to shadow doctors in different fields for an entire summer. I witnessed surgeries, tagged along during oncology rounds, and held tiny babies in the Neonatal Intensive Care Unit, but the most vivid and powerful memory I have of that entire experience was spending an afternoon with an obstetrician. He was doing an external cephalic version on a patient with a breech baby. During an external cephalic version, the doctor pushes on the woman's belly, directing the baby's head from her ribs to her pelvis. It is a fast procedure and often helps a woman avoid a cesarean delivery for an upside down baby. After the procedure was done and the doctor was filling out his paperwork, he explained to me why he loved his specialty, "It is a hard job and I work long hours, but every day I get to be there for the most important moment in someone's life. There is no better job."

In the grueling day to day experience of residency, that simple truth is forgotten by young doctors in training. It is also forgotten by nurses, anesthesiologists, and the attending doctors who take care of these women throughout their entire pregnancy. To the medical staff, the most special and intimate day in a woman's life is just another delivery, section, epi, or cervix to check. We talk of television shows as women are pushing their babies out. We call patients "hun" and their partners "dad" because we cannot be bothered to learn their names. We take their babies the second they are born to suction, stamp, and weigh so the right boxes can be filled out in enough time to accept the next patient. There is nothing sacred. It is just business as usual. Is it any wonder we don't take the time to care about their birth plan?

All residencies are characterized with militaristic terminology, but obstetrics residencies, similar to other surgical training programs, truly function like boot camp. Residents are organized in a hierarchical fashion, usually in teams composed of a member of each resident year, with the more senior team members supervising the lower year residents. Little to no management or teaching training is provided for the senior team members, yet they are held responsible for their team's performance, as well as their patients' well-being. Senior team members care for the higher risk pregnant patients and perform the more complicated surgical procedures, while the junior residents are handed the volume tasks of performing all low-risk deliveries, triaging incoming patients, and managing all postpartum and postsurgical patients on the hospital floors. This creates a stressful dynamic where upper-year residents are being challenged with the sickest patients and most difficult surgeries while attempting to supervise the lower-year residents, with the least knowledge, who are juggling the greatest number of tasks. Mistakes are inevitable and even considered a necessary part of the training process. As one attending put it, "Residents need enough rope to hang themselves, just not enough to hang the patient."[1]

Junior residents report being frequently yelled at by their upper-year residents, while upper-year residents are frequently yelled at by their attending doctors. Sign outs from one shift to another, intended to ensure patient safety by communicating relevant updates on patient status instead often resemble a courtroom, where the outgoing team is adjudicated on each decision they made during their shift. As residents move forward in the program, autonomy and respect increase with experience, but responsibilities and expectations do as well. Fear of making a mistake is pervasive across all training levels.

Sign outs are also a time where residents are frequently "pimped," a method of teaching where the patient being discussed is used as a springboard from which the presenting resident can be grilled on related medical knowledge, with the goal of reaching the point at which the presenting resident no longer has the knowledge base to answer. The pimper then moves on in a sequential fashion to each more senior pimpee. A successful pimping session leaves the entire team demoralized, with each team member having reached the point where their ignorance was displayed for all in attendance.

While attempting to cope with this stress-producing social structure, residents work exceptionally long hours with little to no rest for prolonged periods of time. All residents report extreme sleep deprivation, though it tends to be worse among lower-level residents. In one study, 84% of residents who were evaluated by the Epworth Sleepiness Scale scored at a level which would indicate a need for clinical intervention. Those residents reported significant impairment in their learning ability, job performance, professionalism with colleagues and patients, and personal life.[2] Limitations on work hours meant to address some of these concerns have not had the intended effect, with residents reporting no change in overall fatigue level or frequency of fatigue-related errors after the implementation of the 80-hour work week restrictions.[3] A review of 135 studies from 1980 to 2013 showed similar results, with no improvement in resident wellness, training quality, and patient outcomes with work hour restrictions.[4] However, this is understandable, given that even after the work hour restrictions, residents are still working twice as much as the typical American work week.

The nature of the work itself also produces extreme emotional distress. Most choose the field because of its healthy patients and primarily happy outcomes, but when bad outcomes occur, they are particularly traumatizing because they occur in a young women and their babies, where death is as unexpected as it is incomprehensible. It is most often the resident in the triage unit who diagnoses an intrauterine demise, or stillbirth, and, without training in trauma or grief counseling, is the one that is tasked with informing the expectant mother that her baby is gone. Every resident can describe the very specific wail of grief, horror, and disbelief that fills the room at that moment and no one is emotionally prepared for it. Furthermore, very few receive any counseling to help them cope with the repeated times they will be exposed to this in their training. Residents are on the front lines when a placenta detaches or a fetal heart rate goes down and will not come back up, racing the woman to the operating room. They are the primary surgeons performing the needed crash cesarean, delivering the baby in under 1 minute. Residents are also the ones bedside pushing the antihypertensive medications preventing a severely preeclamptic patient from having a stroke and they are the doctors responsible for discovering, as quickly as possible, if a postsurgical patient on the gynecology ward with low-oxygen levels has a pulmonary embolism so that lifesaving blood thinners can be administered. At the end of a bad shift, labor and delivery feels like a war zone where doctors and nurses wage battle against the very real possibility of maternal and fetal death inherent in every birth.

This method of training does prepare resident obstetricians well for their future roles as attendings and most emerge from residency confident in their delivery and surgical skills. However, a deterioration of empathy is observed the further one advances in their medical training. This erosion of empathy begins in medical school, tragically upon entering third year, when medical students begin their clinical rotations and have first exposure to actual patient care.[5] By the time their training is complete, 36% of obstetricians report high levels of emotional exhaustion and those with self-reported low levels of empathy are the most likely to report frequent conflicts with patients (65%).[6] Ultimately, it is that difficult to maintain empathy that is so essential to the doctor-patient relationship, with perceived doctor empathy affecting patient satisfaction, their likelihood to adhere to physician-recommended treatment, and their likelihood to make a malpractice claim.[7] Empathy is also essential in understanding a patient's birth preferences and working with women through an unpredictable labor process to achieve a safe and satisfying outcome. Unfortunately, programs designed to decrease resident burnout and improve empathy toward patients, such as Balint training, which are widespread and efficacious in family medicine residency programs, have not demonstrated similar efficacy among obstetrical residents.[8] Despite the recognition that process of residency is damaging both personally for those going through it and professionally in regards to the doctor-patient relationship, there are currently no good proposed solutions for problem. Women are left with highly skilled but emotionally battered physicians who have built up psychological walls to survive the rigors of their training.

HISTORICAL BARRIERS

Some even argue this emotional disconnect among obstetricians goes back to the origin of the specialty itself. For most of history, childbirth occurred in the home, attended by community midwives who had likely been known to the women they delivered for much of their lives. Friends and family members would also be present for the birth, providing emotional and physical support for the laboring mother, as well as maintaining her household while she was unable to do so. The first challenge to this tradition of female led, social childbirth, occurred in seventeenth-century England, with a family of apothecaries, the Chamberlens, who entered the midwifery business with a "secret instrument" unknown to the female midwives. Highly successful, this family of male midwives brought a new skill to delivery room and safely delivered infants in situations where often both mother and child were lost. They were said to operate in a clandestine fashion, entering the birthing room with their instrument hidden in an ornate box and working under a sheet. Peter Chamberlen attended the wives of both King James I and King Charles I and delivered King Charles II. Their secret instrument was the obstetrical forcep, which is credited with beginning the transition of birth from the home under the care of women to the hospital under the care of physicians and the subsequent professionalization of delivering babies.

In the United States, however, birth remained in the home, with female midwives, for over 95% of women until the early 1900s. The developing groups of professional physicians in the nineteenth century dedicated themselves exclusively to the study of pregnancy complications and treatment of problem deliveries, rather than normal birth, fostering within the physician community what many midwives came to regard as a warped view that all birth was inherently dangerous and a potential for disaster. Physician-supervised birth became an increasingly physician-controlled event, in an attempt to protect women from the perceived danger it was felt to represent. Yet physician-supervised hospital birth was actually more dangerous than home birth at that time, with higher maternal mortality rates, and maternity hospitals throughout the 1800s mainly served poor, homeless, or working-class women without access to home birth midwives. It was not until the late 1800s that doctors discovered the cause and means to prevent puerperal fever, the main culprit in the increased rate of hospital birth-related maternal deaths. After that time, hospitals came to be seen as safer, cleaner alternatives to home birth. Women also began to strongly desire and have marketed toward them the pain relief offered by hospital-based doctors at the turn of the century. By 1939, half of all American women delivered within the hospital, with even higher rates observed in women who lived in urban centers. While in Europe, midwives were incorporated into this move from home to hospital and maintained their influence over normal, uncomplicated births; in the United States, midwives were excluded from hospital birth and physicians assumed care over the majority of births.

For the 50 years that followed, hospital birth became the norm with the forcep as the primary tool of obstetrical delivery, accompanied by strong anesthesia. The goal was for the mother to literally feel nothing. Initially, the anesthesia provided was a so-called "twilight sleep," that left women relatively unconscious and without memory of their children's birth. Later, as doctors began to worry that this level of anesthesia was unsafe for women and babies alike, it was replaced with spinal anesthesia, which enabled women to remain conscious, though still unable to physically push their babies out, still leaving women dependent on their physician's skill to operatively deliver the child. Doctors were regarded with reverence and practiced unchallenged and with little concern for their patients' preferences for several decades.[9]

A significant shift occurred during the 1960s and 1970s, with two developments: the epidural and the natural birth movement. Epidurals, the so-called "Cadillac of Childbirth," were a form of anesthetic which provided effective pain relief throughout labor, but unlike twilight sleep and spinal blocks, enabled women to remain alert and able participants in both their labor and the actual delivery of their children. Suddenly the dynamic between doctor and patient began to change, buoyed by the women's rights movements and the increasing numbers of women entering the medical field. Alert and able bodied laboring women quickly realized that they did not necessarily want their babies extracted with metal instruments or large episiotomies cut into their perineum. Books emerged, such as *Our Bodies Ourselves*, which called into question much of what was standard practice in the labor and delivery room and encouraged women to take charge of their births. Articles in popular women's magazines also detailed mistreatment and traumatizing hospital birth experiences.

Women increasingly began to insist that their husbands be allowed behind the curtain to support and protect them during labor and witness their children's birth. Slowly, hospitals relented but insisted that fathers wanting into the delivery room attend childbirth education with their wives, so they would not be a hindrance to the birth process. Lamaze, a method that encouraged unmedicated births, came to fill that education need and, unintentionally, with that education came more informed parents with opinions about how their babies were being brought into the world. More and more women wanted labor and childbirth the "old fashioned way," but within the safety net of the hospital. Women began talking about their birth experience and seeing the process of labor and delivery as more than something that gets a baby out. Many came to feel that it was an important part of the passage from maiden to mother and endued labor itself with more and more significance.

Physicians, however, were not trained on how to relate to this new empowered patient and manage labors without the control of the medications and procedures that had been the standard of care to which they were accustomed. The concept of a "birth experience" was very far down on the priority list. "Natural birth," for those within the medical community, quickly became equated with anti-medical hippy nonsense. Furthermore, as epidurals became better and better throughout the 1980s and 1990s, most within the medical community felt confident that they had mastered the birth process with effective, safe pain relief and regarded those choosing to forgo it as foolish and ill-informed at best and difficult and subversive at worst.

Today, doctors and nurses continue to be educated in that same tradition that views all birth as potentially pathologic and, in their day-to-day work, they are confronted with the very real danger that birth can represent. Whether it is the stress of that reality or a product of the rigors of their training, the desire to remain behind the sheet was strong and still remains strong. Most simply cannot understand why a patient would choose "warm and fuzzy" or "natural" over the safety and reliability of their machine.

THE CHICKEN COOP: LABOR AND DELIVERY NURSING CULTURE AS A BARRIER TO NATURAL BIRTH

I own a small flock of hens and I learned very quickly in the process of raising them that hens develop a pecking order, even from a young age. There is always a dominant hen who eats first, chooses where she lays her eggs, and exerts control over the other hens in the flock. Every hen learns where they stand in the flock and, while there may be some pecking from time to time and other verbal and physical displays of dominance, in order to coexist in the small coop, the pecking order must be respected.

As I walked into Labor and Delivery, birth ball under my arm and pulling a large suitcase filled with items to make a hospital room more like home, there they were…the nurses in their station. They all turned their gaze on me. I could almost hear the low throated "clucking" sound. I immediately felt threatened. The dominant one called out to me, "Are you a doula?" Total silence followed, along with eye rolling and exchanges of meaningful glances and obvious suppression of laughter.

"Yes. I am," I declared proudly and knew immediately that the pecking order had been threatened. The mother I was supporting was already in her room, having arrived a few minutes before me, and I joined her there. Her assigned nurse soon followed. She directed her attention only to the mother, refusing to even speak to me. As the soon to be mom pulled out her birth plan and handed it to the nurse to read, the nurse quickly folded it in four and informed the mother that she would not even read it because she wouldn't want to jinx her, but that she could "try" to achieve a natural birth. She rattled off a few instructions, "rules" for patient and certainly for me, and turned on her heal, headed back out to the coop, clucking as she went.

In the many births I supported at that same large teaching hospital in the years which followed, I discovered that there was definitely a culture in place, with unwritten laws as stringent as the rules of my chicken flock. Unfortunately, that culture often had nurses pushing down the "inferior" patient who was simply too "uppity" or "too stupid to know better" when asking for or planning something which the nurse did not think was a good idea or did not care to provide. As a doula trying to advocate for my patient, I was lower than the dirt marring the laminate floor. I also observed nurses yelling at each other, complaining about their work load, mocking patients within ear shot, and bad mouthing doctors and midwives, especially the few doctors and midwives who would actually take care of and support the patients that wanted to naturally birth. The nurses were the ones who told the patient what they were allowed to do, they told them when to get the epidural and whether they needed pitocin or other medicines, and they decided when the women were ready to push and how. It's interesting, but everyone in the natural birth community always complains about doctors this, or doctors that, but what I have observed is that it is the nurses who are really in charge and often determine whether a woman, especially a naturally birthing woman, has a positive birth experience or not.

What had happened to some of these women, most of them mothers, who had entered a profession as a caretaker and ended up so jaded and mean? From what I have seen during the many hours I have spent visiting the Labor and Delivery units in various hospitals, I believe that many of these nurses have become disconnected from their patients, avoiding the real personal connection the profession demands, and are more preoccupied by what is going on at the nursing station than what is going on in their patient's room. They are more obsessed with keeping a baby on the monitor than helping their patient manage their contractions. Any patient that asks more from them, that isn't just quietly laying in bed, is simply a nuisance. I have gained a deep understanding of why more and more women are paying for their own labor support in major hospitals and why women who arrive without support are very likely to be intimidated away from their desired birth experience. I imagine there are many women who never even feel comfortable enough to pull their birth plan out of the bag.

—C. G., certified doula

There is a common myth that is often perpetuated by books, movies, and television shows of the benevolent labor and delivery nurse of old who sits by her patient's bedside, helping the laboring mother through each contraction, teaching her how to breathe, placing a cool cloth on her head, offering her sips of water, and comforting her as the masked doctor hangs behind the sheet until the moment a screaming baby is lifted into view. Many patients expect to meet that nurse when they enter the hospital in labor, but most are disappointed. Undoubtedly there are many nurses who were inspired to enter the profession by such images and admirably strive to fill that role, despite all the forces working against them, but, in reality, that has not been the history of labor and delivery nursing nor is it likely achievable in modern labor and delivery units today. When birth moved into hospitals, nurses were the enforcers of the controlled labor management prescribed by physicians. While serving that role in the multi-bed labor wards of the mid-twentieth century, labor and delivery nurses were frequently called out for inhumane treatment of women, such as verbal abuse, restraining patients on delivery tables for prolonged periods of time, and withholding even water. Nursing staff isolated women from their families and often did not allow them to see their babies for days under the rationale of preserving sterility. Labor and delivery units were about order and efficiency, often described as assembly lines rather than care centers.[10]

Thankfully, today's labor and delivery units are much more mother-friendly and the vast majority of nurses treat their patients with kindness, even if they do not personally like their birth plan. However, nurses remain as the enforcers of the physician's orders and, given the busy nature of labor units and the small percentage of the time physicians actually spend with women in labor, nurses are often seeking the orders they feel are indicated and interpreting those orders in the way they wish. Ninety percent of maternity wards in the United States are run with a "nurse-managed labor model," meaning nurses assume a semi-autonomous role with intermittent communication with an off-site obstetrician or midwife.[11] Patients are overwhelmingly kept in private rooms, behind closed doors, where there is surprisingly little oversight of their care by either the physician or other nurses. This gives each individual nurse enormous power over their patient, as she (labor and delivery nurses are overwhelmingly female) may very well be the only care provider the woman sees until delivery is imminent and their doctor or midwife arrives. For example, a doctor may order that a patient has ambulation privileges during labor, but it is up to the nurse to determine if the monitoring of the baby and the vital signs of the mother really permit that. A patient may have orders permitting food or drink during labor, but the nurse may withhold these if she feels the patient is not stable enough to eat or she may tell the patient eating will make her nauseous, less directly restricting her diet but nonetheless restricting it. For a patient receiving a medication such as pitocin to promote contractions, once the medication is ordered, the nurse sets the rate of the medication and can independently turn the medication up or down, on or off, based on her judgment of the baby's well-being and contraction frequency. Their influence over the labor and delivery process is actually significant enough to affect cesarean section rates, with cesarean section rates varying greatly between individual nurses within the same institution, working with the same doctors and midwives.[12]

Exactly how that nurse exerts her influence over the labor process depends on a number of factors, including the nature of the hospital where she works, the way she was trained, and her own personal childbirth experiences and philosophy about birth. There has been an increasing trend toward centralization of maternity services, meaning the majority of births in any geographical area are performed in large regional centers, where high-risk perinatology, high-level NICU care, and advanced gynecological surgical services are all provided in one hospital. This enables one institution to provide care for all types of patients, from the simple, healthy low-risk vaginal birth to the highest risk premature or surgically complicated births. Centralization of services is cost effective and ensures proper resources without the need for transfer in the rare event that a low-risk patient experiences a high-risk complication. However, there are negative consequences of this organization structure as well. Centralization makes for increasingly hectic, less personalized labor and delivery units. For example, a healthy woman can be laboring in the room next door to a premature patient with severe preeclampsia who suddenly needs an emergency cesarean. She can hear the commotion that ensues when multiple staff members rush the woman to the operating room and the uncomplicated laboring woman likely does not get the same time and attention she would receive if there was not a simultaneous emergency going on. After the stressful event, the nursing staff who dealt with that emergency understandably have less energy and emotional stamina for the other patients they are caring for. They likely have less patience as well. Nurses frequently complain that the current labor and delivery structure leaves them overworked and unable to provide the care they want to provide because they are responsible for too many patients at one time and often these patients are extremely sick and emotionally draining to care for.[13] Centralization also means that all nursing staff are routinely exposed to high-risk situations and poor outcomes, creating the feeling that birth is more dangerous than it actually is, particularly for low-risk mothers. This may make individual nurses less inclined to support what she may deem too high risk of a birth request, not on the basis of evidence, but on her own subjective experience.

The design of a unit and charting demands can also impact the way a nurse interacts with her patients. Many labor and delivery units are organized around one central nursing station, with a single bank of fetal monitors and a board for tracking each patient's progress. Charting, which occupies an ever increasing percentage of working hours as documentation requirements increase, is most often electronic and usually completed in this same station. Hence, nurses are spending most of their time with other nurses, rather than with the patients themselves. This close working environment often fosters frequent and open discussion about the patients among the labor and delivery staff. This can be a positive thing, as all the members of the team are aware of each patient and can potentially step in to help care for that patient, but it can also create a breeding ground for venting and complaining about frustrations with other team members and the patients they are caring for. This is particularly true when the individual team members are stressed and overburdened with work and emotionally difficult cases. More senior and dominant nurses, who may have trained and practiced in a time when labor and delivery care was even more controlled than it is now, can also influence the way other nurses take care of their patients, either in a positive or negative way, as the management is discussed and debated at the nursing station. In units where many members are not very fond of natural birth, this is often the setting where birth plans are passed around and joked about among staff. This can either consciously or subconsciously impact the way that particular naturally birthing patient is treated, as well as future patients who desire a natural birth, as patients with birth plans become labeled as "one of those" in the minds of nursing staff. Once the patient is "one of those," instead of a complete person with understandable fears and desires worthy of respect, how can her preferences be sufficiently honored?

FINANCIAL BARRIERS

Many patients and nonmedical critics of the American maternity system mistakenly believe doctors make more money on cesarean sections and this is why they are reluctant to adopt practices that may reduce the cesarean section rate. While there are studies that demonstrate an association between higher cesarean reimbursement rates and higher cesarean section rates in hospitals, individual physicians tend to have similar cesarean section rates across differing hospitals and reimbursement structures. Yet, when physicians care for patients with medical knowledge, a lower cesarean section rate is observed, even when controlling for other factors including education. This supports the opinion that non-medical factors do impact physician decision making.[14]

Certainly money does factor into the problem but not frequently in the simplistic fashion that has been discussed. Most physicians who participate with insurance companies, which is over 80% of the obstetricians in practice, are paid according to a global fee schedule for the entire pregnancy, delivery, and postpartum care. This means they make the same amount of money whether their patient has an induction or goes into labor spontaneously, whether she has a long or short labor, or whether she has a vaginal delivery or cesarean section. Reimbursements for providing this care vary from state to state but are uniformly decreasing. For example, in the Mid-Atlantic region of the United States, a global fee may be as low as $2600 for a privately insured patient, whereas $6000 used to be the standard rate and is still the rate received in certain areas. In that same geographical area, malpractice costs an average of $80,000 annually, meaning an obstetrician has to deliver 30 patients annually just to break even with their malpractice expense.

This impacts care in several ways. First, physicians must take on more obstetrics patients in order to cover their overhead costs and still earn a reasonable income. Many physicians have joined together in larger and larger group practices to help manage this volume and centralize administrative office functions and lower overhead. In large group settings, patients may only see the same provider a few times and any provider may be the one on call the day of delivery. Thus, many patients do not have a strong personal relationship with the doctor delivering their baby and may or may not have had an opportunity to discuss their intentions for their birth with them. Large group practices also tend to promote a shift mentality among their members, so the individual doctors often do not have as much invested in the birth experience of any one particular patient.

Among physicians that have decided to remain in solo practice or in small groups, the increased patient volume necessitated by the financial demands of current practice must be spread over a smaller number of doctors. Consequently, the individual doctors have less time to spend with each patient, both in the office and in labor and delivery. Usually doctors and patients know each other better in this setting, due to the greater number of appointments spent with that physician, but it is more likely that their doctor may need to be caring other patients while their patient is in labor, as most small practices do not have set call days that are devoid of other responsibilities. Hence, the laboring woman may not have ready feedback from their doctor during the labor process, as they are often not available until the very end of labor when delivery is imminent, and most of the in labor care is provided by nurses, residents, or laborists. Smaller practices may also be more inclined to manage their practice in an efficient way, by scheduling inductions that will not interfere with scheduled office hour times, and when the doctor in a solo office takes time off, usually the patient has never met the covering physician. There is simply no perfect way to provide continuity of care 24 hours per day, 365 days per year, yet continuity of care is what every woman wants and is considered an important part of supporting a naturally laboring woman in today's maternity care climate.

Further complicating the situation is the fact that, given lower reimbursements and an all-in-one payment setup, patience in labor may simply not seem cost effective for many physicians. For example, assume an individual obstetrician receives a global fee of $2600 for a delivery. That fee can be broken down into an hourly rate of care for the patient as follows. First, one must calculate the amount of work hours an obstetrician completes for each obstetrics patient outside of delivery care (Table 2-1).

When this total is added to the time spent caring for the patient in labor, it becomes apparent that once a labor approaches 12 hours, the actual hourly rate a physician earns caring for any one patient is lower than any standard outpatient physician hourly fee, even before expenses are taken into account. As labor approaches 24 hours, the hourly rate more closely resembles the hourly rate of nurses, counselors, and even

TABLE 2-1: TIME SPENT WITH PATIENT OUTSIDE OF LABOR AND DELIVERY CARE

Visit Type	Visit Number	Length of Visit	Total Work Hours
Outpatient antepartum	13	15 min	3.25
Inpatient post delivery	2	30 min	1
Outpatient postpartum	1	15 min	.25

Total work hours outside of labor and delivery: 4.5 hours.

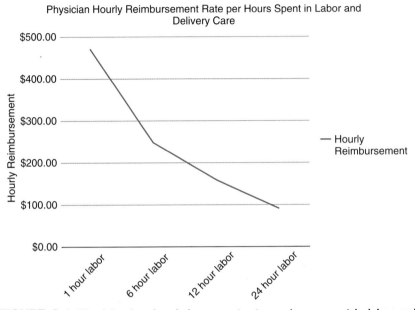

FIGURE 2-1. Physician hourly reimbursement rate per hours spent in labor and delivery care.

massage therapists, rather than that of a highly trained surgeon. How much this plays into decision making in labor and delivery is difficult to quantify, but certainly the less time a patient spends in labor and delivery the better for the doctor from a purely financial standpoint. When one considers the personal cost to physicians of caring for women through long labors, the scales become even more heavily weighted against the woman needing more time to bring her baby into the world (Figure 2-1).

Insurance companies are attempting to financially motivate physicians to achieve better outcomes. However, these proposed policy changes are mostly punitive. One proposal would offer different reimbursement tiers to hospitals and physicians dependent on cesarean section rate. Other proposals would simply hold back a percentage of reimbursement once a physician or hospital exceeded a certain cesarean section rate. There has not been any reevaluation of the global fee for obstetrics care or suggestions that obstetricians could earn higher reimbursements for vaginal deliveries or caring for a woman through a longer labor.

While it has not been demonstrated in the scientific evidence that unmedicated births take significantly longer than medicated births, there is a widespread belief among obstetricians that they do. Obstetricians also commonly have the misperception that women forgoing pitocin or an epidural are more likely to end up in a cesarean. With this mentality among care providers, proposed changes in reimbursement that aim to decrease unnecessary and costly medical intervention may serve only to lessen support of women who present to labor and delivery with natural birth plans.

THE LITIGATION BARRIER AND THE ISSUE OF CUMULATIVE RISK

The average cost of medical malpractice coverage varies greatly from state to state. In some states that have implemented tort reform, legal restrictions on the amount that can be rewarded for noneconomic damages in a malpractice case, annual rates are as low as $16,000. However, in states without any legal limitations on malpractice awards, annual malpractice costs for obstetricians can exceed $150,000.[15] Studies have shown an association with higher malpractice rates and more intervention heavy medical practices, such as higher rates of cesarean section and fewer VBACs; however these associations are more modest than one might expect. Nonetheless, physicians themselves admit that fear of litigation, particularly fear of a large suit that would restrict future practice, affects their decision making routinely, with 93% of physicians in high-risk litigation specialties reporting "defensive medicine" practices.[16] Defensive medicine takes many different forms, including referring patients to specialists, ordering additional blood tests and imaging, recommending inductions and cesareans, and avoiding high-risk procedures and complicated patients.

The most common reasons obstetricians are sued for delivery-related incidents include poor outcomes, such as a neurologically impaired infant, stillbirth, or neonatal death, and complications resulting from shoulder dystocias, VBACs, and operative deliveries, such as a vacuum or forceps delivery.[17] Legally speaking, a successful malpractice suit is supposed to include three components: an adverse outcome, deviation of the medical provider or institution from standard practice, and evidence that the deviation from practice caused the adverse outcome. In the actual courtroom, however, the adverse outcome is often the most heavily weighted of these components, particularly when an injured child is presented to the jury. This reality leaves obstetricians feeling that a suit is

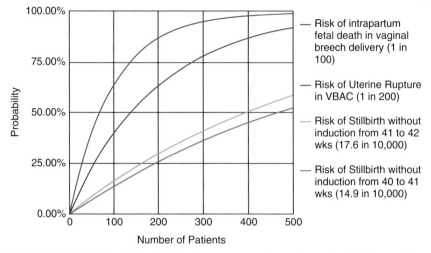

FIGURE 2-2. Probability of at least one poor outcome in a physician's practice over a given number of patients.[18,19]

inevitable and indefensible when any bad outcome occurs, regardless of the care they provide. Hence, most obstetricians rigidly avoid any risk of an adverse outcome and often see a liberal application of both induction and cesarean delivery as the most reasonable way to reduce that risk. One common line of advice handed down from older attendings to their more junior partners and residents is "you never regret the C-section you do, only the one you don't do."

A consideration of the probability that a physician will experience a poor outcome offers some understanding of why physicians choose to practice this way. For example, consider some of the examples of possible poor outcomes discussed previously. A woman considering a VBAC knows there is a 1 in 200, or less than 1% chance, of a uterine rupture, with an even lower chance that rupture will result in the loss of her baby (1.6 in 1000). With an 80% chance of being successful in that VBAC attempt, it seems very reasonable from her perspective to choose a trial of labor instead of a repeat cesarean. However, for the physician deciding whether to perform VBACs in general, he or she must consider that after performing less than 150 VBACs, there is a 50% chance that one of their patients will have a uterine rupture, basically the flip of a coin (Figure 2-2).

Put another way, if an obstetrician performs one to two VBACs per month, after 10 years in practice it is very likely they will be responsible and liable for the outcome of a uterine rupture. Given that many doctors feel something like this will almost certainly lead to a lawsuit and potentially jeopardize their career and livelihood, it also seems very reasonable that any individual doctor would not want to perform a VBAC.

However, when the risk of a less likely poor outcome is taken into account, such as that of stillbirth from 40 to 41 weeks as compared to the risk from 41 to 42 weeks, the argument is not nearly as strong. As seen in the chart above, the probability of stillbirth is fairly similar whether a physician induces all patients by 41 weeks or by 42 weeks. However, the fear of doing anything that is higher risk, even marginally, is still strong. Furthermore, even when these low probability poor outcomes are considered, it is also easy to understand how general population recommendations develop a very liberal application of induction, as it only takes 500 women going past either 40 or 41 weeks to reach that critical 50% mark where at least one patient will experience a stillbirth. Hence, what makes sense to recommend from a public health perspective may be much more medically aggressive than what seems warranted when considering any one woman's individual risk of a poor outcome.

Sadly, this means that women and their doctors are often considering risk and making decisions from a very different perspective. However, doctors must remember that they should not be making recommendations based on their own probability of a poor outcome. Doctors should be advising and caring for only the woman in front of them and that woman is entitled as an autonomous person to make her own independent decision reflective of the way that risk applies to her, particularly when the risk being discussed is the risk of nonintervention. Doctors can with confidence refuse to perform a procedure when they determine the benefits do not outweigh the risks. However, "permitting" a woman to spontaneously labor and have a vaginal delivery is not a procedure, though it has come to be seen this way. Labor followed by a vaginal delivery is the natural and spontaneous conclusion of a pregnancy. Inductions and cesareans are the procedures that doctors offer in order to try to improve upon that natural process.

Doctors should recommend care in accordance with their personal judgment and guidelines, as these are put in place to ensure the best outcomes for the greatest number of people, but each individual patient has the right to decide if that recommendation is appropriate for them and physicians are obligated to discuss the risk that those recommendations are based on as it pertains to that patient. Given the facts, most patients will agree that the recommendation for a cesarean in the setting of a breech baby makes sense for them personally, that the risk of something happening to their baby is just too high. However, they may not agree that a recommendation to induce by 41 weeks makes the same sense, as their personal risk is not that high and their desire for a spontaneous start to labor may be greater than their concern about the small risk of stillbirth, especially if all indicators of fetal well-being are reassuring. As long as doctors are having open and honest conversations, they should feel comfortable sharing in decision making with their patients.

REFERENCES

1. Fogelson N. On resident autonomy and getting yelled at. The Academic OB/GYN Blogcast. Available at https://academicobgyn.com/2010/09/03/on-resident-autonomy-and-getting-yelled-at/. Accessed 2/2017.
2. Papp KK, Stoller EP, Sage P, et al. The effects of sleep loss and fatigue on resident physicians: a multi-institutional, mixed method study. *Acad Med.* 2004;79(5):394-406.
3. Biller KC, Antonacci AC, Stephen Pelletier S, et al. The 80-hour work guidelines and resident survey perceptions of quality. *J Surg Res.* 2006;135(2):275-281.
4. Ahmed N, Devitt KS, Keshet I, et al. A systematic review of the effects of resident duty hour restrictions in surgery: impact on resident wellness, training, and patient outcomes. *Ann Surg.* 2014;259(6):1041-1053.
5. Hojat M, Vergare MJ, Maxwell K, et al. The devil is the third year: a longitudinal study of the erosion of empathy in medical school. *Acad Med.* 2009;84(9):1182-1191.
6. Yoon JD, Rasinski KA, Curlin FA. Conflict and emotional exhaustion in obstetrician-gynaecologists: a national survey. *J Med Ethics.* 2010;36(12):731-735.
7. Frankle R. Emotion and the physician-patient relationship. *Motiv Emot.* 1995;19(3):163-173.
8. Ghetti C, Chang J, Gosman G. Burnout, psychological skills, and empathy: Balint training in obstetrics and gynecology residents. *J Grad Med Educ.* 2009;1(2):231-237.
9. Wertz RW, Wertz DC. *Lying In: A History of Childbirth in America.* New Haven, CT: Yale University Press; 1989.
10. Shah NS. *Forced Labor: Maternity Care in the United States.* Elmsford, NY: Pergamon Press; 1974.
11. Morton CH. Preventing cesarean delivery, What is the nurse's role? Available at https://www.scienceandsensibility.org/blog/preventing-cesarean-delivery-what-is-the-nurses-role. Accessed January 2016.
12. Edmonds JK, O'Hara M, Clarke SP, et al. Variation in cesarean birth rates by labor and delivery nurses. *J Obstet Gynecol Neonatal Nurs.* 2017. pii:S0884-2175(17)30259-9. doi:10.1016/j.jogn.2017.03.009.
13. Simpson KR, Lyndon A, Wilson J, Ruhl C. Nurses' perceptions of critical issues requiring consideration in the development of *Guidelines for Professional Registered Nurse Staffing for Perinatal Units. J Obstet Gynecol Neonatal Nurs.* 2012;41(4):474-482. doi:10.1111/j.1552-6909.2012.01383.x.
14. Johnson E, Rehavi M. Physicians treating physicians: information and incentives in childbirth. *Am Econ J.* 2016;8(1):115-141.

15. Medical Liability Monitor. Annual rate survey. 2013;37(10):1. Available at http://www.medicalliabilitymonitor.com/rate-survey.php.

16. Minkoff H. Fear of litigation and cesarean section rates. *Semin Perinatol.* 2012;36(5):390-394.

17. Shwayder J. Liability in high-risk obstetrics. *Obstet Gynecol Clin North Am.* 2007;34(3):617-625.

18. Menacker F, MacDorman MF, Declercq E. Neonatal mortality risk for repeat cesarean compared to vaginal birth after cesarean (VBAC) deliveries in the United States, 1998–2002 birth cohorts. *Matern Child Health J.* 2010;14(2):147-154.

19. Rosenstein MG, Cheng YW, Snowden JM, Nicholson JM, Caughey AB. Risk of stillbirth and infant death stratified by gestational age. *Obstet Gynecol.* 2012;120(1):76-82.

Are Midwives the Solution?

CHAPTER 3

When my midwife entered the room during our first visit, she was not at all what I had been expecting. I think I imagined a friendly granny or a long haired hippy in a skirt down to her ankles. Instead, Lisa entered the room with her short, spiky red hair, wearing thick purple glasses and blue jeans. She warmly greeted me, immediately setting me at ease, and spent the better part of the next hour reviewing my health history, discussing my usual diet and exercise and making suggestions for improvement, and exploring how I was planning to deliver this baby, my second child, and integrate him into our family. We talked about what had gone right in my last pregnancy and delivery and what I hoped would be different this time around. I was struck by how different this type of care felt from that I received previously with my obstetrician. In my initial visit with my OB, we had reviewed my bloodwork, discussed testing options, and I left with a list of do's and don'ts and when to call. My midwife did those things too, but they were not the focus. I felt like the focus was much more on me as a person this time around. The visits that followed, while less time consuming, were still more personal and by the time my labor started, I felt like Lisa really understood me. She was calm and reassuring during the labor, which this time I had decided to do without any medication. She really let me know that I could do it and I had a smooth, easy all natural delivery. I don't know if it was that way because it was my second time or because of Lisa, but I would choose a midwife again if I had a third child. The entire experience was better all around.

—L. A., new mother

THE MIDWIFERY MODEL OF CARE

With the increasing awareness of the problems afflicting the American maternity system, many have begun to question whether, at this point, we are too far gone along the path of intervention as standard of care to ever change course. It seems particularly unlikely that change is possible when we continue to apply the same philosophy of care, birth in the same locations, and utilize the same providers. How many generations of doctors will it take before the main tide of opinion favors low intervention and natural options for childbirth. This is because, as profoundly stated by Akileswaran and Hutchinson,[1] "what is missing is a reference point of what is normal; the concept of normalcy is secondary in the medical model of health, in which suspicion of pathology is often the lense for each interaction or decision."

The midwifery model of care offers that reference point, by beginning with view that pregnancy and childbirth are normal life events. This does not mean midwives believe childbirth is devoid of any danger. That would be a denial of the high rate of maternal mortality (608 in every 100,000 births) observed less than century ago in the United States and still seen in some parts of the world today.[2] However, the midwifery model of care attempts to find that elusive middle ground of avoiding bad outcomes without subverting the normal process of birth. The manner in which this is done is through the establishment of close personal relationships with patients, which promote a partnership mentality and shared decision making. Noninterference in normal processes and continuous hands-on support of the laboring mother are standard and there is a judicious use of technology and medical interventions. Referral to obstetrics services is employed only when complications arise or a woman is at sufficient risk of a complication. Healthy lifestyle choices are encouraged in order to minimize complications and the physical, psychological, and social well-being of the mother are monitored throughout pregnancy.[3]

This care philosophy appears to have excellent results. In the most recent *Cochrane Review* of 15 separate trials, involving 17,674 predominantly low-risk women who were cared for and delivered by certified midwives in a hospital setting, midwife-led care demonstrated multiple advantages over standard physician-led care. Patients cared for by midwives utilized epidurals at a lower rate, had lower rates of operative deliveries and premature birth, and lower rates of perinatal death. Midwifery-led care was also less likely to include episiotomies, pitocin use, and artificial rupture of the membranes or amniotomy. Furthermore, patients cared for by midwives were more satisfied with their care.[4] A reduction in the risk of cesarean section was not observed in the *Cochrane Review*, but alternative reviews have also found a decreased rate of cesareans among patients cared for by midwives.[5] From this data, it seems expanding the availability and utilization of midwives would be a simple way to increase the number of providers applying a low-intervention approach and offer more women a supported natural birth.

Expanding midwifery care also seems like the path of least resistance. Why not direct women to the care providers who already support natural birth to the degree that it forms the basis of their mission statement and care philosophy? Many in the media have come to this same conclusion and a public doctor versus midwife debate has raged in print, social media, and on television. Articles such as "Are Midwives

Safer than Doctors?," "Doctors versus Midwives: The Birth Wars Rage On," and "Pregnancy Is Way Better Without an OB/GYN," are just a small sampling of the polarized discussion that has ensued.[6-8] Unfortunately, this has created the impression in the minds of many that midwives are somehow outside of the medical system, rather than operating with a different philosophy within it. It also has presented doctors and midwives as two equivalents that a woman must choose between, rather than presenting the midwifery model of care as something that should be broadly adopted for all low-risk women by doctors and midwives alike. This is problematic because there are a number of challenges preventing the widespread transition of maternity care from doctor to midwife.

CHALLENGES TO WIDESPREAD MIDWIFERY CARE IN THE UNITED STATES

Lack of Midwife Accessibility

Many women in the United States who may wish to receive care from a midwife simply do not have that option. According to the American Midwifery Certification Board, as of 2016, there were 11,475 certified nurse midwives and 103 certified midwives in practice, mainly in the hospital setting.[9] According to the National Association of Certified Professional Midwives, there are an additional 2,454 certified professional midwives also providing care, mainly in the home or birth center setting.[10] Even when the addition of non-nurse midwives, who are not currently supported by the American College of Obstetrician and Gynecologists, are taken into account, there are not enough midwives to provide care for all the low-risk women within the United States who may desire it. In comparison, there are 33,316 practicing obstetricians in the United States as of 2010, which is in itself insufficient to provide care for the number of women requiring it, 49% of whom live in a county without a single obstetrician.[11]

Besides inadequate numbers of midwives, regulation of midwives also limits their accessibility. Many states require certified nurse midwives to have either direct supervision of a physician or a written collaborative agreement in order to even obtain licensure and many hospitals require collaboration in order to obtain hospital privileges. If a midwife is unable to find a physician in her area who is willing to provide that supervision or collaboration, she is unable to practice. Some states also restrict midwives' ability to prescribe medications or specifically prohibit even nurse-midwives from attending out-of-hospital births. Furthermore, even if a state does not restrict midwifery practice through licensing limitations, hospitals may use their own discretion when deciding whether or not to grant admitting privileges and few states have laws in place preventing them from discriminating against midwives.

Another accessibility barrier is financial. Insurance companies have been slow to contract with midwives for in-network maternity care or be willing to offer reimbursement for out-of-hospital births. This means many patients desiring midwifery care have been forced to go out-of-network or pay out-of-pocket for services, which is financially prohibitive for many women. The situation has improved with the passage of the Affordable Care Act, which mandated insurance coverage for out-of-hospital birth, but with the future of that law in political jeopardy, many worry that insurance companies will not even be mandated to provide maternity benefits, let alone coverage for midwifery or out-of-hospital birth. Even when insurance companies are willing to reimburse for midwifery care, sometimes that reimbursement is lower than that of physicians. Hence, most midwives find themselves in the same financial struggle obstetricians find themselves in: low reimbursement for the care provided and high liability insurance overhead. They are further financially handicapped by lost reimbursements when they must refer care to an obstetrician due to the development of a complication. Consequently, midwives are often forced to play the numbers game and increase the number of patients they see, limiting their ability to practice according to the midwifery model of care. Many midwifery practices struggle to simply stay afloat.

TRADITION AND ACCEPTANCE

When I turned eighteen, I started having issues with my period. My mom took me to see one of the younger partners of the doctor she had seen for twenty years, the doctor who had delivered both me and my brother. She was a really nice doctor and talked me through my first pelvic exam. I kept seeing her every year when I came home for summer break during college. Eventually, I moved back home and got married. The same practice took care of me throughout my first pregnancy and it was actually my mom's doctor, the same doctor who had delivered me, who delivered my daughter. It was pretty cool. I didn't have any real birth plan and I didn't ever think about going anywhere else. I felt comfortable with that practice that had quite literally brought me into the world.

—*M. B., new mother*

Obstetricians have dominated the birthing business for so many generations that few American women have a member of their family who was cared for or delivered by a midwife. Most women receive their routine gynecologic care in adolescence and young adulthood from an OB/GYN as well. Consequently, when they become pregnant, few women even think to seek care elsewhere. Most equate doctor-supervised hospital birth with safety and often mistakenly believe midwife care is synonymous with home birth or birth center birth. There is also a misperception that only women who want natural births see midwives and, if a woman plans on an epidural, she should see an obstetrician. While many women come into their first pregnancy with the idea to try and do things as naturally as possible, most are open to an epidural and want the option. Unless they have been exposed to other women who have used midwives or they have received information regarding natural birth and midwives in their childbirth education, it is usually only after their first birth does not go as planned that women begin exploring other options and learning about the medicalization of birth. It will take several generations of increasing percentages of women being cared for by midwives before the majority of women see midwifery care as commonplace and familiar.

There is also a huge barrier of tradition and acceptance to overcome in the medical community. Good midwifery care depends on strong collaboration with obstetricians, as will be discussed. Few obstetricians have ever trained or worked with midwives, so they have not been exposed to their philosophy of care and had the opportunity to grow comfortable with their approach. There are also large numbers of obstetricians with strong biases against midwives, who view them as undertrained and often dangerous in their anti-medical extremism. This bias is generated by stories of midwifery births gone wrong that are passed along at conferences and on labor and delivery units and supported by the limited exposures that obstetricians have to midwife-supervised births, which unfortunately are predominantly excluded to those births which have not gone according to plan. If a midwife-supervised birth has gone well, the obstetrician need not ever lay a hand or eyes on the patient. It is only when problems arise which the midwife is unable to handle that the obstetrician is called in. This supports the obstetrician held view of the midwife as an inferior care provider, especially when the midwife seeking assistance has been managing the labor in a manner different from that which the obstetrician is accustomed.

For example, an obstetrician may be called in after a woman with a protracted labor has a prolonged and unsuccessful pushing stage. Perhaps she never received pitocin or an epidural, things this doctor would have standardly encouraged, and the patient has been permitted to push longer than this doctor would have typically allowed. The obstetrician inherits a swollen, exhausted patient who now needs a cesarean that is likely to be more complex, due to the engorged tissues and low station of the baby in the pelvis from the extensive pushing. She is more likely to have extensive bleeding and a uterine injury in this situation than she would have been if the surgery had been performed sooner. In the mind of the doctor, this patient would have been a lot better off if she had just gotten pitocin and an epidural. She would have reached fully dilated more rapidly and either discovered the baby was undeliverable sooner or been able to vaginally deliver because she would have been less tired. Her surgery would have been less complicated and her recovery easier because she would not have been exhausted from the long, tortuous labor. Perhaps in this situation the obstetrician is correct, as hindsight always is. However, what the obstetrician does not see are the other 10 deliveries this woman's midwife has cared for in the exact same manner who went on to have healthy vaginal deliveries and never required the obstetrician's services.

DIFFERENCES IN TRAINING

I have always looked "too young to be a doctor." When I first graduated residency and entered private practice, I would often be asked by new patients and their families how many babies I had delivered. I would laugh and say I had lost count long ago. They would be surprised, but it was true. I was required to keep track of all my vaginal deliveries until I reached 500. After that, we could stop counting and I had reached that number two years into my training. I was also required to keep track of how many cesareans I had performed and I had completed over 400 by the time I graduated and I had stopped counting those at some point as well. I hired a newly graduated midwife when I was roughly four years into practice and I was beyond shocked when I learned she had only been required to deliver 40 babies to graduate from her midwifery program and had just reached that number. I had completed 40 deliveries by the end of my first month of residency and I would not have felt confident enough to deliver a baby by myself at that point. It wasn't really until I was in my third year that I felt like, yeah, I have this. I don't need my attending to be here.

Another part of the reason there is hesitation in accepting midwives as the primary providers of low-risk maternity care, particularly in an independent capacity, is because there are significant differences in the training of midwives when compared to obstetricians. Obstetricians are exponentially more experienced by the time they complete residency and enter private practice and they are well prepared to recognize and handle the vast majority of complications that may occur in pregnancy, labor, and delivery without referral to another provider. Many women feel comforted by knowing their doctor is well trained and able to provide care for them regardless of the situation. Table 3-1 delineates the differences in training and skill level between the two professions.[12,13]

Many advocates of midwifery argue that this imbalance in training is appropriate, that obstetricians are surgeons first and foremost, demanding a higher level of education and training, and the level of training for midwives is more than adequate for the type of care they provide, as indicated by the outcomes in the research. However, the research that is currently available does not indicate the experience level of the midwives studied, meaning those positive outcomes could be the work of midwives with many years of experience, rather than a mere 40 births. The current reviews also reflect varying levels of physician involvement in the care. In some studies midwives were the lead provider with possible consultation with a physician, while in others the care was primarily physician-led with midwife involvement only at the hospital level during labor, delivery, and postpartum under the supervision of the physician. In still other studies, the care was shared, with the midwife and physician alternating as lead care provider throughout pregnancy, labor, and delivery. Regardless, midwifery input into maternity care appears to have had a positive effect; however, just how much physician involvement was contributing to the safety of that care is not well defined.

There is also some flaw in the argument that midwives are more knowledgeable about normal low-risk birth than obstetricians, as obstetricians graduate residency having performed many more normal vaginal deliveries than midwives perform during their training. Midwifery advocates would counter that those vaginal deliveries are not "normal births," as they are performed in the medical model; however, midwives are training in the same medicalized environment as obstetricians, with over 94% of midwife births occurring in hospital. Even members in the midwifery community have questioned whether their midwives are really training within the midwifery model of care,

TABLE 3-1: COMPARISON OF MIDWIFERY AND OBSTETRICS EDUCATION, EXPERIENCE, AND SKILL SET[12,13]

Provider	Certified Nurse Midwife	Obstetrician
Undergraduate requirements	*4-year* Bachelor of Nursing: Classroom health science, general education, and clinical hours in all medical specialties required	*4-year* undergraduate degree in any background, minimum requirements in general sciences, English, and math required for medical school
Pre-graduate clinical experience	*1 year*, preferably in field related to OB/GYN	*None required*, however, most successful applications have some clinical medicine exposure
Graduate education requirements	*2 years* for master's degree (86% of CNM), combines clinical and classroom hours	*4 years* for MD or DO degree, with 2 years spent in classroom and 2 years spent in clinical rotations
Postgraduate specialty training requirements	*None required*	*4 years* of clinical training specifically in OB/GYN
Minimum number of procedures performed to complete training	Varies by institution, average: 40–60 vaginal births as primary midwife No surgical or ultrasound training required	Defined by ACGME, most graduating residents far exceed this number: *200 vaginal births* as primary physician *15 operative vaginal deliveries* *145 cesarean sections* *100 ultrasounds*
Obstetrical procedures providers are able to perform	• Prenatal and intrapartum care for low-risk women • Vaginal delivery • Repair 1st and 2nd degree perineal lacerations • Postpartum mother and infant care	• Prenatal and intrapartum care for low- and high-risk women • Ultrasounds • Vaginal delivery • Operative vaginal delivery • Cesarean section • Repair all laceration types • Hysterectomy and other lifesaving techniques in the event of hemorrhage • Postpartum mother care

THE BATTLE FOR NATURAL BIRTH

particularly when so many midwives come to the profession through labor and delivery nursing, with the view of medicalized birth as the norm and standard.[14]

Furthermore, with such limited clinical experience and an education focused on "normalcy," how can midwives recognize when normal becomes abnormal, when low risk becomes high risk, if they have not been exposed to either. There is a common saying in medical education that "the eyes cannot see what the brain does not know." It is why one is always said to be practicing medicine, having never truly mastered it. Each new clinical experience has something to teach the practitioner; there is something to learn in every birth. How many of those opportunities are midwives missing when they enter independent practice?

Confusion in Midwifery Credentials

Further complicating the issue of midwifery acceptance is the fact that there are actually five types of midwives practicing within the United States, each with vastly different education requirements, experience levels, and philosophies. Many people, even within the medical community, are not aware of this fact and believe all who go by the name "midwife" are equivalent. However, in America, truly not all midwives are equal.[15]

- Certified nurse midwives (CNMs)
  Certified nurse midwives, as shown in Table 3-1, hold both a bachelor's degree in nursing and master's degree in midwifery. They have the most extensive education of all midwives. They are licensed to practice in all 50 states, with varying degrees of physician collaboration. Most CNMs attend births exclusively in a hospital or birthing center setting and seek to find a balance between supporting physiological birth and utilizing medical intervention to ensure healthy outcomes.
- Certified midwives (CMs)
  Certified midwives are midwives who have a bachelor's degree in a field other than nursing and a master's degree in midwifery. Like CNMs, they are highly trained medical providers and must pass the same certification exams; however, not all states license CMs. They also are primarily hospital and birth center based and support a low-intervention approach to maternity care.

- Certified professional midwives (CPMs)
  Certified professional midwives are midwives who are credentialed through the North American Registry of Midwives, which will credential midwives on the basis of an apprenticeship with a qualified midwife and completion of an entry-level portfolio evaluation process or graduation from a midwifery school accredited by the Midwifery Education Accreditation Council. CPMs are not required to hold a bachelor's degree. They must perform 20 births as the primary midwife under supervision, 20 births as the assistant under supervision, and observe 10 additional births in order to be credentialed.[16] They advocate for as few technological interventions as possible and mainly deliver in the homes or birth centers. The safety of the care they provide, particularly in the home birth setting, has been questioned and they are not licensed to practice independently in all states.
- Direct entry midwives (DEMs)
  Direct entry midwives are midwives who are not credentialed by any given body of midwives, but have been licensed by their given state according to that state's legal requirements. Education and experience requirements vary from state to state and DEMs deliver exclusively in the home or in freestanding birth centers. Like CPMs, they typically advocate for as little technological interference in the birth process as possible.
- Lay midwives
  Lay midwives, like DEMs, are uncredentialed and usually lack any formal education. Most are taught via apprenticeship or self-study. While some states have begun to license lay midwives with the intention of gaining more oversight and accountability for them, most states do not offer lay midwives licenses and they practice rouge. They exclusively deliver in the home.

Unfortunately, when poor outcomes occur, usually in the home birth or birth center setting, this confusion over "who is the real midwife" often places the blame for births gone wrong and anti-medical extremism at the feet of the midwifery profession as a whole. There are many in the medical and public health community that believe that the CPM and DEM credentials should be abolished, which require significantly less experience and education than the CNM or CM credential and do not meet international standards of midwifery care. Critics of these non-medical midwives strongly argue that the existence of these credentials offers women false comfort that they have a qualified birth attendant and prevents the integration of midwifery and home birth into the obstetrics system, which makes childbirth in America less safe.[17]

However, proponents of these midwives counter that few CNMs and CMs attend births outside of the hospital and most "med-wives" do not truly embrace the midwifery model of care. They argue that maintaining licensure for an alternative midwifery pathway outside of the medicalized system is essential and, without it, women will lack licensed care providers who really offer an alternative to techno-medical birth. This will lead to more women giving birth unassisted at home, without any care provider, as women will continue to seek out home birth whether there is a licensed care provider or not. According to their argument, banning the CPM credential will drive more women to more extreme birth options, not less.

The consideration of all of these challenges, as well as the many barriers to natural birth in general, begs the question: just what is the solution? Are midwives the solution? Certainly, the argument can be made that midwives are an important part of the solution, but they are not the solution. Reeducation of obstetricians and hospital nursing staff and reevaluation of the medicalized maternity system in general is necessary, as obstetricians outnumber midwives seven to one and will be the primary providers of low-risk maternity care for some time to come. Simply writing article after article encouraging women to choose midwives does not help the many women who are geographically or financially restricted from midwifery care or who culturally only feel comfortable with a doctor involved in their care.

Furthermore, do we really want to define normal, physiological vaginal birth as a specialty procedure, something only a midwife is able to do? There is no magical secret whispered in hushed tones in the halls of midwifery schools or taught at the elbow of seasoned midwives that renders them uniquely able to support a woman through natural birth. Support of natural birth requires only patience, respect for the autonomy of the laboring mother, and a relaxation of the DEFCON 1 status that has come to define labor and delivery units in America today. However, as has even been stated by the leaders of the American College of Obstetrics and Gynecology, midwives do offer the best chance to provide both needed obstetrical services to the many women who geographically find themselves without a local care provider and low-intervention, natural options for the women who desire that approach.[18] In order to effectively do this, obstetricians and midwives need to begin to embrace a true collaborative care model, an integrative collaboration model, which would minimize many of the barriers to midwifery practice and better merge the midwifery model of care into the modern maternity system.

INTEGRATIVE COLLABORATIVE CARE MODEL

There are many ways for obstetricians and midwives to collaborate. Midwives and physicians can work together in a hospital-based team setting, providing acute care for labor and delivery according to each member's skill set and expertise. They can work in outpatient private midwife-physician practices, either with two separate patient loads or with some cross consultation between groups of patients, or they can work in more of a segregated manner, with separate outpatient practices in which the obstetrics practices act only as consultants or backup for high-risk patients and complicated labors. However, the ideal model, the model that offers all women the benefits of each group's unique strengths and minimizes duplication of services, is a true integrative model where obstetricians and midwives share responsibility for all the patients in a practice through pregnancy, labor, delivery, and postpartum.[19]

In this model of care, obstetricians and midwives are not in competition. They are working together to provide comprehensive care that best serves the needs of their patients. In one sample structure of this type of integrative model, all patients would have their initial obstetrics appointment with a midwife in the practice, who has the time to complete a thorough history and provide significant education about warning signs in pregnancy, diet, exercise, and what to expect in the weeks to come. Based on risk factors, follow-up care could be scheduled predominantly with either midwife or obstetrician, but all patients would have some visits with both providers. If significant complications arose, consultation with a perinatologist could also be arranged. Labor and delivery care of low-risk women and appropriate higher risk women could be either alternated between obstetricians and midwives or managed primarily by the midwife, with regular consultation with the obstetrician and obstetrician assistance if indicated by labor complications. However, unlike the segregated collaborative care models that currently predominate in the United States, if the obstetrician needed to assist in a labor initially managed by the midwife, the patient would still have continuity with both the providers and philosophy of care, as all care providers would be known to the patient and they would be working together toward the best outcome for the patient.

This model also offers each group of providers the opportunity to learn from each other. Midwives would gain more exposure to high-risk patients and complications and, thus, learn to more readily recognize and initially manage them. Obstetricians would gain exposure to alternative delivery techniques they may not have learned in their training, such as hands and knees positions or birthing stool deliveries, as well as comfort with less aggressive management styles. In an ideal integrative model, both groups would have opportunities to work together even at the training level to help build professional camaraderie and respect from the onset of practice.

The integrative model would also help reassure patients that they can have the best of both worlds. More natural minded patients would not have to feel afraid of the obstetrician who works hand in hand with their trusted midwife. Patients who are happy with the medicalized birth model as it is would also benefit from more extensive antenatal counseling and a lower intervention approach of midwives, even if ultimately they desire an epidural, induction, or even an elective cesarean, and their obstetrician can be freed from some of the responsibility of these low-risk patients who might not have otherwise had any care from a midwife. This allows the OB/GYN more time with higher risk obstetrics patients and gynecology care that might otherwise be neglected if the schedule is inundated with routine obstetrics visits.

In terms of the CPMs and other midwives serving women desiring out-of-hospital birth, currently these midwives are serving women who are not being served by the doctors and midwives in the medical field. To deny that there are women who will seek out home birth no matter how many times AGOG states its opposition to the practice is again setting women up for extremes of care. In the same way obstetricians can say they do not recommend a breech vaginal delivery but must still be willing to provide the best care they can for the woman who refuses a cesarean in that situation, so too should midwives and doctors be able to say they do not recommend a home birth but they respect a woman's right to choose one and help her to have the safest home birth possible. It would be wise to integrate the midwives who are already providing this care into the medical system by creating a national credential for non-nurse midwives, which meets a standard agreed upon by the obstetrics and nurse-midwifery communities, and license these midwives to provide home births with appropriate nurse-midwife and obstetrician supervision and integration. Midwives who are currently in practice who do not meet this standard could be granted a grace period to obtain the additional necessary training they needed. This would provide accountability and prevent dangerous midwives from practicing outside of their scope of care, without leaving women with only hospital birth or unassisted home birth as options for care.

REFERENCES

1. Akileswaran CP, Hutchison MS. Making room at the table for obstetrics, midwifery, and a culture of normalcy within maternity care. *Obstet Gynecol.* 2016;128(1):176-180.
2. Singh GK. Maternal mortality in the United States, 1935–2007: substantial racial/ethnic, socioeconomic, and geographic disparities persist. A 75th anniversary publication. Health Resources and Services Administration, Maternal and Child Health Bureau. Rockville, MD: U.S. Department of Health and Human Services; 2010.
3. The Midwives Model of Care. Midwifery task force. Available at http://cfmidwifery.org/mmoc/define.aspx. Accessed 1996-2008.
4. Sandall J, Soltani H, Gates S, et al. Midwife-led continuity models versus other models of care for childbearing women. *Cochrane Database Syst Rev.* 2016;4(1):CD004667. doi:10.1002/14651858.CD004667.pub5
5. Newhouse RP, Stanik-Hutt J, White KM, et al. Advanced practice nursing outcomes 1990-2008: a systematic review. *Nurs Econ.* 2011;29(5):1-22.
6. The Editorial Board. Are midwives safer than doctors? *The New York Times.* December 2014:A26.
7. Kluger J. Doctors versus midwives: the birth wars rage on. Available at http://content.time.com/time/health/article/0,8599,1898316,00.html. Accessed May 2009.
8. Bregel S. Deciding between a midwife or OB/GYN was a no brainer for me: pregnancy is way better without an OB/GYN. [Web log post]. Available at http://www.mommyish.com/midwife-or-obgyn/. Accessed April 21, 2014.
9. Essential facts about midwives. American College of Nurse Midwives. Available at http://www.midwife.org/acnm/files/ccLibraryFiles/Filename/000000005948/EssentialFactsAboutMidwives-021116FINAL.pdf. Accessed February 2016.
10. Who are CPMs. National Association of Certified Professional Midwives. Available at http://nacpm.org/about-cpms/who-are-cpms/. Accessed 2/2017.
11. The Workforce Studies and Planning Group of the American Congress of Obstetricians and Gynecologists. The Obstetrician-Gynecologist Distribution Atlas. American Congress of Obstetricians and Gynecologists. Available at https://www.acog.org/Resources-And-Publications/The-Ob-Gyn-Workforce/The-Ob-Gyn-Distribution-Atlas. Accessed 2/2017.
12. Ciotti M. Minimum thresholds for obstetrics and gynecology procedures. American Council for Graduate Medical Education. Available at https://www.acgme.org/Portals/0/PFAssets/ProgramResources/220_Ob_Gyn%20Minimum_Numbers_Announcment.pdf. Accessed July 2012.
13. Midwifery programs for aspiring midwives to consider: admissions requirements and programs structure. American College of Nurse Midwives. Available at http://www.midwife.org/Midwifery-Programs-for-Aspiring-Midwives-to-Consider. Accessed 2/2017
14. Walker D, Lannen B, Rossie D. Midwifery practice and education: current challenges and opportunities. *OJIN.* 2014;19(2):Manuscript 4. Available at http://www.nursingworld.org/MainMenuCategories/ANAMarketplace/ANAPeriodicals/OJIN/TableofContents/Vol-19-2014/No2-May-2014/Midwifery-Practice-and-Education.htm. Accessed 2/2017
15. What is a midwife, CNM, CM, CPM, and DEM. Available at http://www.graduatenursingedu.org/careers/certified-nurse-midwife/what-is-a-midwife/. Accessed 2/2017

16. Updates to CPM eligibility requirements. Available at http://narm.org/entry-level-applicants/. Accessed 3/2017.

17. Teuter A. Why is American home birth so dangerous. *The New York Times*. April 30, 2016:SR7.

18. Rayburn W. The obstetrician-gynecologist workforce in the United States: facts, figures, and implications, 2017. American Congress of Obstetrician Gynecologists. Available at https://www.acog.org/Resources-And-Publications/The-Ob-Gyn-Workforce/The-Obstetrician-Gynecologist-Workforce-in-the-United-States. Accessed 3/2017.

19. Waldman R, Kennedy HP, Kendig S. Collaboration in maternity care. *Obstet Gynecol Clin*. 2012;39(3):435-444.

The Evidence in Support of a Natural Birth Plan

The first step to change is awareness. The second step is acceptance.

—Nathaniel Branden

THE MEDICAL BIRTH PLAN

When I went into labor with my first baby, I had no idea what to expect. I had done the hospital birthing class, so I knew the mechanics of labor and had learned some breathing, but my doctor didn't really talk to me about anything except to call her when my water broke or when my contractions reached the 5-1-1, five minutes apart, lasting a minute, for an hour. I arrived at the hospital at six in the morning after my contractions had kept me up all night. They put me in a little triage room and then put the baby on the monitor. Some doctor I didn't know checked me and luckily I was 4 cm dilated, so I got to stay. The nurse drew blood, started an IV, and asked me if I was ready for my epidural. By that point I was because the stretcher I was on was really uncomfortable. They moved me to a labor and delivery room, I got my epidural, and then fell asleep. At some point the nurse came in to give me some medicine to keep my labor going because I guess my contractions had stopped and a different resident doctor broke my water. They kept having to turn the medicine on and off because the baby's heart rate was going up and down. I felt like I was on some assembly line that kept moving forward and then backing up, but eventually I got to 10 cm dilated and they called in the doctor who was covering for my doctor to come for my delivery. It took a while for me to push the baby out because I was pretty numb from the epidural, but eventually he was born. The doctor told me she needed to make a little room to get his head out, so while she was busy sewing me back up, the nurse was doing all the weighing and stamping of the baby at the baby warmer. Finally they brought him back to me so I could try and breastfeed. I don't know what I expected but it wasn't quite that.

—L. P., new mother

It is no secret that most members of the medical community despise natural birth plans. To quote a few anonymous doctors and nurses:

A birth plan is the fastest ticket to the OR. You know what my birth plan is: get the baby out!
Patients shouldn't confuse their google searches with my medical degree!
All birth plans should be burned.
Babies make their own birth plans.

However, what the medical community rarely acknowledges is that a birth plan exists for every woman who enters the hospital in labor whether they took the time to write one or not. It may not be printed on pretty paper, accessorized with cute pictures, or laminated to signal its inflexibility to the staff, but it is every bit as detailed and defined as the birth plan provided by women who wish to labor naturally. For a significant percentage of women, this birth plan is put into place before they even arrive at the hospital, with a scheduled induction or cesarean section. For the remainder of women, the medical birth plan is initiated as they enter the hospital in labor and is finalized when their admission orders are written. All laboring women are triaged upon arrival, which consists of being placed on a fetal monitor and a pelvic exam to confirm that labor has indeed begun, evaluate the labor progress, and determine if membranes have ruptured. If it is determined that a woman's labor is far enough along to remain in the hospital, blood will be collected, an IV will be placed, and intravenous fluids will be initiated, as eating and drinking in labor are not permitted in most labor and delivery units.

After the initial admission procedures, women are moved from triage to their labor and delivery rooms, as it is now standard for a woman to both labor and deliver in the same room, instead of being moved to an operating room or separate space for the actual delivery of the infant. Most women are confined to the bed from this point forward, both out of concern about the safety of ambulation and to enable continuous monitoring of the fetal heart rate and contraction frequency. Active management of labor is typically ordered by the private attending obstetrician and is carried out by the nurses, resident doctors, and laborists, who are certified obstetricians, without private practices of their own, who stay "in-house" and provide care and oversight for all laboring women admitted to the hospital. Active management of labor consists of manually rupturing the amniotic membranes, if they have not ruptured spontaneously, and routine augmentation of the labor with intravenous pitocin, the synthetic version of the natural hormone oxytocin that produces contractions. The dosing of pitocin is done gradually, increasing until a stable contraction pattern consisting of contractions every 2 to 3 minutes is established. Cervical exams are performed every 2 hours to demonstrate the efficacy of the pitocin augmentation and, if labor progression is found to be insufficient, an internal uterine contraction monitor may be placed in order to demonstrate that the strength and frequency of contractions are adequate and permit better titration of pitocin, if needed.

Epidural anesthesia is the preferred and assumed mode of pain relief in the medical birth plan and, in most labor and delivery units,

THE NATURAL BIRTH PLAN

anesthesiologist are staffed 24 hours a day in order to be able to provide it. After the epidural is placed, a woman is unable to ambulate, as epidurals contain both a numbing and paralytic component that renders the recipient immobile from the waist down. A bladder catheter is also typically placed because these same medications make it difficult to know when the bladder needs to be emptied and to physically empty it.

Once full dilation of the cervix is achieved, if the woman's private physician is not at the hospital already, they will be notified to come for the delivery. The woman will be coached on how to push, which usually consists of a valsalva push style, with the woman positioned on her back or semi-reclined in the delivery bed and her legs pushed back with the assistance of stirrups or a combination of the nurse and the woman's labor support partner. An episiotomy may be cut to facilitate delivery, usually based on what is the preferred delivery technique of the attending physician. A vacuum or forceps may also be used to facilitate delivery if the woman is having difficulty pushing the baby out on her own.

Once the baby is born, the mouth and nostrils are cleared of fluid with a bulb suction, the umbilical cord is clamped by the delivering doctor, and then the cord is cut by the woman's labor support partner, if they wish to. The baby is then passed off to the nurse, for further suctioning, stimulation, and assessment. Vitamin K, to assist with blood clotting, and antibiotic eye ointment, to prevent eye infections transmitted via the vaginal bacterial flora, are administered. The baby is weighed, diapered, and wrapped and footprints are collected. When these admission tasks are completed, the baby is returned to the mother for bonding and breastfeeding. Some hospitals are beginning to change this portion of the delivery experience and hand the baby immediately to the mother for bonding, in order to better facilitate breastfeeding; however, that is still not the standard of care in the majority of hospitals in the United States.

While the baby is being cared for, any vaginal tears or episiotomy that occurred during the delivery are repaired. The placenta is delivered and the uterus is massaged and manually cleared of any retained clot or membranes. An additional bolus of pitocin is also typically provided through the IV, in order to minimize post-delivery bleeding. After 1 to 2 hours of observation, the mother is moved to her postpartum room, where she will stay for 2 days. The baby, in most hospitals, is taken to an admission nursery where further assessment is performed and the baby is bathed. Once the baby is deemed stable, he or she will be returned to the mother in the postpartum unit.

This sequence of events is so standard that few in the medical community question either its benefit or necessity. Several aspects of the medical birth plan are supported by quality medical evidence; however, much of what is done is simply a result of the manner in which doctors and nurses were trained to manage labor and their subjective determination of what is or is not safe. Their resistance toward the natural birth plan often comes, not from a place of malice, but from a lack of experience working with women laboring in a different way and a fear that what a woman is asking for may be dangerous or completely ineffective. Also, given that much of what is detailed in a natural birth plan is the avoidance of a medical intervention, instead of an implementation of an intervention, often there is not a wealth of research to "prove" natural birth as a management technique, from either an efficacy or safety standpoint. The following chapter will examine the motivation for the most common components of a natural birth plan and explore their comparability to the medicalized birth model in terms of risk profile and outcome.

THE NATURAL BIRTH PLAN

CHAPTER 4

The Environment for Birth

I felt the first signs of my labor in the early evening and by midnight my contractions were strong enough that I had to breath through them and I was beginning to feel myself tense up in anticipation of each one. They were still too far apart to go to the hospital, so I woke my husband up for some support. He could see I was really stressed, so he turned down the lights, lit some candles, and played some music. I began to feel better though the contractions kept coming. By three it was time to go to the hospital. The ride was hard and when we arrived everything was so loud and bright. They asked me a lot of questions and I realized my body was really tense and cold. My contractions had spaced out too. Luckily we had hired a doula and the first thing she did when she arrived was to turn down all the lights, put on some battery candles and music, and I felt like I was at home again. My labor picked back up but it was more manageable in a calm space. I definitely feel like mood of the room changed the mood of my labor.

—*E. P., new mother*

I would like to birth in the comfort of my home or a freestanding birth center

The debate surrounding out-of-hospital birth either at home or in a free-standing birth center could very well fill a book on its own; however, it is impossible to discuss birth plans without acknowledging the small percentage of women who, no matter how much hospital birth changes, will never be comfortable with hospital-based care. Several studies have examined the reasons women decide to birth out-of-hospital, even if it means a skilled attendant is not available to deliver their child. Some common motivations expressed by many women who have had out-of-hospital births were a strong desire to maintain control over their birth, as well as avoid a traumatizing hospital experience and remain in a loving, supportive family friendly environment. Many women expressed more fear of hospital interventions than complications during childbirth, with a common theme being that they wanted to trust their body and the process of birth.[1-3]

The question is whether or not it is safe. Until recently, there was little research available on the safety of home birth in the United States, as it was only in 1991 that nonmedical midwives formed a credentialing organization and registry of nonmedical midwives and their outcomes began to be tracked.[4] Home birth was also such a rare event prior to the last two decades that it generated little attention for study, as it had no significant contribution to public health outcomes and was regarded as simply a fringe practice. Furthermore, the research that did exist out of countries where home birth was more common was reassuring. For example, in the Netherlands where one-fourth of the deliveries occur in the home, no difference in perinatal mortality, which includes fetal loss after 20 weeks, intrapartum fetal death, and neonatal death up to 28 days after birth, or other significant complications were observed in the over 400,000 women who planned a home birth, compared to over 250,000 who planned to deliver in hospital.[5] Research out of the United Kingdom, where home birth represents 8% of the total births, showed similar results.[6] Even in Canada where home birth is less common, the most recent study by Hutton et al.,[7] comparing 11,493 planned home-births and 11,493 planned hospital births, showed no significant difference in rates of perinatal mortality or significant morbidity and need for resuscitation with intended birth location and a lower rate of obstetrical interventions in the planned home delivery group.

In the United States, as home birth rates have been increasing and more data about American home birth has become available, there has been much debate about whether home birth is as safe in the United States as it appears to be in other countries. Data released by the Midwives Alliance of North America (MANA) in 2014, which analyzed the outcomes of 16,924 women who intended home birth, cared for by non-medical midwives, was initially determined to be consistent with the European and Canadian data on home birth, demonstrating low rates of obstetrical intervention without an increase in adverse outcomes.[8] However, reexamination of this data with a logistic regression of risk factors to maternal and neonatal outcomes found significant increases in perinatal mortality, especially in the setting of home birth among first-time mothers, mothers with a previous cesarean, mothers with a breech baby, and mothers with multiple gestations.[9] A separate retrospective cohort study of all Oregon births from 2012 and 2013 examining planned out-of-hospital births and planned in-hospital births demonstrated higher rates of perinatal mortality in planned out-of-hospital births (3.9 vs. 1.8 deaths per 1000 deliveries). It also showed higher rates of neonatal morbidity for home births, including neonatal seizures consistent with neurological injury and admission to the neonatal intensive care unit.[10]

There are many explanations for why American home birth is more dangerous than home birth in other countries and approximately three times more likely to result in perinatal death than hospital birth. As discussed previously, home birth is not integrated into obstetrical system. It is predominantly performed by non-nurse midwives with varying

THE NATURAL BIRTH PLAN

degrees of experience, education, and expertise. In the countries where home birth has comparable safety to hospital birth, out-of-hospital births are performed by nurse midwives who follow strict risk stratification guidelines and have specific protocols for transfer. In Canada, that transfer rate is as high as 25% and approaches 50% for first-time mothers. In the United States, in part because obstetricians have been so reluctant to offer any validation of homebirth, there are no such guidelines or transfer protocols, and MANA has been equally reluctant to define any limitations to home birth, instead stating those decisions should be between each woman and her midwife. Consequently, as the MANA data shows, there are significant numbers of high-risk births being performed at home, contributing to poorer outcomes.[11]

However, despite these facts and ACOG's strong statement opposing home birth, there are many who feel home birth should be considered a reasonable option for women, including the American College of Nurse Midwifery.[12] This is because the absolute risk of home birth is small, even if higher than hospital birth, and is comparable to other risks that obstetricians would consider acceptable, such as VBAC.[13] Thus, in the same manner that personal autonomy and reasonable representation of risk should be promoted in maternity care in regards to other non-interventions, home birth should be regarded and presented in a balanced way. As long as patients are being counseled about the small but increased risk, they should not be unduly pressured out of a planned home birth and providers should instead work to make home birth rare, but as safe as possible. Efforts toward that goal should include standardization of midwife credentialing and training, proper physician oversight of midwifery care, clearly defined inclusion criteria for home birth and indications for transfer, and integration of home birth into the maternity system.

In terms of out-of-hospital delivery within freestanding birth centers, this is generally less controversial. Freestanding birth centers are staffed with certified nurse midwives to a much greater degree than home births, thus minimizing some of the concerns surrounding this type of out-of-hospital birth. Furthermore, certified freestanding birth centers must meet state licensing standards, as well as standards set by the American Association of Birth Centers, the Joint Commission, and the Accreditation Association for Ambulatory Health Center. While there are certainly emergencies that can occur even in low-risk births that could be more appropriately treated in a hospital, with the ability to perform an emergency cesarean, the regulations over birth centers offer proper risk stratification as well as guidelines and protocols concerning transfer to hospital that home births lack. For this reason, both ACOG and the ACNM support birth within certified freestanding birth centers.[12]

I would like lights to be kept dim, voices to be kept quiet, personnel to be kept to a minimum, and the music of my choice to be played

A calming birth environment is a goal listed in nearly every natural birth plan. Interestingly, it is only within the more recent history of hospital births that this could even be addressed or determined by women, as it is only within the last thirty years that private labor and delivery rooms became widespread. Prior to this, women labored in large wards or shared rooms, alongside other laboring women and without the support of their spouse or family. Women were only taken to a private space when delivery was imminent. There was little concern for the labor experience and birth, like any other hospital function, was handled in a utilitarian manner. Today, having babies has become big business. Hospital administrators have discovered that where a woman delivers her children has a large association with where her entire family will seek future care, as women typically direct health care utilization in most families. Women will readily seek out the hospital which can provide the nicest maternity environment and, to attract women to their hospitals, maternity units are frequently updated and renovated and hospitals are increasingly providing private rooms throughout a woman's stay. Hospitals also invest generously in large marketing campaigns where decor is emphasized as much as quality of care. Women often make the choice of hospital based on appearance, privacy, and perceived comfort. Interestingly, hospital choice frequently trumps the decision regarding their care provider, with women often specifically selecting doctors or midwives who deliver at their preferred hospital.

Wood paneling and nice art work on the walls may professedly have little to do with quality healthcare and conversations about labor and delivery ambiance perhaps seem better suited to playgrounds and mommy blogs than medical journals. Nonetheless, multiple studies have been performed exploring the effect of environment on laboring women. For example, the PLACE pilot trial in Canada demonstrated that women who labored in an "ambient clinical setting," where the hospital bed was not a center of focus in the room and additional design features that promoted relaxation, mobility, and calm were implemented, were less likely to receive pitocin augmentation for labor dystocia and reported less time spent in bed and greater overall satisfaction.[2] Another recent study showed that women who viewed nature images throughout their

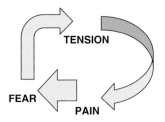

FIGURE 4-1. The Fear-Tension-Pain Cascade.

labor had higher patient reported quality of care scores, lower heart rates throughout labor, and higher APGAR scores in their infants.[3] While the studies to date have been small in scale, they support what women themselves have been saying: environment does matter.

The extent that environment is thought to benefit or inhibit the labor process is related to the perception of safety, comfort, and sense of personal control that it evokes in the laboring woman. Most natural labor texts discuss this in the context of the fear-tension-pain cascade, a concept that originated in the 1940s with Dr. Grantly Dick-Reed and his book *Revelation of Childbirth*, which was retitled *Childbirth without Fear*. According to Dr. Dick-Reed, when women anticipate pain in childbirth and fear the process, their muscles become constricted in response to the sensations of labor and that tension produces pain, which then justifies and reinforces the woman's fear response, promoting an endless cycle of suffering. Through his observations of patients who expressed little discomfort during labor, he proposed that if women could be taught to relax during labor and not be fearful, much pain during labor could be prevented as well (Figure 4-1).[14]

Ina May Gaskin, in her book *Spiritual Midwifery*, and Marie Mongan, who originated the HypnoBirthing Method, expanded on this idea. They theorized that the elimination of fear not only prevented pain in childbirth, but was also essential to the process of cervical dilation. They proposed that the cervix functions in pregnancy and labor like sphincters, which are structures in the body composed of circular smooth muscles that perform the dual functions of constricting a body passage and relaxing to permit the flow of liquids and solids through that passage as required for natural physiological functioning. In the case of the cervix during pregnancy, the circular smooth muscles remain constricted to maintain the pregnancy, while during labor they relax in response to longitudinal muscle contractions in the body of the uterus to effect the release of the baby.[15,16]

In fulfilling these dual functions, Gaskin holds that the cervix obeys several "Sphincter Laws." In her laws, Gaskin states that the cervix needs privacy and intimacy to open and that the process is hindered by time limits and commands. She describes several situations where the cervix can open only to close again if the mother is stressed and also where a closed cervix opened easily in response to positive emotional stimulus after a long, protracted labor. She also observes a connection between a relaxed, open jaw and cervical and vaginal stretching and opening.

While many of Gaskins observations about the cervix may be true, her theory of the cervix as sphincter is inherently flawed and simplifies an incredibly complex process. The cervix is actually composed mostly of connective tissue, with only 8% of the distal portion of the cervix being composed of circular smooth muscle.[17] The strength of the cervix during pregnancy is determined by the extracellular matrix of collagen fibers, rather than the level of contraction of the smooth muscle. When the cervix begins to ripen, the process by which the cervix softens and thins in the days and weeks that precede active labor, it is due to a decrease in the collagen concentration rather than a relaxation of the smooth muscle. This change in cervical composition is caused by a relative increase in hydrophilic glycosaminoglycans and non-collagenous proteins which increase the tissue's hydration and, in turn, break up the collagen fibers which create the cervical tensile strength. What exactly initiates this process is still poorly understood.

However, if a woman's psychological state is not impacting the cervix directly, as Gaskin proposes, then what is going on? Why is the emotional state of laboring women observed to impact labor progress? Likely, relaxation of the other muscles in the abdomen and pelvis contribute to the process by allowing for more optimal descent of the fetal head into the pelvis. That descent and resultant pressure on the cervix is what is aiding the labor process in the ways that Reed, Gaskin, and Mongon observe in their texts. Though there are no direct studies that demonstrate this, epidurals in the later stage of labor have been shown to aid in the labor process in this manner, so it is a reasonable to theorize that muscular relaxation in an unmedicated birth would function in a similar fashion. The psychological state of the laboring mother also impacts the intricate balance of hormones that bring about labor, as it does in other mammalian species. Mammals universally seek out environments of darkness and safety for birthing and the labor process can be observed to halt or speed up in response to external stimuli that produce stress or comfort. Hormones, such as adrenalin and cortisol, which are released when a laboring woman enters a "flight or fight" stress response, inhibit the release of oxytocin and, by extension, slow the progression of labor. Vasopressin, also released during a stress response, directs blood flow away from the uterus, contributing to fetal distress and preventing the muscles from contracting effectively.[18]

Interestingly, the light in the room may also impact the hormones of labor. Melatonin has been shown to synergize the effects of oxytocin, enhancing the contractility of myometrial smooth muscle cells. This promotes more coordinated and forceful contractions necessary for parturition.[19] Blue light, produced in large quantities by fluorescent and LED lights, has been shown to inhibit melatonin production.[20] Low lighting may not just promote maternal relaxation and contribute to the ambiance of the birthing environment, it may be essential to the proper functioning of the uterine muscle. This effect is thought to explain why a higher proportion of labors are observed to begin in the nighttime. It may also be why labor frequently seems to slow down upon entry of a laboring woman into the bright lights of the hospital.

Music therapy, specifically, has not been studied in relation to labor pain and maternal psychological well-being. However, it has been examined as a complementary approach to pain relief in other medical specialties. It has been shown to reduce pain perception in burn patients during treatments, as well as reduce their heart rate and anxiety levels.[21] It has also been shown to reduce pain levels in patients recovering from spinal surgery and to aid in maintaining stability and easing the postanesthetic transition among patients undergoing general anesthesia for abdominal surgery.[22,23] This suggests that music may also have similar effects on pain and anxiety perception in laboring mothers, in addition to supporting the overall tranquility of the laboring space.

However, the importance of a calm labor environment for the woman laboring without the aid of medication or an epidural extends beyond whatever small benefits may be demonstrated in medical studies in regards to labor speed and efficacy or pain scale ratings. All instructional methods of non-pharmacologic childbirth preparation, whether HypnoBirthing, Bradley Method, or Lamaze rely upon deep focus and an intentional breathing technique. Quiet, minimal staff, music, and dimmed lights all aid in minimizing distraction of the laboring mother, which is essential for women to effectively utilize their chosen labor preparation techniques. A quiet, relaxed space for birthing allows the mother to remain composed and centered, while also conveying to staff that enter the room to slow down and respect the woman's process.

Yet, perhaps the strongest argument for helping create this nest of comfort for the laboring woman to deliver her baby within is simply that women want it so and that should be honored. The process of welcoming a child into a family is a sacred one, irrespective of one's particular faith background. Parents remember the moment their child was born as one of the single most important moments in their lives. It is understandable that they would want that moment to look a certain way and feel as non-clinical as possible, as it is deeply personal event. The structure and equipment of the hospital birthing room exists as a safety net for the process, it need not dominate it. Personnel should be kept to the absolute minimum number needed to effectively aid the woman in the labor process and provide care for her infant upon delivery. Labor and delivery should not be a spectator sport for every student doctor, nurse, or aid. Conversations should be centered on the woman and care should be taken when to avoid anxiety-producing volume or language. If staff requires more lighting for needed monitoring or procedures, it should be the minimal amount required and lighting should be returned to the patient's preferred level when the task is completed. Consideration of rheostat lighting should be part of any labor and delivery redesign, though flashlights can be utilized in units that do not have the ability to modify the intensity of lighting. Delivery itself is primarily done by feel and bright light is not needed; it is more of a habit. If care is taken to respect the sanctity of the moment, women will have more satisfying birth experiences and will be less likely to seek out-of-hospital alternatives.

I want my partner, doula, another support people of my choosing in my labor and delivery room

When forming their labor plan, most women will also give special attention to the people in the room. The people present during the labor and delivery are an integral part of the laboring woman's birth environment and can have a profound effect on her emotional state. As mentioned previously, it is now standard to permit a woman's partner into the delivery room. Most hospitals, however, restrict the number of people besides the father or partner to one or two additional people and ban children under a certain age from labor and delivery. This small support base for the laboring woman and even the inclusion of the father in the delivery room is, however, a relatively recent development in the history of birth in America. Traditionally, when birth occurred exclusively within the home, birth was a social event confined to the female sphere. Female family and friends of the woman's choosing would come to the laboring woman's home to attend the birth, provide physical and emotional support, and attend to the domestic responsibilities that the laboring woman was unable to complete, while a midwife would perform the actual delivery. Even when families began employing physicians to perform

THE NATURAL BIRTH PLAN

deliveries, the tradition of female support for the laboring mother continued. It was only when childbirth moved into the hospital that women began to labor and deliver in isolation from their family and friends and it was this aspect of hospital birth that was the first to be challenged by women wanting a different experience.[24]

However, women in hospital birth settings in the past did receive more continuous, hands on support from nursing staff than women do in modern birth settings. Labor and Delivery units today are typically organized with two to one nursing ratios, meaning one nurse is responsible for two laboring patients at a time. Nurses are required to enter a note in the chart every 15 minutes that a typical patient is on the labor floor and, upon delivery, nurses have extensive documentation to complete regarding the events of the birth. This leaves little time for nurses to complete any of the activities that would be part of what is termed continuous support of the laboring woman: emotional reinforcement, comfort measures, informing and teaching, establishment of breastfeeding, and patient advocacy. Many women expect that their nurse will be helping them manage contractions and provide needed support through the labor process. These women are often surprised and disappointed to find that their nurses rarely have time to do much more than check on them periodically and take their vital signs once per hour.

This is unfortunate as companionship, in and of itself, has been shown to impact a laboring woman's experience significantly. Even the simple presence of an untrained volunteer in the labor room has been shown to reduce patient reported pain and anxiety, increase the perception that patients coped well with their labors, and reduce their need for analgesia.[25] The presence of partners and companions from the women's social networks have also been shown to benefit laboring mothers in a similar fashion, however the best outcomes have been demonstrated with continuous support provided by professional doulas.

Doulas are defined by DONA INTERNATIONAL, the largest doula accreditation group in the United States, as "trained professionals who provide continuous physical, emotional and informational support to a mother before, during, and shortly after childbirth to help her achieve the healthiest, most satisfying experience possible." Doulas must complete a minimum of 28 hours of structured classroom instruction, attend breastfeeding support education, and apprentice for at least three births in order to become certified.[26] Doulas are typically in near daily contact with the mother from 36 weeks of pregnancy until delivery. They stay with the mother throughout her entire labor process, supporting her through each contraction, and assist with breastfeeding in the postpartum period. In 2013, the *Cochrane Review* performed the largest systematic review of doula care and continuous labor support, which included 23 trials from 16 different countries and involved data from 15,000 women laboring in different circumstances. This review showed many benefits of continuous labor support, in general, and doula care, in particular. Specifically, when patients receiving doula care were compared to patients receiving standard hospital care, the following was demonstrated[27]:

- thirty-one percent decreased incidence of pitocin use
- twenty-eight percent decreased risk of cesarean section
- thirty-four percent decreased incidence of being dissatisfied with the birth experience
- twelve percent increase in spontaneous, non-operative, vaginal delivery rates

Unfortunately, most women do not have the benefit of doula care, as it is not covered by most insurance plans, restricting doula access to those that can afford to pay out of pocket for their services. Doula fees vary according to geographical region and doula experience but average $1200 and may exceed $2000 in certain areas. Hence, the majority of doula clients are well-educated, upper-middle class women. Critics suggest that the benefits of doula care have been overestimated due to the demographics of the patients who use their services, however, the results of the *Cochrane Review* have been replicated, even among low-income, Medicaid beneficiaries, who come from more diverse racial and ethnic backgrounds.[28] In fact, the American College of Obstetricians and Gynecologists and the Society for Maternal-Fetal Medicine stated in their joint committee opinion on cesarean prevention in 2014 that continuous labor support is among "the most effective tools to improve labor and delivery outcomes" and is likely underused.[29] While insurance coverage of doula care was not mandated by the Affordable Care Act, it was suggested that doula care could be a means of achieving its defined goals.[30]

Despite this overwhelming evidence in support of doula care, doulas are often met with resistance on labor and delivery units themselves. Nurses and physicians often see the doula's role as patient advocate to be confrontational and challenging their expertise. There is a misperception that doulas are overcompensated for their work, despite the fact that doulas are on call for their clients 24 hours a day, can spend over

24 hours awake, on their feet, continuously supporting a woman in labor, and are limited in the number of clients they can accept due to the time and physical restraints of their work. Members of the medical staff are also often resentful and distrusting of the close personal relationship that most doulas develop with their patients throughout labor, which often stands in sharp contrast to the impersonal relationship they have with the patient. There are even obstetrical practices and hospitals that forbid patients from hiring doulas or create such restrictive visitor policies on labor and delivery that women must choose between having a doula and having their partner or other close family members present.

These types of practices and attitudes are unnecessarily divisive and have no basis in the medical evidence. Continuous support of the laboring mother has no associated negative birth outcomes. The decision about who is in the room during labor and delivery should belong to the mother and the mother alone. Hospital visitor policies should exist only to prevent one patient's visitors from disrupting another patient and should be fluid enough to accommodate for the varied wishes patients have while laboring. Strict hospital protocols about numbers of visitors, doulas, and age of visitors depersonalize care and institutionalize what should be a family inclusive event.

REFERENCES

1. Rigg EC, Schmied V, Peters K, Dahlen HG. Why do women choose an unregulated birth worker to birth at home in Australia: a qualitative study. *BMC Pregnancy Childbirth*. 2017;17:99. doi:10.1186/s12884-017-1281-0.
2. Hodnett ED, Stimler R, Weston JA, McKeever P. Re-conceptualizing the hospital room: the PLACE (Pregnant and Laboring in an Ambient Clinical Environment) pilot trial. *Birth*. 2009;36(2):159-166.
3. Aburas R, Debajyoti P, Casanova R. The influence of nature stimulation enhancing the birth experience. *HERD*. 2016;10(2):81-100.
4. History of the development of the CPM. North American Registry of Midwives. Available at http://narm.org/certification/history-of-the-development-of-the-cpm/. Accessed March 2017.
5. de Jonge A, Geerts CC, van der Goes BY, Mol BW, Buitendijk SE, Nijhuis JG. Perinatal mortality and morbidity up to 28 days after birth among 743,070 low-risk planned home and hospital births: a cohort study based on three merged national perinatal databases. *BJOG*. 2015;122(5):720-728.
6. Brocklehurst P, Hardy P, Hollowell J, et al. Perinatal and maternal outcomes by planned place of birth for healthy women with low risk pregnancies: the Birthplace in England national prospective cohort study. *BMJ*. 2011;343:d7400.

7. Hutton EK, Cappelletti A, Reitsma AH, et al. Outcomes associated with planned place of birth among women with low-risk pregnancies. *CMAJ.* 2016;188(5):E80-E90. doi:10.1503/cmaj.150564.

8. Cheyney M, Bovbjerg M, Everson C, Gordon W, Hannibal D, Vedam S. Outcomes of care for 16,924 planned home births in the United States: the Midwives Alliance of North America Statistics Project, 2004 to 2009. *J Midwifery Womens Health.* 2014;59(1):17-27. doi:10.1111/jmwh.12172.

9. Bovbjerg ML, Cheyney M, Brown J, Cox KJ, Leeman L. Perspectives on risk: assessment of risk profiles and outcomes among women planning community birth in the United States. *Birth.* 2017; 44(3):209-221 doi:10.1111/birt.12288.

10. Snowden J, Tilden E, Snyder J, Quigley B, Caughey A, Cheng YW. Planned out-of-hospital birth and birth outcomes. *N Engl J Med.* 2015;373:2642-2653.

11. Teuter A. Why is American home birth so dangerous. *The New York Times.* April 30, 2016:SR7.

12. ACNM Home Birth Position Statement. Planned Home Birth Committee Opinion No. 476. American College of Obstetrics and Gynecologists. *Obstet Gynecol.* 2011;117(1):425-428.

13. Wilbur MB, Little S. Szymanski LM. Is home birth safe? *N Engl J Med.* 2015;373(27):2683-2685. doi:10.1056/NEJMclde1513623.

14. Dick-Reed G. *Childbirth Without Fear.* London: William-Heinemann; 1942.

15. Gaskin I. *Spiritual Midwifery.* Summertown, TN: Book Publishing Company; 1975.

16. Mongan M. *Hypnobirthing: The Mongan Method.* Deerfield Beach, FL: Health Communications, Inc.; 1992.

17. Schwalm H, Dubrauszky V. The structure of the musculature of the human uterus—muscles and connective tissue. *Am J Obstet Gynecol.* 1966;94:391-404.

18. Foureur M. Creating birth space to enable an undisturbed birth. In *Birth Territory and Midwifery Guardianship: Theory for Practice, Education, and Research.* London: Elsevier Limited; 2008.

19. Sharkey J, Puttaramu R, Word A, Olcese J. Melatonin synergizes with oxytocin to enhance contractility of myometrial smooth muscle cells. *J Clin Endocrinol Metab.* 2009;94(2):421-427.

20. Brainard G, Hanifin JP, Greeson J, et al. Action spectrum for melatonin regulation in humans: evidence for a novel circadian photoreceptor. *J Neurosci.* 2001;21(16):6405-6412.

21. Mondanaro JF, Homel P, Lonner B, et al. Music therapy increases comfort and reduces pain in patients recovering from spine surgery. *Am J Orthop.* 2017;46(1): E13-E22.

22. Kahloul M, Mhamdi S, Nakhli MS, et al. Effects of music therapy under general anesthesia in patients undergoing abdominal surgery. *Libyan J Med.* 2017;12(1):1260886.

23. Li J, Zhou L, Wong Y. The effects of music intervention on burn patients during treatment procedures: a systemic review and meta-analysis of randomized controlled trials. *BMC Complement Altern Med.* 2017;17(1):158. Available at https://www.ncbi.nih.gov/pmc/articles/PMC5356403. Accessed April 2017

24. Bishop EH. Pelvic scoring for elective induction. *Obstet Gynecol.* 1964;24:266-268.

25. Hofmeyr G, Nikodem V, Wolman WL, Chalmers BE, Kramer T. Companionship to modify the clinical birth environment: effects on progress and perceptions of labour, and breastfeeding. *Br J Obstet Gynaecol.* 1991;98(8):756-764.

26. DONA International. What is a doula. Available at https://www.dona.org/what-is-a-doula/. Accessed 2017. Accessed April 2017

THE NATURAL BIRTH PLAN

27. Hodnett ED, Gates S, Hofmeyr G, Sakala C. Continuous support for women during childbirth. *Cochrane Database Syst Rev.* 2013;(7):CD003766. doi:10.1002/14651858. CD003766.pub5. Available at http://www.cochrane.org/CD003766/PREG_continuous-support-for-women-during-childbirth. Accessed April 2017

28. Kozhimannil KB, Hardeman RR, Attanasio LB, Blauer-Peterson C, O'Brien M. Doula care, birth outcomes, and costs among Medicaid beneficiaries. *Am J Public Health.* 2013;103(4):113-121.

29. Caughey AB, Cahill AG, Guise JM, Rouse DJ. Safe prevention of the primary cesarean delivery. *Am J Obstet Gynecol.* 2014;210(3):179-193.

30. Nan Strauss JD, Giessler K, McAllister E. How doula care can advance the goals of the affordable care act: a snapshot from New York city. *J Perinat Educ.* 2015;24(1): 8-15.

Labor
Management

CHAPTER 5

I want labor to begin on its own

I had really hoped for a natural labor, but when I went to the doctor for my 39wk visit, he told me that he induced all of his patients if they hadn't gone into labor by three days after their due date. Unfortunately, my labor did not start on it's own and so I went to the hospital for my induction. My cervix was only dilated one centimeter, so they first had to soften it. They put a pill in my vagina every few hours and then, once I was dilated enough, they broke my water and started pitocin. The contractions were really intense and so I ended up asking for the epidural after about eighteen hours into the induction. After twenty-four hours, I hadn't dilated past six centimeters and my doctor said it had been going on too long and my baby was in danger of an infection, so they took me back for a cesarean. I often wonder what would have happened if we had just waited.

—P. S., new mother

SPONTANEOUS LABOR PROCESS

Spontaneous labor is best described as the gradual process by which the cervix goes from being a strongly contracted structure that holds the baby within the uterus to a completely relaxed structure that lets the baby out. It is helpful to think of the circular smooth muscles and collagen of the cervix as a tightly bound spool of ribbon, forming a thick, firm base for the uterus. As the longitudinal muscles of the body of the uterus contract, the structure of the cervix relaxes, causing the cervix to slowly thin and open, just as a spool of ribbon unwinds (Figure 5-1).

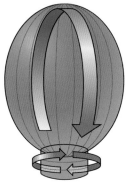

FIGURE 5-1. Uterine Muscle Structure.

The melting away of the firm structure of the cervix, until it is flush against the baby's head, is referred to as effacement and as the cervix both opens and effaces, the baby is able to descend lower and lower into the pelvis. Once the cervix has completely relaxed and retracted behind the baby's head, the woman uses her abdominal muscles to push the baby down through the lower bony structure of the pelvis and out through the soft tissues of the vagina.

For most women, the first signs of labor are subtle. The baby engages in the pelvis, with increasing sensations of pressure along the pubic bone and lower pelvis. The mother may feel cramping sensations in the upper thighs and lower back pain and shooting vaginal discomfort. The cervix will begin to soften and open, frequently indicated by more significant amounts of vaginal discharge and the passage of the mucus plug, a thick collection of cervical mucus that is yellow or brown in color, occasionally containing small streaks of pink or red blood as well. The gastrointestinal tract may become irritable, as the same hormones that stimulate the uterus stimulate the bowel, resulting in nausea, loose stools, or both. Emotionally, women frequently report a general sense of restlessness.

Uterine activity begins to increase as a woman's labor process advances. In the early stages of labor, often called latent labor, uterine contractions are mild, short, and irregular. Typically referred to as Braxton Hick's contractions, many women are not even aware that these contractions are occurring, beyond noticing a periodic tightening of the abdomen. However, once a woman moves toward a more active labor pattern, uterine activity becomes both progressive and persistent, with shorter intervals between contractions, building in both their intensity and duration of the contractions themselves. Once contractions are strong enough and frequent enough to significantly dilate the cervix, most women will find that they need to pause, focus, and breath through the contractions, while in the earlier stages of labor many women are able to continue their daily activities while experiencing contractions. As the cervix further thins and opens, often women will notice mucusy red or brown discharge, referred to as bloody show or birth show.

The latent phase of labor varies greatly in its length, taking only a few hours for some women and lasting days to even weeks for others. It is usually a shorter process for women who have labored in the past, while first-time mothers generally experience a significantly longer period of early labor symptoms before their labor pattern becomes active. Women who experience longer, more symptomatic latent labors frequently express frustration and fatigue with the process and many ultimately elect to have the process medically hastened. However, this gradual process of cervical opening and thinning, referred to as cervical ripening, and fetal descent is important for active labor to proceed in a normal fashion.

This was first examined in the 1960s by Dr. Edward Bishop. He developed a pelvic scoring system, taking into account cervical dilation, effacement, consistency, position, and station, which could be used to predict the likelihood of an induction of labor being successful.[1] While he initially only applied the system to women who had a previous vaginal delivery, more recent studies have replicated his findings in first-time mothers, using a simplified system that only looks at cervical dilation, cervical effacement, and the baby's station.[2] These studies have demonstrated that a woman is less likely to have a vaginal delivery if this process of cervical ripening is not complete, whether her labor is induced or begins spontaneously. However, even among women with the least ripe cervixes, a spontaneous labor in an uncomplicated, first-time mother is more than two times more likely to result in a vaginal delivery than an induction, regardless of induction type.[3] Fear of ending up in a cesarean section is one of the most common reasons that women cite when indicating why they want to avoid induction.

METHODS OF INDUCTION

As discussed previously, induction is incredibly common in the United States, with one in five women being induced. The exact process of induction depends on whether or not a woman's cervix is ripe at the beginning of the induction. For women with ripe cervixes, most doctors simply start pitocin, which is given intravenously in gradually increasing doses. The amniotic membranes are also routinely ruptured during an induction to aid in the process.

For women without a ripe cervix, the process is more challenging and the preferable method to initiate that process is a subject of frequent study and much debate among medical professionals. Various prostaglandins, physiologically active lipid compounds with hormone-like effects, are used to artificially achieve cervical softening and early dilation, in a process that can take 24 hours or more. These agents can also initiate active labor, but often subsequent pitocin use is necessary to continue active labor progression. The most common agents used in the United States are misoprostol or Cytotec, which can either be administered orally or vaginally, and dinoprostone or Cervidil, which is administered via a vaginal insert. The dosage of Cytotec, unlike Cervidil, is not standardized and studies demonstrating efficacy of Cytotec vary accordingly. However, both Cytotec and Cervidil have been shown to be effective at bringing about delivery within 24 hours, in comparison to pitocin induction alone. Both agents, however, have higher rates of uterine hyperstimulation and meconium fluid, where the baby has a bowel movement while still inside the uterus and can be associated with respiratory distress upon delivery. Cervidil has the benefit of being able to be taken out if too many contractions are noted or the baby does not tolerate the labor. However, Cervidil administered independently as an induction agent is more likely to require subsequent pitocin administration, whereas misoprostol can often achieve full dilation independently. In order to improve the efficacy of both these agents, a balloon dilator may be placed within the cervix to aid in the process by mechanically opening it. Using a balloon dilator can help speed up the ripening process and decrease the incidence of uterine hyperstimulation and meconium fluid, but it does increase maternal discomfort during the induction (Table 5-1)[4,5]

TABLE 5-1: SUMMARY OF PHARMACOLOGICAL AND NONPHARMACOLOGICAL AGENTS OF INDUCTION[6]

Agent	Mode of Administration	Benefits	Risks
Pitocin	IV drip	• Efficacious • Can be used in VBAC • Adjustable dosing	• Hyperstimulation • Stronger, more painful contractions • Fetal distress
Misoprostol (Cytotec)	Oral or vaginal tablet	• Efficacious • Less need for subsequent pitocin	• Increased meconium • Cannot be removed after administration • Cannot use in VBAC • Hyperstimulation
Dinoprostone (Cervidil)	Vaginal insert	• FDA approved • Can be removed after administration • Efficacious	• Often requires subsequent pitocin • Cannot use in VBAC • Hyperstimulation
Balloon dilator	Cervical placement manually or with speculum	• Can be used in VBAC • Faster ripening • Nonpharmacologic • Less hyperstimulation	• Often requires additional induction agent • Maternal discomfort

INDICATIONS FOR INDUCTION

The number of medical indications for induction has increased in recent years. Induction is considered medically indicated when it is determined that the risk of continuing the pregnancy is higher to the mother or the baby than the risks associated with induction itself, such as complications of a premature or early term delivery or cesarean section. Some common indications for induction are given in Table 5-2.

In general, the earlier the gestational age, the stronger the risk criteria must be to warrant an induction. Once the 39-week threshold is crossed, induction carries no recognized increased risk to the baby and the indications for induction are significantly more liberal. Some studies even suggest improved neonatal outcomes for induction at 39 weeks when compared to waiting for spontaneous labor up to 42 weeks. The main risk of induction that is considered after this point is the risk of cesarean section however the evidence connecting induction to cesarean is confusing and heavily debated. For patients with a previous vaginal delivery, the risk of a cesarean is small whether they are induced or go into labor on their own, 4.5% versus 2.5%. The main concern about inductions and higher cesarean risk is for first-time mothers, so most of the recent studies focus specifically on this group of patients. The data for many years overwhelmingly cautioned against elective induction in

TABLE 5-2: INDUCTION INDICATION BY GESTATIONAL AGE[6]

Preterm Delivery (<37 weeks)	Early Term Delivery (>37 weeks, <39 weeks)	Term Delivery (>39 weeks)
• Severe preeclampsia • Severe fetal growth restriction • Preterm premature rupture of membranes • Multiple gestations • Uncontrolled maternal health conditions (hypertension, diabetes)	• Mild preeclampsia • Moderate fetal growth restriction • Prelabor rupture of membranes • Multiple gestations • Controlled maternal health conditions (hypertension, medication controlled-diabetes) • Cholestasis of pregnancy • Oligohydramnios (low fluid)	• Elective • Ripe cervix/Advanced prelabor dilation • Advanced maternal age (>40) • Obesity • Diet-controlled diabetes • Prelabor rupture of membranes • Post dates (>41 wks gestation) • Large for gestational age

first-time mothers prior to 41 weeks, demonstrating a twofold increased incidence of cesarean in induced patients when compared to those who entered labor spontaneously. However, more recently this evidence has been called into question, as these studies were comparing groups of patients, those that were induced at a certain gestational age and those who went into labor spontaneously at that gestational age, but not really a management decision. Patients cannot choose to go into spontaneous labor at any specific gestational age and thus the decision women and their providers must make is between induction now or waiting until labor begins spontaneously or a medical indication for induction occurs at a later date, when the risk of a cesarean may be higher simply due to larger fetal size and poorer fetal tolerance of the labor process. That decreased tolerance of labor may be due to placental maturation or the complication of pregnancy itself that necessitated the induction. Recent studies comparing women who were electively induced at 39 weeks to women who went into spontaneous labor or had a medical indication for induction at 40 week or beyond demonstrate that the induced groups had similar, or in some studies, lower rates of cesarean than the groups who waited and delivered at later gestational ages.[7] These newer studies have even led some to suggest that *all* women should be induced at 39 weeks.[8] This certainly has not become standard practice and many labor and delivery units actually prohibit elective inductions prior to 40 weeks, but it does raise the question of why women wanting a natural birth are so opposed to induction when it may actually decrease their risk of a cesarean. Are they simply misinformed?

IMPACTS OF INDUCTION ON THE NATURAL BIRTH PLAN

While vaginal delivery rate is the principal outcome that is considered when induction is evaluated by the medical literature, the desire for a physiological start to labor among women wanting an unmedicated birth goes beyond the risk of cesarean section. Virtually all components of a natural birth plan are dependent on a spontaneous labor process. This is because all induction agents carry the risk of uterine hyperstimulation and fetal distress and continuous fetal monitoring is nearly universally recommended whenever pharmacologic agents are being utilized for induction. Continuous fetal monitoring is often problematic for naturally laboring women because it confines a woman to bed positions for labor, unless her hospital utilizes mobile monitors. However, as will be

TABLE 5-3: EFFECTS OF INDUCTION ON LABOR MANAGEMENT

Common Complications of Induction	Typical Consequential Change in Labor Management
• Increased hyperstimulation • Increased fetal distress	• Continuous monitoring • Decreased mobility • Possible decreased access to hydrotherapy depending on hospital protocol
• Increased risk of cesarean	• Restriction of food and/or drink
• Increased maternal discomfort	• Increased analgesia/Epidural use
• Increased meconium	• Possible increased need for infant suctioning, inhibiting delayed cord clamping, and skin-to-skin • Possible need for NICU care

discussed further, continuous monitoring is frequently challenging even with the aid of mobile monitors, so women frequently find their movement restricted even when out-of-bed monitoring options are available. Due to the increased frequency of fetal distress and surgical delivery during inductions, intravenous hydration is commonly prescribed and food and drink are typically restricted or withheld, even if the provider and hospital would otherwise be willing to permit oral intake. The experience of an induction for the mother is also vastly different from a spontaneous labor. Induced labors are significantly longer, increasing the level of maternal fatigue. Higher levels of discomfort are consistently reported in women undergoing induction and, unsurprisingly, the rates of pharmacologic pain relief utilization are increased in response. Even providers supportive of natural birth will often counsel their patients that an unmedicated birth is ill conceived in the setting of an induction. Many feel that because induction is not a natural process, it is nearly impossible to utilize natural methods for coping with the pain of an induction (Table 5-3).

WHO REALLY *NEEDS* TO BE INDUCED?

The majority of women intending to naturally birth prefer to only be induced if truly necessary. It is the defining of what is truly necessary that is the subject of so much debate and disagreements among members of the medical community itself and between patients and their providers.

For the purposes of this discussion, only the common indications for induction in low-risk pregnancies will be discussed, as high-risk patients desiring unmedicated births are a separate consideration.

Unpleasantly, the usual reason induction is recommended is because of the concern that if the pregnancy were to continue, the risk of loss of the baby in utero would be too great. Thus, to really understand if induction is necessary, parents are forced to contend with the unfortunate and tragic reality that babies can and do die prior to birth. It is a horrific fact that no one wants to think about and can be used to heavily influence a patient who is attempting to avoid a medical induction. Another albeit less significant reason inductions are recommended is to lower the risk of cesarean or development of complications of pregnancy. However, there is a lot of gray in the data surrounding these common indications for induction and ultimately many parents find themselves just agreeing to "the safest thing for the baby," when in reality they may have been choosing between two safe options for the baby, just depending on how we define safe.

Post Dates

Pregnancies that extend beyond the due date are common, with one in three deliveries in the United States occurring after 40 weeks, according to data analyzed by the CDC.[9] The number of pregnancies extending beyond 42 weeks, pregnancies that are defined as post term, is approximately 7%. However, in the United States, this rate has been dropping, due both to improved dating of pregnancies with the widespread adoption of early first trimester dating ultrasounds and broader, earlier induction policies, such that only 10% of pregnancies extend to 41 weeks and only 4% extend to 42 weeks.[10] Post dates is the most common indication for induction of labor, accounting for up to one-third of all inductions performed.[11,12]

As previously discussed, the risk of stillbirth remains fairly constant throughout pregnancy but begins to slowly increase in the last month of pregnancy until 41 to 42 weeks of gestation, when the rate of loss begins to exponentially rise. The absolute risk of stillbirth through the 42 week is relatively small, however, this exponential rise in poor outcomes continues past the 42-week point and approaches 3 per 100 by 43 weeks, a risk most feel is unacceptable. This is why the 42-week cutoff for induction is so universally applied (Figure 5-2).[13]

The larger debate has been whether induction should be routine at 41 weeks or even earlier, though throughout the United States many

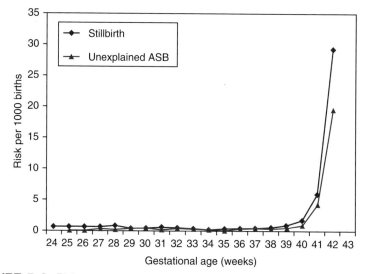

FIGURE 5-2. Risk of stillbirth by gestational age (per 1000 ongoing pregnancies). (Reproduced with permission from Sutan R, Campbell D, Prescott GJ, et al. The risk factors for unexplained antepartum stillbirths in Scotland, 1994 to 2003. *J Perinatol*. May 2010;30(5): 311–318.)

practices routinely induce all patients by this gestational age. The reason the 41-week point has become the new cutoff is due to a number of studies that have demonstrated a lower risk of both cesarean and perinatal mortality with this induction threshold. A large randomized trial compared induction at 41 weeks to expectant management up through 44 weeks and found a lower risk of cesarean and higher patient satisfaction with induction.[14] A systematic review that included 22 trials of varied quality involving over 9000 women also demonstrated lower cesarean rates with earlier induction and lower rates of perinatal mortality and meconium aspiration.[15]

From this data, induction at 41 weeks seems reasonable and should be considered by women and their providers when pregnancies are prolonged. However, the data certainly does not support mandatory inductions by 41 weeks. Furthermore, there has not been significant study into whether antepartum testing may mitigate some of the risks of going into the 42nd week of pregnancy and beyond, but the current information available suggests this.[10] Antepartum testing is typically performed in the outpatient setting one to two times per week and consists of short durations of electronic fetal heart rate monitoring and/or ultrasounds to evaluate amniotic fluid and other signs of fetal well-being. There also have been newer conflicting studies specifically examining first-time mothers with uncomplicated pregnancies which did show higher rates of cesarean with induction as compared to allowing patients to wait until 42 weeks for spontaneous labor.[11] Ultimately, each woman should feel able to decide for herself whether the potential benefits of an induction outweigh the negative impacts induction will have on her labor process.

Prelabor Release of Membranes

Prelabor release of membranes (PROM) is when the amniotic membranes release or waters break before any regular uterine activity or cervical dilation occurs. Water breaking is a common first sign of labor, affecting anywhere from 5% to 10% of pregnancies. Some known risk factors for the development of PROM include maternal yeast and bacterial infections, membrane sweeping, and weekly vaginal exams in the last month of pregnancy.[16–18] It is also a very common indication for induction. The motivation for induction is to prevent maternal and neonatal infection, both of which increase in incidence when the barrier provided by the amniotic membranes is breached for prolonged periods of time, exposing the sterile environment of the uterus to the unsterile, bacteria colonized, environment of the vagina. Most obstetricians perceive rupture of membranes as the starting of the clock on the labor process and aim for delivery within 24 hours.

This perception and the routine recommendation for induction in the setting of PROM is based on early studies in the 1960s and 1970s which showed concerning rates of neonatal infection and mortality of up to 5% when the time from rupture of membranes to delivery exceeded 24 hours.[19] However, these studies were conducted at a time when antibiotics were limited both in terms of their efficacy and application, meaning many women and babies were not appropriately treated when they demonstrated signs of infection and, when they were treated, often those antibiotics were not good at treating the infections present. During this time, there was also no screening or treatment for maternal colonization with group B streptococcal bacteria (GBS), which is a significant risk factor for both maternal infection (chorioamnionitis) and neonatal sepsis and meningitis. Despite these notable differences in infection prevention and treatment, the "24-hour clock" on ruptured membranes has remained a standard part of the obstetrical mindset and labor management.

More recent studies have tried to determine whether routine induction makes sense today, when there is better screening for GBS and better treatment for infection should it occur. A large, randomized

THE NATURAL BIRTH PLAN

trial by Hannah et al. in 1996 compared induction at the time of membrane rupture, using either pitocin or prostaglandins, versus waiting up to 4 days for labor to begin. Interestingly, this study showed no significant difference between the two groups in terms of neonatal infection rates, neonatal mortality, or cesarean section rates. The study did demonstrate, however, an increased rate of maternal infection or chorioamnionitis in the patients who were not induced; however, critics have pointed out that this study did have a relatively liberal definition of maternal infection, possibly over diagnosing infection in the expectant management group. Furthermore, at the time this study was completed, screening and treatment for GBS colonization was still not routinely performed, which could have contributed to the higher rate of infection observed.[20] Another more recent observational study of over 6000 women, which included routine screening and treatment of GBS colonization, examined women who were expectantly managed for up to 48 hours rather than induced in the setting of PROM. This study showed low rates of neonatal infection and cesarean in both groups of women, as well as significantly lower rates of maternal infection in the expectantly managed group than in Hannah's randomized control trial (2.8 vs. 6.7).[21]

The American College of Obstetrics and Gynecology has been flip flopping on their recommendations on PROM for the last 20 years. In 1997, as a result of the Hannah trial, they concluded that either induction or expectant management were reasonable options. However, in 2007, they reversed this position recommending induction on the basis of strong scientific evidence, though the cited sources were no different than in 1997. They repeated this recommendation in 2013, but acknowledged that it was based on limited and inconsistent evidence. Finally in 2017, in the Committee Opinion regarding ways to minimize intervention during labor and birth, they stated that women could be supported in expectant management for 24 to 48 hours, provided no other indication for delivery arose.[22]

Interestingly, all the debate over whether to induce actually turns out to be unnecessary for the vast majority of women who find themselves with prelabor rupture of membranes. As was shown in the Hannah trial, when nature is allowed to take its own course, half of women will labor within 5 hours and 95% of women will deliver within 28 hours. Without any evidence to show that induction is necessary from the standpoint of either risks to the baby or maternal risks of cesarean, it would seem all the anxiety and strong armed induction policies are out of place. Women do not "need" to be induced the minute their water breaks; however, they should be counseled about the possible benefits of induction and they may reasonably choose to do so, especially if their hospital has strict policies regarding NICU admission in the event of a maternal fever. They should not be afraid that induction in this setting will increase the risk of a cesarean, but should be aware of the ways in which induction will impact their plans for a natural birth. However, waiting it out is also a safe alternative that doctors and hospitals should support without making women afraid for their infants' well-being.

Advanced Maternal Age

At my first prenatal appointment, before we even did the ultrasound to confirm I was pregnant, I was told I would need to be induced by due date, because I was 41. This was really frustrating because I was really hoping for a natural birth. Between that and all the craziness about down syndrome, I felt like a ticking time bomb. I just worried all the time that something would go wrong with my baby. Of course, with all that stress, labor never started but I felt like I had no choice but to be induced because otherwise I could lose my baby that I had been waiting for my entire life.

—K. O., new mother

The average age of women giving birth has risen in the last 50 years. Today, roughly 15% of women giving birth are over 35 and one in five women has their first baby after the age of 35.[23] Women over 35 are known to be at increased risk for a number of pregnancy complications, including gestational diabetes, preeclampsia, chromosomal abnormalities, abnormal placental location and fetal position, and cesarean section.[24] They are also at an increased risk of stillbirth when compared to women under 35, with the highest rates observed in women over 40, even when no other complications of pregnancy are present. The cumulative risk of loss from 37 to 41 weeks in older mothers is considerable, occurring in 1 out of 382 women age 35 to 39 and 1 out of 267 women 40 or older.[25] Rates of stillbirth in women over 35, as in younger women, have also been shown to increase exponentially in the last weeks of pregnancy, with older women demonstrating higher rates of loss at all gestational ages. However, when recent data is examined, the risk is not nearly as shocking in any given week of gestation and is comparable to younger women at later gestational ages when expectant management is still considered reasonable. For example, from 38 to 40 weeks gestation, the risk of stillbirth in women under 35, between 35 and 40, and

THE NATURAL BIRTH PLAN

over 40 is 0.65/1000, 1.1/1000, and 1.39/1000, respectively. After the due date and extending up to 42 weeks, those rates rise across all age groups, but remain relatively low overall, with a risk of stillbirth of 0.84/1000, 1.91/1000, and 1.61/1000 for women under 35, between 35 and 40, and over 40, respectively.[26]

Nonetheless, given the overall risk of stillbirth for women of advanced maternal age, several interventional strategies have been proposed and adopted with the aim of reducing the incidence of still-birth in older mothers. Some of the strategies that have been suggested for women starting at either age 35 or 40 include antepartum testing beginning in last month of pregnancy, with induction or cesarean in those with nonreassuring testing, and/or routine induction somewhere between 39 and 41 weeks gestation.[27] However, the only randomized trial to date analyzing the strategy of induction, the 35/39 trial, did not include enough women to accurately assess whether induction reduced stillbirth rates in older mothers. It did demonstrate that there was no difference in the rates of cesarean or other complications of delivery in women over 35 who were induced or expectantly managed until the 42nd week and there were no stillbirths in either group, though only around 600 women were studied.[28] While this study did not answer the question of whether women over 35 *should* be induced to decrease the incidence of stillbirth, it certainly supported the argument that induction is a reasonable option for women of advanced maternal age which does not significantly increase their risk of cesarean. Another observational study comparing approximately 1500 mothers over 35 to approximately 3000 mothers under 35 demonstrated that a strategy of antepartum testing starting at 36 weeks and delivery by 41 weeks resulted in similar rates of stillbirth in both groups of women. While this study type was not sufficient to reliably prove this strategy, it lends support to the argument that the risk of stillbirth in mothers of advanced maternal age can be effectively reduced and provides comfort to those mothers who may desire expectant management and a natural start to labor, at least until 41 weeks of pregnancy.[29] To date, neither the American College of Obstetrics and Gynecology nor the Society for Maternal Fetal Medicine recommends either routine antepartum testing or specific induction guidelines for women over 35.

Obesity

Rates of obesity in pregnant mothers, similar to rates of advanced maternal age, are steadily increasing in the United States. Currently, 31.8% of women of reproductive age have a BMI in the obese range.[30] Also similar to older mothers, women with elevated BMIs are at increased risk for a number of pregnancy and delivery complications, including diabetes, preeclampsia, cardiac problems, and cesarean. In addition, they are 40% more likely to have a stillbirth than non-obese pregnant mothers, though the absolute risk is still small.[31] In a large cohort study examining over 2 million women, women with obesity had an overall risk of loss of 3 in 1000 births, with higher rates of loss at all gestational ages when compared to non-obese women and a similar rapid rise in the rate of loss past the 39th week. The highest rates of overall loss and most rapid increases in loss rates in the later weeks of pregnancies were observed in women with the highest BMIs. For example, women with a BMI greater than 50 were observed to have a 5 and 13 fold increase in the rate of stillbirth when compared to non-obese women at 39 and 41 weeks respectively.[32] Antepartum testing and early induction have also been proposed as means to reduce risk in this group of patients, however, at this time, there is insufficient evidence that these strategies effectively reduce that risk and are not currently recommended by the American College of Obstetrics and Gynecology. Induction may be particularly problematic in these women, as they are known to have longer labors, greater likelihood of induction failure, and higher rates of cesarean, with increased complications associated with those cesareans, most notably infections.[6,33,34] Ultimately, mothers with elevated BMI, similar to mothers who are over 35 or go past their due date, should be free to consider induction in the context of their own goals and concerns, rather than be pressured into induction, as the current evidence does not show induction has clear benefit and it may have higher costs for these women.

Concern for a Big Baby

My pregnancy had been progressing normally until I went for my 36 week appointment. When my doctor entered the room, he rudely asked, "What have you been eating? That baby looks huge." He then measured my belly and said my belly was measuring three weeks ahead of schedule. He arranged an ultrasound that said my baby was already eight pounds. Each appointment after that was pretty much focused on the size of my baby and my doctor's concerns about it. He told me her shoulder could get stuck and that it was really unlikely that she would come out vaginally, because I was so small. They repeated an ultrasound at thirty-nine weeks that now said my baby was over nine pounds and could be as big as ten pounds.

My doctor strongly recommended a cesarean, which we scheduled a few days later. The baby came out big, but only eight pounds, ten ounces. I think I could have pushed her out. My mom had a nine pound baby vaginally, but they just scared me so much, the C-section seemed like the best thing.

—M. L., new mother

Large babies, babies weighing over 8 pounds and 13 ounces, occur in approximately 8% of births within the United States, with only 1.1% of all babies weighing 9 pounds and 15 ounces or more.[35] However, two out of three women have an ultrasound near the end of pregnancy to estimate fetal size and one out of three women are told their baby may be too big. Of those women who are suspected of having a big baby, two out of three reported that induction was discussed as a means to prevent the baby from getting bigger and one out of three reported that a scheduled cesarean was suggested.[12] Interestingly, the average size of those suspected big babies was 7 pounds and 13 ounces.

Providers and ultrasounds are similarly bad at predicting which babies will actually be born large for gestational age or macrosomic. A review of 14 studies examining whether ultrasound could predict birth weights found that in most studies, the predictive value of an ultrasound measurement of weight was less than 50%, meaning it was incorrect in the weight estimate as often as it was correct. Ultrasound's accuracy in predicting very large babies, those weighing more than 9 pounds and 15 ounces was less than 30%.[36] Doctors and midwives fare no better at predicting which babies are going to be over 8 pounds and 13 ounces, with those estimates being correct roughly only half the time. In the best-case scenario, an ultrasound is accurate within 1 pound of the actual birth weight, meaning if a baby is estimated to be 8 pounds on ultrasound, it could be as large as 9 pounds or as small as 7 pounds.[37] When a woman is told she has a "big baby" based either on a clinical exam or ultrasound, she can basically flip a coin and be as accurate at predicting whether that is true.

However, her provider's suspicion that she has a big baby can, in and of itself, be a negative thing. Several studies have demonstrated that suspicion of a large baby is associated with higher rates of cesarean, more inductions, and increased labeling of stalled labor. Two interesting studies compared outcomes in mothers who delivered large babies and were suspected to have big babies prior to labor to mothers who also delivered large babies but were not suspected of having a large baby prior to delivery. In the mothers with large babies who were suspected of being so, the rates of induction, cesarean, and maternal complications were significantly higher than those mothers who had surprise big babies, demonstrating that the suspicion of the big baby was more dangerous than the big baby itself.[38,39]

Adding to the frustration surrounding this "big baby" obsession is that the interventions that aim to reduce the risks associated with big babies are not significantly effective. The main goal of induction and cesarean with suspected big babies is to reduce the likelihood of a shoulder dystocia, a complication of delivery where the head of the infant delivers, but the shoulder is stuck under the pubic bone, delaying the delivery of the baby and potentially restricting oxygen flow and injuring the nerves to the arm and hand. Shoulder dystocia occurs in 6.7% of deliveries of infants weighing between 8 pounds and 13 ounces and 9 pounds and 15 ounces and occurs in 14.5% of babies weighing 9 pounds and 15 ounces or more at birth.[40] However, the rate of significant injury, either due to nerve injury or oxygen deprivation, as a result of a shoulder dystocia is less than 1%.[41] While a recent *Cochrane Review* of four randomized control trials comparing early induction of suspected macrosomic infants with waiting for spontaneous labor did show a small decrease in the incidence of shoulder dystocia among women who were induced early, there were no differences in rates of cesarean or severe maternal or neonatal complications, including shoulder dystocia related nerve injury or oxygen deprivation.[42] No randomized trials have been performed analyzing cesarean as a preventative strategy, but in an analysis by Rouse and associates, it was estimated that 3695 cesareans for suspected fetal weights of 9 pounds and 15 ounces or greater would have to be performed in order to prevent one shoulder dystocia related nerve injury. Using the 8 pounds and 13 ounces cutoff, 2345 cesareans would have to be performed to prevent one case of nerve injury.[40] Despite this underwhelming evidence that estimating fetal weights and intervening in response to them makes any sense in low-risk women, these practices are widespread. Some doctors are even mandated by their malpractice insurance providers to perform a CALM shoulder screen, a computerized risk assessment which purportedly can identify mothers at risk for shoulder dystocia though this has not been proven accurate, and counsel their "at-risk" patients about alternative delivery options in response to that supposed risk. The American College of Obstetricians and Gynecologists clearly states in their most recent Committee Opinion that suspected macrosomia is not an indication for induction, but leaves the door open to offering cesarean delivery for babies suspected to weigh 9 pounds and 15 ounces or more.[43]

THE NATURAL BIRTH PLAN

OTHER CONSIDERATIONS OF THE EVIDENCE RELATING TO INDUCTION AND CESAREAN

It is worth noting that all the studies regarding induction and its impacts on cesarean rates have been conducted within a medically managed model. Many in the natural birth community argue that there is not truly a nonintervention "control" to which induction is being compared, because those in the non-induction groups are likely being restricted to bed, with continuous monitoring, and receiving pitocin for augmentation, having their water broken, and receiving epidurals. Consequently, much of the labor management in the induced groups is similar to the non-induced groups. To really know if induction increases cesarean rates and rates of other complications in all of the situations discussed, women who are induced should be compared to women who are being managed according to a low intervention model, with intermittent monitoring, freedom of movement, continuous hands-on support, oral intake, and access to hydrotherapy. Until then, we are likely only comparing types of apples, not apples and oranges.

I want freedom of movement during labor

Being able to move was really important to me. Every time I had to get in the bed, I just felt like the contractions were so much worse. It was like there was just so much energy moving through my body and I just had to get it out. Moving my hips, leaning over the bed, bouncing on the ball...it all helped. I think if they had made me stay in the bed, I would have asked for an epidural. I just can't imagine doing it that way.

—S. L., new mother

One of the most common fears expressed by women prior to childbirth, particularly among women planning an unmedicated birth, is that they will be "strapped to the bed," unable to move in the ways they wish. Their concerns are not unfounded. In the Listening to Mother's survey, 76% of mothers reported that they were restricted to bed throughout their labors.[44] Freedom of movement is a standard request made in any natural birth plan.

There are numerous reasons why unrestricted movement is desirable in labor. Women report less pain, especially less continuous back pain in upright and ambulatory positions. This has been demonstrated in multiple studies of women throughout the first stage of labor.[45–47] Additional studies have also demonstrated less incidence of operative delivery when women are permitted freedom of movement in labor, shortened duration in the time needed to reach complete dilation by 1 hour, less need for pitocin, and less epidural use, with no adverse outcomes observed.[48] Even in studies where these benefits were not observed, 99% of women randomized to ambulation groups indicated that they would want the option of ambulation in future labors.[49] An additional benefit of freedom of movement that is not so easily studied, but that women frequently discuss, is an increase in the feeling that they are in control of their labor process, able to move and cope with it in the way their body is telling them to. Furthermore, given the historical context of bed rest, being restricted to bed psychologically conveys the message that one is sick and labor is dangerous, increasing fear and anxiety throughout the labor process which, as shown previously, initiates a hormonal cascade that is counterproductive to the labor process.

Why, given the benefits and the lack of any evidence to suggest a downside to ambulation, is the practice so widely restricted? Unfortunately, much of the reason for confining women to bed lies in the same reason women want to avoid it: control. Keeping patients in bed and on continuous fetal heart rate monitoring makes it easier to monitor both patients and their babies from one central location. Nurses can observe both the mother's vital signs and the baby's heart rate from the nursing station and complete their charting uninterrupted. When patients are ambulating, it is simply more time consuming to complete these monitoring tasks. Restriction to the bed also eliminates the concern that the patient will progress suddenly and deliver their baby outside of the bed, in a manner that is less conducive to a provider controlled delivery. Bed rest in labor also makes for a more controlled general labor and delivery environment, with patients contained in their rooms rather than roaming the halls.

Another concern that is frequently cited by labor and delivery staff is that ambulation increases the risk of an umbilical cord prolapse, especially in the setting of ruptured membranes. As discussed previously, the risk of umbilical cord prolapse is low, occurring in 1 in 1000 births. The most significant risk factors are malpresentation, prematurity, and artificial rupture of membranes. There is no evidence supporting this belief held by nurses and doctors alike and yet, the practice persists and women asking to get out of bed are frightened needlessly that the "cord will fall out" if they walk. This is essentially just an old wife's tale, or old nurse's tale, preventing a beneficial practice from becoming the standard of care for laboring mothers. It is also interesting to note that the benefit in terms of decreased time spent in the first stage of labor with ambulation is the same as the benefit of routine pitocin augmentation, without any of the adverse outcomes associated with artificial augmentation. Perhaps that fact alone may be enough for efficiency minded labor and delivery units to update their practices in an evidence-based way.

I would like intermittent monitoring

I think the most frustrating part of my natural birth was the monitoring. My doctor was pretty good overall, but she insisted that the baby be monitored the entire time I was in the hospital. Even though they had those mobile machines, every time I would move in a certain way, the bands would slip and the nurse would come running in to find the baby. That always freaked me out and I would hold my breath until I heard that little horse trotting sound again. At some point, I guess they thought the heart rate was going down and I got really scared. They made me get in the bed then so they could make sure they were tracing the baby. The baby was fine, of course, but I wish someone would just invent a better way to keep tabs on the baby during labor.

—J. R., new mother

FETAL MONITORING TYPES

Electronic fetal monitoring (EFM) is the most common type of fetal monitoring used in labor and delivery. It measures the response of the fetal heart rate to contractions via two receivers, the external tocometer and the external doppler monitor. The tocometer measures the change in abdominal curvature, indicating when a contraction is occurring, but not the intrauterine intensity of the contraction, a common misperception. The doppler continuously measures the fetal heart rate. The two devices are held in place on the mother's abdomen using elastic bands and wires connect the devices to the fetal heart rate machine, which records the two measurements simultaneously on a graph, either on paper or digitally. Most women undergo what is termed continuous EFM, where the laboring mother is connected to the fetal heart rate machine for the duration of her labor and delivery.

An alternative to continuous EFM is intermittent auscultation, where the fetal heart rate is observed either with a special stethoscope, a fetoscope, or a portable handheld doppler device at various points throughout the labor. There is no standard, evidenced-based protocol, for intermittent auscultation, but most professional organizations of obstetricians and midwives recommend listening to heart rate every 15 to 30 minutes during active labor and every 5 minutes during pushing, for up to 1 minute at a time, and increasing the frequency if abnormalities are observed and modifying care if there is indication of distress.[50]

Another, supposedly middle of the road approach is what is termed intermittent EFM, where the electronic fetal monitor is used to assess fetal well-being, just not continuously. Different protocols exist, but most commonly monitoring is performed approximately 20 minutes for every hour a woman is in labor and, provided no abnormalities are observed, the monitor is removed for the remainder of the hour. Usually continuous monitoring is still performed during the pushing stage of labor.

More consistent, but also more invasive, means of monitoring also exist, but are only used when satisfactory monitoring cannot be achieved with less invasive means. These include intrauterine pressure catheters (IUPCs), which are capable of measuring both frequency and strength of contractions, and fetal scalp electrodes, which are small, curved wires with a sharp end capable of puncturing the skin, and are applied directly to the fetal head. Fetal scalp electrodes can measure the fetal heart rate continuously regardless of maternal positioning or body habitus. Risks of invasive internal monitors include maternal or fetal infection, uterine injury, or injuries to the baby, including burns and bruising.

THE NATURAL BIRTH PLAN

THE HISTORY OF ELECTRONIC FETAL MONITORING IN LABOR

Continuous EFM has become the standard of care on labor and delivery units in the United States. Its utilization is based on the principle that low oxygen levels during labor eventually lead to the changes in the fetal nervous system that can be identified by changing characteristics of the fetal heart rate patterns, which are a product of sympathetic and parasympathetic outflow. Exploration into EFM was initiated in the 1960s with the goal of decreasing morbidity and mortality in both the mother and the newborn. Prior to its introduction, fetal well-being was assessed using a combination of intermittent auscultation of fetal heart tones and fetal scalp ph sampling. In 1969, Kubli and his associates published data showing a correlation between fetal heart rate patterns and fetal pH. Myers and colleagues, 4 years later, demonstrated a correlation between fetal heart rate patterns, specifically late decelerations, and fetal death in Rhesus monkey fetuses. In the same year, a separate group observed decreased perinatal mortality in their patients with EFM, and a number of multiple randomized trials were initiated comparing EFM to the previous standard of intermittent auscultation. These subsequent trials included both high- and low-risk women and, surprisingly, did not demonstrate a significant improvement in neonatal outcomes. They did show, however, an increase in cesarean rate among patients with EFM. Consequently, by the 1980s, with no obvious benefit of continuous EFM demonstrated scientifically, researchers began to wonder whether it would be more appropriate to apply continuous EFM to higher risk pregnancies and labors. Subsequent studies were done comparing universal EFM to "selective monitoring," where only patients with specific, though admittedly liberal, indications were continuously monitored. These studies also failed to show a significant benefit to continuous EFM.[51]

Despite this lack of evidence and a recommendation by the US Preventative Task force in 1996 that EFM should not be used in low-risk pregnancies and that there was even insufficient evidence to recommend its use in high-risk pregnancies, EFM was broadly adopted. By the late 1990s, 70% of labors had continuous monitoring, and by the late 2000s over 80% of women received continuous monitoring, affecting over 3 million women per year. In 1997, the National Institute of Child Health and Human Development worked to clarify the definitions of abnormal fetal heart rate tracings and adopt a common language for discussing tracings that could better guide future research and clinical practice. They also concluded from the existing research that a normal tracing was a reliable indicator of a normally oxygenated baby and that certain patterns were uniformly nonreassuring.[52] However, further research working to clarify the link between abnormal tracings and neurological injury in neonates, mainly neonatal encephalopathy and cerebral palsy, demonstrated that abnormal fetal heart rate tracings were present in roughly half of babies who eventually developed cerebral palsy, but that only 1 in 1000 babies with an abnormal fetal heart rate tracing went on to develop cerebral palsy. This called into serious question the assumption that the majority of poor neurological outcomes were even due to a hypoxic event in labor, much less that EFM could actually prevent those poor outcomes. Certainly, no study to date has demonstrated that EFM saved babies' lives. In 2009, the American College of Obstetricians and Gynecologists issued a practice bulletin acknowledging these realities regarding EFM. Most notably they stated[53]:

- EFM increases cesarean delivery rate and operative vaginal deliveries.
- EFM does not reduce overall perinatal mortality, though this may be shown with further research with larger sample sizes.
- Nonreassuring fetal heart rate tracings are not predictive of poor neurological outcomes and EFM does not decrease the rate of poor neurological outcomes.
- EFM or intermittent auscultation are acceptable forms of monitoring.
- Continuous EFM should be used in patients with high-risk conditions.

So why does EFM remain the most common medical intervention in labor management? For one, most clinicians believe EFM still has potential to improve outcomes if properly studied and utilized. The other reasons are probably more to do with clinical habit and provider and nursing anxiety and perceived need to guarantee fetal well-being throughout the labor process rather than the actual science itself. Undoubtedly, the medical-legal environment also discourages providers from abandoning universal continuous EFM, as a normal fetal heart rate tracing or acting on an abnormal fetal heart rate pattern may be their only defense in a lawsuit regarding a poor neurological outcome, despite the evidence to the contrary.

HOW DOES CONTINUOUS ELECTRONIC FETAL MONITORING AFFECT NATURALLY LABORING MOTHERS?

The desire to be ensured of their baby's well-being throughout the labor process is nearly universally expressed by laboring women. Unfortunately, the technology currently available renders providers unable to honestly provide that reassurance with 100% certainty, though the overall risks of labor and delivery in low-risk women are perhaps low enough to warrant that reassurance unnecessary. However, the technology does negatively impact mothers, particularly mothers laboring without the aid of pharmacological pain relief, in many ways.

First, the mechanics of fetal monitoring are, in themselves, challenging. The tocometer and fetal heart rate monitoring device are small, flat circular disks that are placed on the curved surface of the mother's abdomen. Slipping and flipping of these devices are a persistent frustration on labor and delivery units. The fetal heart rate device sends and receives sound waves in a straight, vertical fashion, requiring the device to sit rather precisely over the fetal heart. This can be an onerous enough task when the mother is laying flat in bed, let alone when she is standing, walking, or bending over. The fetal heart rate monitor also requires a gel medium to transmit and receive the sound waves, which quickly melts away in water or maternal sweat. Furthermore, the majority of labor and delivery units still utilize stationary monitor machines, meaning the laboring mother can never venture further than 3 feet from the large central monitoring machine. Even when a mother has access to a mobile monitor, these monitors frequently have narrow ranges from which they are able to receive input and the mothers are still burdened with the wire attachments to the portable units, posing tripping risks, and many simply find the mobile units cumbersome. Hence, insistence on continuous EFM predictably restricts mobility in laboring mothers, which, as noted previously, is a critical component of a natural birth.[54] It also limits laboring mothers' ability to utilize other effective methods of nonpharmacologic pain relief, including hydrotherapy.[55] Other frequently cited irritations with monitoring include discomfort from the elastic bands, which typically must be pulled quite tight to maintain the position of the monitoring disks, and the continuous presence of gel on the abdomen, which many woman feel is uncomfortable.

Another possible effect of EFM is on the laboring mother's psyche. This has not been studied but warrants consideration, given what we know about the effect of maternal stress on the labor process. Continuous fetal monitoring, however subtly, sends the psychological message to women and their partners that birth is dangerous, that the baby is at risk. This, in and of itself, can be anxiety producing for women. When changes in the fetal heart rate are observed, this effect is only further exacerbated. While a normal fetal heart rate tracing may have a positive, reassuring effect for many women, given the large percentage (52%) of normal labors of healthy babies where some abnormal fetal heart rate pattern is observed, it seems more likely that continuous monitoring is generating some degree of anxiety during the labor process for a large number of women.[56]

However, even more importantly, changes in the fetal heart rate tracing are a frequent reason that other requests in a woman's birth plan may begin to be denied. Most hospital policies restrict access to hydrotherapy if any abnormalities in the fetal heart tracing are observed. Most nurses will also insist that patients remain in bed for more reliable monitoring if some concern arises. Abnormalities in the tracing also usually lead to restriction of oral intake, due to a heightened concern that a surgical birth may be indicated. IV fluids are often initiated when fetal heart rate abnormalities are observed, further restricting mobility and possibly affecting labor in other ways, and more invasive monitoring may also be initiated, including internal pressure catheters and fetal scalp electrode monitors, even more effectively confining the woman to bed. Finally, abnormalities in monitoring increase the likelihood that a woman wanting a natural birth will deliver in an operating room instead. Nurses, doctors, and midwives surely feel these interventions are indicated in the setting of possible fetal distress and they may indeed be, but if the current research does not demonstrate the benefit of monitoring to begin with, it is difficult to justify the level of interventions initiated as a consequence of it. Is our technology perceiving a cry of fetal distress that is not really there and are women suffering as a result? Women deserve an honest and critical examination of all medical interventions, including fetal monitoring. EFM is more than simply being hooked up to the monitor.

I want my water to break on it's own

One of the first things they did when I got to my labor room was break my water. The resident told me my doctor had ordered it, that it was standard, and would just help me along. I think I was maybe four or five centimeters at that time. Well, my labor stalled and then they said it had been too long that my water had been broken and they needed to do something. So I ended up getting pitocin and an epidural.

—L. G., new mother

Artificial rupture of the membranes (AROM), known by the technical term amniotomy or in lay terminology as breaking the waters, is one of the most common medical interventions performed. It is done with the intent to speed up labor, strengthen contractions, and allow the fetal head to descend further into the pelvis. It is also thought that AROM releases prostaglandins which aid in the labor process. It is performed during a vaginal examination, either digitally by the examiner or through the aid of a crochet-like long handled hook. In some countries, such as the United States, it is performed routinely in all women, while in other countries it is reserved for inductions or as a method to augment a slowed labor.

In 2013, a *Cochrane Review* of 15 studies, involving 5583 women with a spontaneous onset of labor, failed to demonstrate that routine

THE NATURAL BIRTH PLAN

amniotomy significantly shortened labor and a possible increase in the rate of cesarean section was suggested by the data.[57] Some of the frequently cited concerns regarding routine amniotomy are that it may increase the risk of umbilical cord prolapse, abnormal fetal heart rate patterns due to cord compression with less fluid in the uterus, and lower Apgar scores. This review did not, however, justify those concerns, as rates of these complications were similar in women who had routine amniotomy and those that did not. However, other independent studies have shown an association with amniotomy and umbilical cord prolapse, with cord prolapse rates highest in populations where routine amniotomy is the standard practice.[58] Additionally, amnioinfusion, a technique where fluid is returned to the uterus after membrane rupture, has been shown to decrease repetitive fetal heart rate decelerations, so it stands to reason that fluid cushioning the fetus and the umbilical cord from the external forces of labor is important to the labor process and fetal wellbeing. The American College of Obstetrics and Gynecology also supports women wanting to avoid this routine intervention, stating in their 2017 Committee Opinion that there is no need for routine amniotomy in women with normally progressing labors.[22]

Beyond this, however, naturally laboring women may wish to avoid routine amniotomy because there is a perception that once the water has broken, there is effectively a time clock on the labor. Providers routinely express concern about the length of time that has past since membranes ruptured given that longer durations of rupture are associated with an increase in the risk of neonatal infection and chorioamnionitis. Failure of labor progression after rupture of membranes is a common indication for both pitocin use and cesarean. Other reasons for avoiding amniotomy are the pervasive fears of allowing women with ruptured membranes to ambulate or utilize hydrotherapy, however nonevidenced based this may be. Routine amniotomy often, in practice, limits a woman's mobility and utilization of alternative pain relief methods. Furthermore, many women report that contractions are stronger and labor more painful once the water is broken, though this has not been specifically studied. If a woman had that experience in the past or knows of someone who had that experience, she may wish to spend a greater percentage of her labor without the water broken, especially given the lack of evidence that membrane rupture speeds up the process to any great degree.

Routine amniotomy, like so much that has become routine in labor management, appears to be no more than clinical habit. If a woman wishes to avoid it, there is no reason for that wish to not be respected.

I would like to avoid the use of pitocin

Pitocin was the end of my natural birth. They told me they were going to give me "just a little pit" to help things along, but those contractions were wicked! There was no way to just breath through that stuff.

—N. Z., new mother

Pitocin is a synthetic version of oxytocin, the hormone that naturally generates contractions in the laboring woman. The natural hormone oxytocin is also released during breastfeeding, at the time of the milk let-down reflex, during human orgasm, and during other encounters of emotional bonding.[59] The synthetic version of pitocin has several uses in obstetrics. It is used to induce labor, augment a spontaneous labor with the goal of shortening the process or encourage a slowing labor along, and reduce the risk of hemorrhage after delivery by facilitating stronger and more rapid contraction of the uterus, which compresses the enlarged blood vessels that had been supporting the pregnancy. When used appropriately, it can be lifesaving and help women with medical indications for delivery prior to the onset of labor to avoid cesareans via an effective induction of labor. It can be administered both intravenously and intramuscularly, via injection, however it is only approved for intravenous use during the labor process. The dosage of the medication is increased at small intervals generally in order to achieve a contraction frequency of every 2 to 3 minutes. Its effects, when administered intravenously are nearly immediate, and last up to 1 hour. When given intramuscularly, it takes 3 to 5 minutes to become effective and lasts from 2 to 3 hours.[60]

Routine pitocin use, the administration of pitocin to women without the indications of induction or labor dystocia, an abnormal slowing of the labor, has become both commonplace and controversial. Forty-seven percent of women report its routine application in their spontaneous labor.[44] This practice started back in the 1970s, with a study in Dublin in which women were randomized to early amniotomy, vaginal examinations every 2 hours, and pitocin augmentation if adequate labor progression was not observed on any exam, according to the Freeman curve. The group of women randomized to this "active management of labor" protocol had a shorter duration of labor by approximately 2 hours, with the majority of women achieving delivery within 12 hours of admission in labor, without an increase in cesarean section rate. Epidurals were not available and the women were provided with the continuous hands-on labor support of a midwife at bedside.[61] A more recent study in Dublin, performed in a similar fashion with the exception that participants

THE NATURAL BIRTH PLAN

had ready access to epidural anesthesia, demonstrated similar results.[62] A *Cochrane Review* in 2011 also confirmed a comparable decrease in labor time with routine pitocin use, without an increase in overall cesarean rate, though no other benefit was shown for either mother or baby. This review did show, however, an increased rate of uterine hyperstimulation and changes in the fetal heart rate tracing.[63]

For the naturally laboring woman, however, routine pitocin can be problematic in a number of ways. Pitocin use initiates a number of modifications in labor management due to the higher association of uterine hyperstimulation and fetal heart rate abnormalities. Continuous EFM is nearly universally employed when pitocin is used, with the resultant limitations in mobility and other ramifications discussed above. Additional restrictions in mobility occur as a consequence of IV administration of the medication, where the woman receiving it must be attached to a medication pump for the duration of its use. Diet is most often restricted and most hospitals also prohibit access to hydrotherapy when pitocin is in use. Furthermore, pitocin contractions are different than contractions produced by naturally released oxytocin. Pitocin contractions tend to reach their peak faster and persist at that peak for a longer duration of time.[64] Synthetic pitocin is also administered continuously, whereas naturally produced oxytocin is released in a pulsatile fashion, usually with longer separations between individual contractions and periods of rest during the labor in which no contractions occur. Naturally produced contractions tend to build in strength and increase in frequency progressively through the labor, whereas pitocin produces strong, frequent contractions usually within 1 hour of administration and they persist at this level for the duration of the labor. Hence with pitocin, in any given time spacing, a woman will have a greater number of contractions and spend a greater percentage of time at the peak of a contraction. This results in greater difficulty managing the labor with nonpharmacologic methods, higher levels of maternal fatigue, and increased rates of analgesic use. It is understandable that women thus perceive routine pitocin administration as sabotaging their intent for an unmedicated birth, no different in its repercussions on their birth plan than an induction (Figure 5-3).

There have also been more serious questions about the routine use of pitocin in recent years which are making parents even more reluctant about the medication, particularly in its possible association with autism. Oxytocin has long been understood as the "love hormone," important in human bonding. Oxytocin levels increases substantially in both the fetus and mother during childbirth and the immediate postpartum. Oxytocin crosses the blood-brain barrier, modulating neurotransmitters

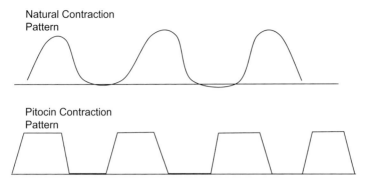

FIGURE 5-3. **Comparison of contraction wave forms with and without pitocin.**[64]

to achieve its various effects on the brain and behavior. However, synthetic pitocin has not been shown to do this and, as it binds the oxytocin receptors, it inhibits further production of natural oxytocin in women receiving the synthetic form. This modification of oxytocin in the central nervous system in the mother and fetus may have several ramifications.[65] For one, maternal oxytocin is transmitted to the fetal brain and causes a neurotransmitter change in the fetal cortical neurons which reduces vulnerability to hypoxic stress during the labor process.[66] Other studies have shown a link between autism and genomic deletion of the oxytocin receptor gene.[67,68] A more recent study out of Duke University in 2013 showed, when 625,000 birth records from 1990 to 1998 were compared to educational records over the following decade, that mothers who underwent induction or had their labors augmented with pitocin were more likely to have a child diagnosed with autism.[69] Oxytocin also appears to be involved in the way the mother bonds with her baby, as female rats given oxytocin antagonists failed to show typical maternal behavior and low levels of oxytocin in human females in the last 2 weeks of pregnancy were associated with higher rates of postpartum depression.[70,71]

While many in the media have been quick to jump to the conclusion that these studies mean pitocin causes autism, which they most certainly do not, they do provide sufficient evidence to give us pause about routine pitocin administration. Without a demonstrable benefit beyond a small decrease in the length of labor, it seems foolish to routinely give women a medication that has so many concomitant effects beyond the labor process. Pitocin has even more immediate negative impacts for the naturally laboring mother and it is important for women planning a natural birth to understand how pitocin may hinder their ability to manage labor in the way they are hoping for. It is also important for doctors, midwives, and nurses to understand that talking a woman into pitocin without an indication is more than just "giving a little pit"; it is an undermining of her entire intention for her birth, with possible disturbances in the delicate biochemistry of maternal-child bonding that we are just beginning to understand.

I want to be free to progress through labor without stringent time restrictions

When I started residency, I was not aware of the concept of labor efficiency. On my first shift, as the intern managing the labor deck, I was informed by my upper year resident that it was our job to "clear the board." We had to make sure every patient had their water broken, had pitocin going, and was making cervical change with each exam, which we performed every two hours. If they were not making cervical change, we would place an internal monitor so we could prove that they were receiving enough pitocin that they should be dilating. If they still did not change their cervix by the next exam, we would notify their attending doctor that they needed to come in and "cut her." If we were not aggressively managing each patient, when we signed out the patients to the next incoming team, we would be eaten alive by our upper years. The attendings seemed to have some of the same anxiety. When it was getting close to the end of their call, they would come section their patient because they did not want to "dump" the patient on the next doctor. When I moved up in the residency hierarchy and tried to give patients more time, attendings would even accuse me of being neglectful and providing bad care.

The definition of what constituted a normal pace of labor was first proposed over 50 years ago by Dr. Emanuel Friedman. In his famous Friedman curve, he divided the first stage of labor into latent and active phases, with active labor initiating at 4 cm dilation. First-time mothers were observed to dilate at a rate of 1.2 cm/h, whereas mothers with a previous vaginal delivery were observed to dilate at a rate of 1.5 cm/h, and failure to dilate for more than 2 hours was termed labor arrest.[72] These expectations for labor progression have governed obstetrical care ever since and deviations from this standard are common indications for medical intervention.

More recent studies, however, have called much of what Dr. Friedman proposed into question. For example, a retrospective study of over 60,000 women demonstrated that dilation from 4 to 6 cm is significantly slower than indicated by the Friedman curve, taking up to 6 hours to progress from 4 to 5 cm and up to 3 hours to progress from 5 to 6 cm. After 6 cm, progression was largely dependent on whether a woman had a previous delivery, with multiparous women actually delivering faster than described by Friedman and primiparous woman taking longer.[73] This study dramatically changed what should be thought of as active labor. Other studies also showed that a rate of dilation as slow as 0.5 cm/h among first-time mothers was normal, without any adverse effect, and that the expectation of a rate of dilation of 1 cm/h likely leads to an overdiagnosis of labor dystocia in first-time mothers (Table 5-4).[74]

Expectations regarding the second stage of labor, the length of time from full dilation until delivery, have also changed from that which Dr. Friedman defined. Previously it was believed that a normal first-time mother would take no more than 2 hours to push their baby out, whereas second-time mothers should be able to deliver with under an hour of pushing. However, the more recent research would suggest that time spent in pushing may be quite longer, especially in the setting of an epidural. The American College of Obstetrics and Gynecology defines a normal "pushing" phase of labor as 1 hour for second-time mothers without an epidural and 2 hours for second-time mothers with an epidural, while first-time mothers can spend up to 3 hours pushing with an epidural and up to 2 hours without. However, giving mothers more time if they are making progress is also recommended. By letting mothers push up to 4 hours, their need for cesarean decreases by half (Table 5-5).[75]

These modified definitions of what establishes an arrest of labor diagnosis are important for both women and their providers to be aware of, given that a third (35%) of primary cesareans in the United States are performed for failure of labor progression and, of first-time mothers who

TABLE 5-4: TIME SPENT IN FIRST-STAGE LABOR[73]

	Latent Labor (<6 cm)	Active Labor (6–10 cm)
First-time mothers	Variable, typically >9 hours	Up to 8 hours (0.5 cm/h)
Mothers with prior vaginal delivery	Variable, typically >9 hours	Up to 2.5 hours (1.5 cm/h)

TABLE 5-5: TIME SPENT IN SECOND-STAGE LABOR (10 CM DILATION TO DELIVERY)[75]

	Without Epidural	With Epidural
First-time mothers	Up to 2 hours	Up to 3 hours, 4 hours is prolonged but safe
Mothers with prior vaginal delivery	Up to 1 hour	Up to 2 hours

undergo a cesarean, nearly half (41.3%) are due to this diagnosis.[76] These improved definitions can also guide women as to when they may want to consider a change in their labor plan, however as long as some progress is being made and mother and baby are doing well, an abnormal labor pattern, in and of itself, is not an immediate indication to change course.

The desire for a rapid labor is shared by women and their care providers, but labor is usually a lengthy process that requires a large amount of patience, especially for first-time mothers. A common saying handed down between obstetricians is that a woman's best friend in labor is her obstetrician's long cigar. While the phrasing may be outdated, the intent behind the saying is more true today than ever. In our fast-paced culture and perception of clean 12-hour working blocks of time that set the rhythm of the labor and delivery units, the appreciation for slowing down and allowing nature to take its course has been lost. Taking the urgency out of the labor process benefits both women and their health care providers. Women are free to labor without staring at the clock and providers are able to care for women without the pressure of "getting them off the board."

Ultimately, in the absence of any other indication of a problem, the decision about how long is too long should belong to the mother. No woman wants to labor indefinitely without making progress. Health care providers should be willing to give women the time and space to come to their own conclusion when labor dystocias occur. Options and guidance can be provided but strict time limits only disrespect the autonomy of laboring women and increase their anxiety and distrust of their care providers.

I would like to minimize vaginal exams during my labor

Vaginal exams to evaluate labor progress are a typical part of the labor and delivery experience for most women. During the exam, the provider, with the protection of a sterile glove, typically inserts two fingers vaginally and feels for the cervical opening against the presenting fetal part. The examiner then subjectively determines how open the cervix is by seeing how far they can separate their fingers across the diameter of that opening. They also assess the thickness of the cervix, or effacement, and how low in the pelvis the baby is resting. They may also assess the cervical consistency and position, as well as whether the amniotic membranes are intact. Without the aid of an ultrasound, vaginal exams are also done to ensure that the baby is head down and to determine which direction the baby is facing by feeling for the sutures on the baby's skull.

Given the subjective natural of cervical exams, their reliability is notoriously poor, with large inter-examiner variations in reports of dilation.[77] Some improvement in accuracy is observed if a consistent examiner performs the cervical assessments throughout the labor, but still the absolute measurement of the cervical dilation at one particular moment is a poor predictor of labor progress.

Nonetheless, most women desire at least some examinations in labor to reassure them of their progress. An initial examination when a woman first presents with labor symptoms is almost certainly necessary to confirm that labor has indeed begun. An examination when the woman has the desire to push is also indicated to ensure that the cervix is fully dilated and the woman is indeed ready to push without the risk of causing a cervical tear. The case can also be made for some follow-up exams during the labor process to ensure the labor is proceeding normally. What most women are opposed to is the more invasive practice of many hospitals and providers of performing scheduled examinations every 2 hours, a by-product of "active management" of labor protocols.

There are many reasons women want to avoid this type of frequent examination, particularly when they plan an unmedicated labor. Many women find examinations uncomfortable and some even find them borderline abusive, especially if they have a history of sexual abuse, which unfortunately affects one in five women. Other women worry that exams will cause unnecessary alarm concerning their labor progress and either they will be pressured to accept medical interventions they do not want or they themselves will become discouraged and be more likely to request alternative forms of labor and pain management. There is also a concern that frequent examinations will increase the risk of intrapartum fever and infection, as several studies have shown an association between the total number of cervical examinations and infection. A recent retrospective cohort study in the United States called this into question, however, this study was limited by adjustments in the overall duration of labor it observed. Finally, there is also research that suggests exams may impact labor progress by increasing maternal anxiety and disrupting their focus.[78]

An alternative to frequent cervical examination is simple observation of the laboring mother. As a woman's labor advances, increased vocalization is often noted, along with skin discoloration and behavioral changes such as alterations in breathing patterns, willingness to continue conversation, and posturing. Duff[79] even proposed a model for labor assessment based on these behavioral cues, though its effectiveness in evaluating labor process has not yet been determined. However, most doctors, midwives, and nurses who frequently work with naturally laboring women report that they can usually judge where a woman is in labor simply by looking at her.

In summary, given the lack of any evidence to guide women or their providers as to the "right" frequency of exams and given the possible concerns about too many exams, it seems prudent to follow the mother's lead. Providers, particularly physicians, often have the urge to just "do something" and, in the case of a natural labor, the only thing they can do is an exam. However, women in labor should ask their care providers and they should ask themselves whether the results of any given examination would be cause to alter the current agreed-on plan of care. If there is nothing the woman is going to want to do differently on the basis of that exam and there is no concern on the part of the provider that the exam is addressing, then it should be considered unwarranted.

I want to eat and drink during my labor

It had always been part of my labor plan to eat and drink in labor if I felt I wanted to. My doctor was supportive of my preference. So when I was admitted in early labor with my water broken and I began to get hungry, I did not think anything of grabbing a muffin I had brought with me. I was about halfway through when my nurse walked in the room and freaked out. She told me I was not allowed to eat, that I could vomit into my lungs and die if I kept doing it. I was so surprised at her reaction, I just kept eating, one muffin bite at a time. That really made her crazy and before I knew it, she had dragged one of the anesthesiologists in to inform me of all the risks of eating in labor. My doctor arrived a bit later and was really upset that they had done that, but I guess old habits die hard.

—B. P., new mother

The withholding of food and drink during labor is commonplace in hospital birth in the United States, though in the past and in other countries, food and drink have been encouraged in labor to the extent that laboring woman wished. The restriction of oral intake in labor was initiated in the 1940s with Mendelson's observation that during anesthesia there was a risk of stomach contents entering the lungs, a phenomenon known then as Mendelson's syndrome and today as aspiration pneumonia. Today, more than 60% of women are confined to ice chips in labor because of this concern.[44]

Is this warranted? To answer this question, one must first consider the risk of aspiration pneumonia for laboring women undergoing general anesthesia. That exact rate is difficult to determine. Some studies show it may be as high as 1 in 650, while others show it may be as low as 1 in 10,000, with modern anesthetic techniques. Regardless, the use of general anesthesia in obstetrics is also low, with less than 5% of elective cesareans and only 15% to 30% of emergent cesareans requiring general anesthetic.[80] The risk of aspiration is further decreased when one considers the likelihood of a true emergency cesarean in a low-risk, naturally laboring woman. The risk of maternal mortality due to aspiration when taking into account all these factors is estimated to be 1 in 1.2 million.[81] The actual rate of overall maternal mortality due to aspiration was 1 in 3.5 million from 1998 to 2008.[82] This is quite literally less than the chance of being struck by lightning.

Policies that restrict the ability of women in labor to respond to normal cues of hunger and thirst are not reflective of the women's preferences.[83] Nor are these policies reflective of the current research, which has lead both the American College of Anaesthesiologists and the American College of Obstetricians and Gynecologists to issue practice guidelines supporting oral intake of clear fluids in labor, at the very least, though they still recommend against solid food in labor.[84,85] A systematic review of over 3000 women, while not powered to assess risk of aspiration pneumonia, did not show any benefit or harm to a liberal diet during labor.[86] In light of the low risks associated with eating and drinking during labor, it would seem in this respect, women are again victims of tradition and fear more than recipients of evidenced-based care. Women should be informed about the small possible risk of aspiration should they require emergency anesthesia and then be free to make their own decision regarding oral intake in a manner that respects their right to make decisions regarding their own body. No woman should "not be allowed" to eat or drink in labor.

One additional note, frequently women are informed by their health care providers, most often their labor and delivery nurses who are perhaps reluctant to clean up a possible mess, that they should not eat in labor because they may become nauseous and vomit. Nausea and vomiting are common symptoms of advancing labor, occurring most often in the transition phase at the end of active labor. Most women will self-restrict solid food and even fluids if nausea becomes a problem, but there is no evidence that withholding oral intake in the absence of nausea decreases a woman's likelihood of experiencing this uncomfortable labor symptom.

I decline IV fluids

I rolled into the hospital fully dilated with my third, ready to push. My nurse was in a panic to "get my IV in." I was uncomfortable, moving a lot, so she kept missing and poking me over and over. It was terrible and distracting and I never really understood the point. They took it out before I went to my postpartum room.

—C. K., new mother

IVs are another standard in hospital birth, with over 80% of women receiving IV fluids during labor. They are initiated for a number of reasons:

- hydration for patients not permitted to eat or drink
- hydration for patients too nauseous to eat or drink
- pre-epidural fluid bolusing to prevent epidural-related blood pressure changes
- establishment of intravenous access for rapid ability to administer medications, blood transfusions, or anesthesia in the event of an emergency

There has also been a suggestion that IV hydration may shorten labor, by decreasing the incidence of maternal dehydration and providing readily available carbohydrate for uterine muscle contraction. This has been shown in two trials which compared IV hydration, with access to oral fluids, to IV hydration alone and, when oral intake was restricted, higher IV hydration rates were associated with more rapid labors. None of the research demonstrated a lower rate of cesarean with IV hydration.[87] Furthermore, there have been other studies that failed to show any benefit to IV hydration when oral fluid was unrestricted.[88]

Women may have a number of concerns with routine IV fluids. To start with, up to 22% of the general population self-reports a fear of needles, often with higher anxiety associated with IV placement than a routine blood draw, given the larger needle and higher levels of associated pain.[89] The time and immobility required to place an IV is often challenging for an actively laboring woman. Once the IV is placed, many women continue to report discomfort at the IV site and find they are unable to move their arm in certain positions because of discomfort. Being connected to IV tubing is often cumbersome and limits mobility. It is also challenging to maintain an IV while utilizing hydrotherapy, as water weakens the securing tape and can lead to displacement of the IV.

Beyond these more technical problems, many women are also concerned that IV hydration will negatively impact their labors and breastfeeding. Often IV fluid bolusing is used to decrease the frequency of premature contractions, though this has not been shown to be an effective way to actually stop premature labor. Nonetheless, women aware of this practice often worry that IV fluids will have the same effect of slowing down their contractions, though no study has shown this to date. Another frequently cited concern is that IV hydration will lead to fluid overload, which will increase the chance of perineal swelling and tearing during delivery. Again, this has not been studied specifically but is a common association listed in natural childbirth texts and classes. Finally, women worry that IV hydration may impact breastfeeding by artificially elevating their babies weights at birth, leading to unwanted formula supplementation if excess weight loss occurs after delivery. This concern is supported by two recent studies that showed if mothers in labor received more than 200 ml/h of IV fluids, their babies were 3.2 times more likely to experience excess weight loss than mothers who received less hydration.[90,91]

There are several alternatives to routine IV hydration. As discussed previously, it is safe for women to orally hydrate throughout labor. If a laboring mother is unable to do so as a result of nausea and vomiting, IV hydration can be considered if and when this occurs. A hep-lock IV, which establishes IV access in the event of an emergency but is not attached to any fluid, medication, or tubing, may also be placed as an alternative, providing a safety net without limiting mobility to the same degree or exposing a mother to the possible negative side-effects of fluid administration. A third alternative is simply to only utilize IV hydration or a hep-lock IV in patients who demonstrate risk of a complication, for example, in response to fetal heart rate changes, nausea or vomiting, vaginal bleeding, or blood pressure changes. Labor and delivery staff are highly trained to obtain IV access when needed and, while it is certainly more convenient to have it before it is needed, this may not be the priority for every women. Many providers and hospitals, unfortunately, insist on routine IV placement for all patients, despite the lack of evidence supporting this practice. This can be anxiety provoking for a patient who really does not want one. Again, respect for a laboring woman's bodily autonomy should be first and foremost in any discussion regarding a medical procedure, even one as seemingly inconsequential as an IV.

THE NATURAL BIRTH PLAN

REFERENCES

1. Bishop EH. Pelvic scoring for elective induction. *Obstet Gynecol.* 1964;24(2):266-268.
2. Laughon SK, Zhang J, Troedle J, et al. Using a simplified Bishop's score to predict vaginal delivery. *Obstet Gynecol.* 2011;117(4):804-811.
3. Davey M, King J. Caesarean section following induction of labour in uncomplicated first births—a population-based cross-sectional analysis of 42,950 births. *BMC Pregnancy Childbirth.* 2016;16(1):1. doi:1186/s12884-016-0869-0.
4. Goetzl L. Methods of cervical ripening and labor induction: pharmacologic. *Clin Obstet Gynecol.* 2014;57(2):377-390.
5. Mozurkewich EL, Chilimigras JL, Berman DR, et al. Methods of induction of labour: a systematic review. *BMC Pregnancy Childbirth.* 2011;11:84. doi:10.1186/1471-2393-11-84.
6. American College of Obstetricians and Gynecologists. ACOG Practice Bulletin No. 107: induction of labor. *Obstet Gynecol.* 2009;114(2 pt 1):386-397.
7. Little SE, Caughey AB. Induction of labor and cesarean: what is the true relationship? *Clin Obstet Gynecol.* 2015;58(2):269-281.
8. Schwenker GL. Why not induce everyone at 39 weeks. Available at http://contemporaryobgyn.modernmedicine.com/contemporary-obgyn/news/why-not-induce-everyone-39-weeks. Accessed May 2016.
9. Martin JA, Hamilton BE, Sutton PD, et al. Births: final data for 2005. *Natl Vital Stat Rep.* 2007;56(6):1-103.
10. Galal M, Symonds I, Murray H, et al. Postterm pregnancy. *Facts Views Vis Obgyn.* 2012;4(3):175-187.
11. Mahomed K, Pungsornruk K, Gibbons K. Induction of labour for postdates in nulliparous women with uncomplicated pregnancy—is the caesarean section rate really lower? *J Obstet Gynaecol.* 2016;36(7):916-920.
12. Declercq ER, Sakala C, Corry MP, et al. Major survey findings of listening to mothers SM III: pregnancy and birth: report of the third national U.S. survey of women's childbearing experiences. *J Perinat Educ.* 2014;23(1):9-16. doi:10.1891/1058-1243.23.1.9.
13. Sutan R, Campbell D, Prescott GJ, et al. The risk factors for unexplained antepartum stillbirths in Scotland, 1994 to 2003. *J Perinatol.* 2010;30(5):311-318. doi:10.1038/jp.2009.158.
14. Hannah ME, Hannah WJ, Hellmann J, et al. Induction of labor as compared with serial antenatal monitoring in post-term pregnancy. A randomized controlled trial. The Canadian Multicenter Post-term Pregnancy Trial Group. *N Engl J Med.* 1992;326(5):1587-1592.
15. Gülmezoglu AM, Crowther CA, Middleton P, Heatley E. Induction of labour for improving birth outcomes for women at or beyond term. *Cochrane Database Syst Rev.* 2012;(6):CD004945. doi:10.1002/14651858.CD004945.pub3.
16. Lenihan JP. Relationship of antepartum pelvic examinations to premature rupture of the membranes. *Obstet Gynecol.* 1984;63(1):33-37. PubMed PMID: 6691015.
17. Velemínský M, Tosner J. Relationship of vaginal microflora to PROM, pPROM and the risk of early-onset neonatal sepsis. *Neuro Endocrinol Lett.* 2008;29(2):205-221. PubMed PMID: 18404134.

18. Hill MJ, McWilliams GD, Garcia-Sur D, et al. The effect of membrane sweeping on pre-labor rupture of membranes: a randomized controlled trial. *Obstet Gynecol.* 2008;111(6):1313-1319. doi:10.1097/AOG.0b013e31816fdcf3. PubMed PMID: 18515514.

19. Gunn GC, Mischel DR, Mortan DG. Premature rupture of the fetal membranes. *Am J Obstet Gynecol.* 1970;106(3):469-483.

20. Hannah ME, Ohlsson AO, Farine D, et al. Induction of labor compared with expectant management for pre-labor rupture of the membranes at term. *N Engl J Med.* 1996;334(16):1005-1010. doi:10.1056/NEJM199604183341601.

21. Pintucci A, Meregalli V, Colombo P, Fiorilli A. Premature rupture of membranes at term in low risk women: how long should we wait in the "latent phase"? *J Perinat Med.* 2014;42(2):189-196. doi:10.1515/jpm-2013-0017. PubMed PMID: 24259235.

22. American College of Obstetricians and Gynecologists. Committee Opinion No. 687: approaches to limit intervention during labor and birth. *Obstet Gynecol.* 2017;129(2):e20-e28. doi:10.1097/AOG.0000000000001905. PubMed PMID: 28121831.

23. Mathews TJ, Hamilton BE. Centers for Disease Control and Prevention. NCHS Data Brief No. 152: first births to older women continue to rise. Available at https://www.cdc.gov/nchs/data/databriefs/db152.pdf. Accessed 4/2017.

24. Jolly M, Sebire N, Harris J, et al. The risks associated with pregnancy in women aged 35 years or older. *Hum Reprod.* 2000;15(11):2433-2437.

25. Reddy UM, Ko CW, Willinger M. Maternal age and the risk of stillbirth throughout pregnancy in the United States. *Am J Obstet Gynecol.* 2006;195(3):764-770.

26. Haavaldsen C, Sarfraz AA, Samuelsen SO, Eskild A. The impact of maternal age on fetal death: does length of gestation matter? *Am J Obstet Gynecol.* 2010;203(6):554.e1-554.e8.

27. Fretts RC, Duru UA. New indications for antepartum testing: making the case for antepartum surveillance or timed delivery for women of advanced maternal age. *Semin Perinatol.* 2008;32(4):312-317.

28. Walker KF, Bugg GJ, Macpherson M, et al. 35/39 trial group. Randomized trial of labor induction in women 35 years of age or older. *N Engl J Med.* 2016;374(9):813-822. doi:10.1056/NEJMoa1509117. PubMed PMID: 26962902.

29. Fox NS, Rebarber A, Silverstein M, et al. The effectiveness of antepartum surveillance in reducing the risk of stillbirth in patients with advanced maternal age. *Eur J Obstet Gynecol Reprod Biol.* 2013;170(2):387-390. doi:10.1016/j.ejogrb.2013.07.035.

30. Ogden CL, Carroll MD, Kit BK, Flegal KM. Prevalence of childhood and adult obesity in the United States, 2011-2012. *JAMA.* 2014;311(8):806-814.

31. Salihu HM, Dunlop AL, Hedayatzadeh M, et al. Extreme obesity and risk of stillbirth among black and white gravidas. *Obstet Gynecol.* 2007;110(3):552-557.

32. Yao R, Ananth CV, Park BY, et al. Obesity and the risk of stillbirth: a population-based cohort study. Perinatal Research Consortium. *Am J Obstet Gynecol.* 2014;210(5):457.e1-457.e9.

33. American College of Obstetricians and Gynecologists. ACOG Practice Bulletin No 156: obesity in pregnancy. *Obstet Gynecol.* 2015;126(6):e112-e126.

34. O'Dwyer V, O'Kelly S, Monaghan B, et al. Maternal obesity and induction of labor. *Acta Obstet Gynecol Scand.* 2013;92(12):1414-1418. doi:10.1111/aogs.12263. PubMed PMID: 24116732.

35. Martin JA, Brady HE, Osterman MJ, et al. Births: final data for 2015. National Vital Statistics Reports, vol 66, no. 1. Hyattsville, MD: National Center for Health Statistics; 2017.

36. Chauhan SP, Grobman WA, Gherman RA. Suspicion and treatment of the macrosomic fetus: a review. *Am J Obstet Gynecol.* 2005;193(2):332-346.

37. Rossi AC, Mullin P, Prefumo F. Prevention, management, and outcomes of macrosomia: a systematic review of literature and meta-analysis. *Obstet Gynecol Surv.* 2013;68(10):702-709. doi:10.1097/01.ogx.0000435370.74455.a8.

38. Sadeh-Mestechkin D, Walfisch A, Shachar R, Shoham-Vardi I, Vardi H, Hallak M. Suspected macrosomia? Better not to tell. *Arch Gynecol Obstet.* 2008;278(3):225-230.

39. Peleg D, Warsof S, Wolf MF, et al. Counseling for fetal macrosomia: an estimated fetal weight of 4,000 g is excessively low. *Am J Perinatol.* 2015;32(1):71-74.

40. Rouse DJ, Owen J, Goldenberg RL, Cliver SP. The effectiveness and costs of elective cesarean delivery for fetal macrosomia diagnosed by ultrasound. *JAMA.* 1996;276(18):1480-1486. PubMed PMID: 8903259.

41. Hoffman MK, Bailit JL, Branch DW, et al. A comparison of obstetric maneuvers for the acute management of shoulder dystocia. *Obstet Gynecol.* 2011;117(6):1272-1278. doi:10.1097/AOG.0b013e31821a12c9.

42. Boulvain M, Irion O, Dowswell T, Thornton JG. Induction of labour at or near term for suspected fetal macrosomia. *Cochrane Database Syst Rev.* 2016(5):1-45. CD000938. doi:10.1002/14651858.CD000938.pub2.

43. American College of Obstetricians and Gynecologists. Practice Bulletin No. 173: fetal macrosomia. *Obstet Gynecol.* 2016;128(5):e195-e209. PubMed PMID: 27776071.

44. Declercq ER, Sakala C, Corry MP, et al. Listening to mothers II: report of the second national U.S. survey of women's childbearing experiences. *J Perinat Educ.* 2007;16(4):9-14.

45. Melzack R, Belanger R, Lacroix R. Labor pain: effect of maternal position on front and back pain. *J Pain Symptom Manage.* 1991;6(8):476-480.

46. Adoach K, Shimada M, Usui A. The relationship between parturients positions and perceptions of labor pain intensity. *Nurs Res.* 2003;52(1):47-51.

47. Regaya BL, Fatnassi R, Khlifi A, et al. Role of ambulation during labor: a prospective randomized study. *J Gynecol Obstet Biol Reprod.* 2010;30(8):656-662.

48. Lawrence A, Lewis L, Hofmeyr, et al. Maternal positions and mobility during first stage labour. *Cochrane Database Syst Rev.* 2009;(2):CD003934. doi:10.1002/14651858. CD003934.pub2.

49. Winslow E, Crenshaw J, Jacobson A. Managing labor: does walking help or hurt? *Am J Nurs.* 2000;100(3):52-54.

50. Intermittent Auscultation for Intrapartum Fetal Heart Rate Surveillance. ACNM Clinical Bulletin No. 11. *J Midwifery Womens Health.* 2010;55(4):397-403.

51. Stout MJ, Canhill AG. Electronic fetal monitoring: past, present, and future. *Clin Perinatol.* 2011;38(1):127-142.

52. National Institute of Child Health and Human Development Research Planning Workshop. Electronic fetal heart rate monitoring: research guidelines for interpretations. *Am J Obstet Gynecol.* 1997;177(6):1385-1390.

53. American College of Obstetricians and Gynecologists. ACOG Practice Bulletin No. 106: intrapartum fetal heart rate monitoring: nomenclature, interpretation, and general management principles. *Obstet Gynecol.* 2009;114(1):192-202.

54. Garcia J, Corry M, MacDonald D, et al. Mother's views of continuous electronic fetal heart monitoring and intermittent auscultation in a randomized controlled trial. *Birth*. 1985;12(2):79-85.

55. Alfirevic Z, Devane D, Gyte GML, Cuthbert A. Continuous cardiotocography as a form of electronic fetal monitoring for fetal assessment during labor. *Cochrane Database Syst Rev.* 2017;(2):CD006066. doi:10.1002/14651858.CD006066.pub3.

56. Spencer JA, Badawi N, Burton P, et al. The intrapartum CTG prior to neonatal encephalopathy at term: a case controlled study. *Br J Obstet Gynaecol*. 1997;104(1):25-28.

57. Smyth RMD, Markham C, Dowswell T. Amniotomy for shortening spontaneous labor. *Cochrane Database Syst Rev*. 2013;(6):CD006167. doi:10.1002/14651858. CD0061.

58. Cohain J. Amniotomy and cord prolapse. *Midwifery Today*. 2013;108:32-33.

59. Carmichael MS, Humbert R, Dixen J, et al. Plasma oxytocin increases in the human sexual response. *J Clin Endocrinol Metab*. 1987;64(1):27-31. doi:10.1210/jcem-64-1-27. PMID: 3782434.

60. "Pitocin." Available at https://www.drugs.com/pro/pitocin.html. Accessed June 2017.

61. O'Driscoll K, Stronge JM, Minogue M. Active management of labor. *Br Med J*. 1973;3(5872):135-137.

62. Bohr U, Donnelly J, O'Connell MP, et al. Active management of labor revisited: the first 1000 primiparous labors in 2000. *J Obstet Gynaecol*. 2003;23(2):118-120.

63. Bugg GJ, Siddiqui F, Thornton JG. Oxytocin versus no treatment or delayed treatment for slow progress in the first stage of spontaneous labour. *Cochrane Database Syst Rev*. 2011:CD007123.

64. Seitchik J, Chatkoff ML. Oxytocin-induced uterine hypercontractility pressure wave forms. *Obstet Gynecol*. 1976;48(4):436-441.

65. Bell AF, Erickon EN, Carter CS. Beyond labor: the role of natural and synthetic oxytocin in the transition to motherhood. *J Midwifery Womens Health*. 2014;59(1): 35-42.

66. Tyzio R, Cossart R, Khalilov I, et al. Maternal oxytocin triggers a transient inhibitory switch in GABA signaling in the fetal brain during delivery. *Science*. 2006;314(5806): 1788-1792.

67. Jacob S, Brune CW, Carter CS, et al. Association of the oxytocin receptor gene (OXTR) in Caucasian children and adolescents with autism. *Neurosci Lett*. 2007;417(1):6-9.

68. Wermter AK, Kamp-Becker I, Hesse P, et al. Evidence for the involvement of genetic variation in the oxytocin receptor gene (OXTR) in the etiology of autistic disorders on high-functioning level. *Am J Med Genet B Neuropsychiatr Genet*. 2010;153B(2):629-639.

69. Gregory SG, Anthopolos R, Osgood LE, et al. Association of autism with induced or augmented childbirth in North Carolina Birth Record (1990-1998) and Education Research (1997-2007) database. *JAMA Pediatr*. 2013;167(10):959-966.

70. Van Leengoed E, Kerker E, Swanson HH. Inhibition of post-partum maternal behaviour in the rat by injecting an oxytocin antagonist into the cerebral ventricles. *J Endocrinol*. 1987;112(2):275-282.

71. Skrundz M, Bolten M, Nast I, et al. Plasma oxytocin concentration during pregnancy is associated with development of postpartum depression. *Neuropsychopharmacology*. 2011;36(9):1886-1893.

THE NATURAL BIRTH PLAN

72. Friedman EA. Primigravid labor: a graphicostatistical analysis. *Obstet Gynecol.* 1995;6(6):567-589.

73. Zhang J, Landy HJ, Branch DW, et al. Contemporary patterns of spontaneous labor with normal neonatal outcomes. *Obstet Gynecol.* 2013;116(6):1281-1287.

74. Neal JL, Lowe NK, Patrick TE, et al. What is the slowest-yet-normal cervical dilation rate among nulliparous women with spontaneous labor onset? *J Obstet Gynecol Neonatal Nurs.* 2010;39(4):361-369.

75. American College of Obstetricians and Gynecologists. Obstetric care consensus no. 1: safe prevention of the primary cesarean delivery. *Obstet Gynecol.* 2014;123(1):693-711.

76. Boyle A, Reddy UM, Landy HJ, et al. Primary cesarean in the United States. *Obstet Gynecol.* 2013;122(1):33-40.

77. Huhn KA, Brost BC. Accuracy of simulated cervical dilation and effacement measurements among practitioners. *Am J Obstet Gynecol.* 2004;191(5):1797-1799.

78. Downe S, Gyte GML, Dahlen HG, Singata M. Routine vaginal examinations for assessing progress of labour to improve outcomes for women and babies at term. *Cochrane Database Syst Rev.* 2013;(7):CD010088. doi:10.1002/14651858.CD010088. pub2.

79. Duff M. *A Study of Labour (PhD thesis).* Sydney: University of Technology; 2005.

80. Bucklin BA, Hawkins JL, Anderson JR, et al. Obstetric anesthesia workforce survey. Twenty year update. *Anesthesiology.* 2005;103(1):645-653.

81. Romano AM. First, do no harm: how routine interventions, common restrictions, and the organisation of our health-care system affect the health of mothers and newborns. *J Perinat Educ.* 2009;18(3):58-62.

82. Chestnut DH, Wong CA, Tsen LC, et al. *Chestnut's Obstetric Anesthesia: Principles and Practice.* Philadelphia, PA: Elsevier; 2014.

83. Pengelley L, Gyte G. Eating and drinking in labour. An update of the NCT briefing paper. *Practising Midwife.* 1998;1:26-28.

84. American Society of Anesthesiologists. Practice guidelines for obstetric anesthesia: an updated report by the American Society of Anesthesiologists Task Force on Obstetric Anesthesia and the Society for Obstetric Anesthesia and Perinatology. *Anesthesiology.* 2016;124(2):270-300.

85. American College of Obstetricians and Gynecologists. Oral intake during labor. ACOG Committee Opinion No. 441. *Obstet Gynecol.* 2009;114(3):714.

86. Sperling JD, Dahlke JD, Sibai BM. Restriction of oral intake during labor: whither are we bound? *Am J Obstet Gynecol.* 2016;214(1):592-596.

87. Dawood F, Dowswell T, Quenby S. Intravenous fluids for reducing the duration of labour in low risk nulliparous women. *Cochrane Database Syst Rev.* 2013: 18(6):CD007715. doi:10.1002/14651858.CD007715.pub2.

88. Coco A, Derksen-Schrock A, Coco K, et al. A randomized trial of increased intravenous hydration in labor when oral fluid is unrestricted. *Fam Med.* 2010;42(1):52-56.

89. Wright S, Yelland M, Heathcote K, et al. Fear of needles—nature and prevalence in general practice. *Aust Family Physician.* 2009;38(3):172-176.

90. Chantry CJ, Nommsen-Rivers LA. Excess weight loss in first-born breastfed newborns relates to maternal intrapartum fluid balance. *Pediatrics.* 2011;127(1):171-179.

91. Noel-Weiss J, Woodend AK, Peterson WE, et al. An observational study of associations among maternal fluids during parturition, neonatal output, and breastfed newborn weight loss. *Int Breastfeed J.* 2011;6(9):1-10.

Pain Management

I'll admit, I am one of those people who really don't like medicine. I rarely even take a tylenol. I am sure that was part of the reason I planned for a natural birth. However, it was more than that. I felt like I was a part of this tradition going back to the beginning of time, where women worked to bring their babies into the world. It may sound strange to a lot of people, but I wanted to experience that. So much of our day to day life is depersonalized and cut off from nature, I just wanted to connect to this very real process of bringing forth life and to see what my body was capable of. I will not say labor was fun, but I am so grateful I chose to do it the way I did. I have never felt more powerful than when, after hours and hours of hard work, breathing through contraction after contraction, I lifted that red, beautiful screaming baby up to my chest. I just looked at her and thought, "I did this, I created this." I really felt like after that, I could do anything. There was no parenting challenge before me that would be too hard. I am sure people have empowering birth experiences other ways as well, but for me the process mattered. It was important. I really felt like I earned my motherhood in that journey.

—L. D., new mother

I would like to avoid an epidural, please don't offer me one

Epidural use for pain management in labor has become standard in the United States, with the number of women selecting this option having tripled since the 1980s. In 2011, the CDC reported that 61% of women delivering vaginally had an epidural, however in individual hospitals, that rate may exceed 90%.[1] During an epidural, a small catheter is threaded into the epidural space, an area between the bones of the spine and the dura mater that surrounds the spinal cord. Two types of medications, a local anesthetic and a narcotic, are then infused into the epidural space continuously throughout the labor until after delivery, providing pain relief, as well as some degree of numbness and immobility, from the breast line down. Overall, epidurals provide effective pain management for the majority of women, with 88% of women who receive epidurals reporting good pain relief. It also is one of the safest forms of pain relief from the standpoint of the both the baby and mother. Rates of permanent maternal injury related to any form of spinal or neuraxial block is low, at 1.2 per 100,000, while the rate specifically with an epidural is 0.6 in 100,000. While all medications cross the placenta to some degree, the amount of medication that enters maternal circulation and thus reaches the baby is low and, when compared to IV narcotics for pain relief in labor, babies do not demonstrate a suppressed breathing response, have higher APGAR scores, and have a lower likelihood of needing medications to reverse the narcotic effect.[2]

EPIDURAL SIDE EFFECTS AND COMPLICATIONS

Given the efficacy of an epidural and the relative safety, many people are incredulous that any woman would want to give birth without one. Common responses women planning to labor unmedicated hear from their family, friends, nurses, and doctors alike are:

- *"You wouldn't have a tooth pulled without anesthesia, why would you have a baby without it?"*
- *"Don't be a hero, having an epidural doesn't make you any less of a mother."*
- *"You say that now, but just wait until labor starts! They don't call it labor for nothing."*
- *"Are you crazy?"*

However, like any other medication or medical procedure, epidurals are not side effect or complication free. Many women would simply like to avoid these possible issues if they are able to manage their labor utilizing other tools, which is far from "crazy"; it is very sensible.

Longer Labors and Increased Chance of Operative Vaginal Delivery

In most of the studies to date, epidurals have been shown to both prolong labor and increase the likelihood of a woman needing instrumentation, either vacuum or forceps, to achieve a vaginal delivery. The studies examining epidurals are numerous and vary greatly in their precise findings, but the largest review on the topic found that epidurals are associated with an increase in the first stage of labor of anywhere from 1 to 4 hours and an increase in the second stage of labor of up to 1 hour. The same review, involving over 8000 women, found that the risk of an operative delivery was 5% greater in patients who received epidurals.[3]

There are several explanations offered for why these variations may exist. One hypothesis is that the large quantities of fluid necessitated by

THE NATURAL BIRTH PLAN

an epidural dilute the hormone concentrations in the blood which are generating the strength and consistency of uterine contractions. While not demonstrated by a study, nearly every provider can describe the phenomenon where a patient enters the hospital with a strong, consistent labor pattern, receives an epidural, and inexplicably her contraction pattern stops. Another theory about the longer labors seen with epidurals, particularly in early epidurals given before full descent of the baby in the pelvis occurs, is that epidural-generated muscle relaxation promotes an inappropriate fetal head extension and increases the rate of malpositions, such as occiput posterior or sunny-side up babies. While not statistically significant according to the *Cochrane Review*, greater numbers of women with epidurals do have malpositioned or occiput posterior babies (18% vs. 13%). When this review is further examined and studies excluded where more than 10% of women grouped in the "non-epidural" category actually received epidurals, the rate of malpositioned babies associated with epidural is even higher (11% vs. 2%).[4] Furthermore, malpositioned babies are also significantly more likely to require an operative delivery. Critics of this theory will argue that rather than epidurals causing malpositioned babies, mothers with malpositioned babies often experience longer, more painful labors and are simply more likely to request an epidural. The evidence to date is insufficient to unravel that chicken versus egg debate, but other factors associated with epidurals that also are thought to increase the second stage of labor and make operative delivery more common are simply the numbness and general muscle weakness generated by the epidural. Given the higher rates of perineal lacerations and neonatal complications observed in operative deliveries, it is understandable that women want to avoid procedures that increase their risk of requiring instrumentation in their delivery.

Increased Rates of Pitocin Administration

Not surprisingly given the longer labors observed in women with epidurals, epidurals are also associated with an increased chance of receiving pitocin.[3] Pitocin may also be more freely given to women with epidurals because, once the epidural is in place, most women will not experience a difference in their labor discomfort as a result of the pitocin and providers may simply want to shorten the labor whether or not the labor is prolonged. Many women have a strong desire to avoid pitocin, for the numerous reasons discussed previously, and this desire alone may be enough for them to want to avoid an epidural.

Hypotension

Hypotension is defined as a 20% drop in systolic blood pressure and is one of the more common side effects of epidural administration, occurring in approximately 10% of women who receive epidurals. Women are given fluid boluses prior to an epidural to decrease the likelihood of this effect and, when they occur, these episodes are typically treated with maternal position changes which displace the uterus off the large vessels of the pelvis and improve blood flow back to the heart, additional fluid boluses, and occasionally vasopressors, medications that increase maternal heart rate and blood pressure. Possible consequences of epidural-related hypotension are maternal nausea and vomiting and feelings of dizziness, as well as fetal heart rate changes and distress as a consequence of poor uterine perfusion. Occasionally, the episodes can be significant enough and the fetal response poor enough to warrant an emergency cesarean.

Pruritus or Itching

Itchiness is the most common side effect experienced with epidurals, occurring in 30% of women, and spinal anesthesia, occurring in 58% of women. It is often mistakenly believed to be due to a histamine release, but antihistamines are ineffective in treating it and can cause decreased milk supply after birth. Opioid antagonists have been shown to help, but are usually not given because they counteract the pain relief benefits.

Maternal Fever

Maternal fever during labor is another common side effect associated with epidural use. The exact rate is not clear, as it is often challenging to isolate the number of women with a fever from another cause from women experiencing fever due to epidural alone. However, one study of over 2500 women receiving epidurals demonstrated that temperatures exceeding 99.5°F occurred in 44.8% of patients, as opposed to 14.6% in the non-epidural group.[5] The association between epidural and maternal fever has also been demonstrated in several randomized controlled trials, though there has been much debate about whether these studies were skewed by compounding variables, such as longer labors, more vaginal examinations, or increased use of additional medications, such as pitocin. It is also unclear whether the etiology of fevers associated with epidurals is inflammatory or a disruption in thermoregulatory processes.

THE NATURAL BIRTH PLAN

The consequences of maternal fever during labor are numerous. Elevated temperatures are associated with an increase in maternal heart rate, cardiac output, and oxygen consumption, which are rarely harmful to healthy laboring women, but can be dangerous in women with cardiac or pulmonary diseases or complications of pregnancy. There is also often an associated change in labor management in response to maternal fever. Women with fevers are twice as likely to undergo either an operative vaginal delivery or a cesarean section than those without fever. It is uncertain whether this is due to an effect of the fever on the labor process or if care providers are more likely to intervene in the setting of a maternal fever for fear of worse complications if delivery is delayed. Maternal fever also typically prompts a sepsis, or infection, evaluation in the newborn, which can mean something as minor as simple blood tests and observation or as significant as automatic admission to the Neonatal Intensive Care Unit and prophylactic antibiotic administration, depending on the hospital protocol. There are conflicting studies addressing whether fever itself is dangerous for babies, with most studies indicating permanent neurological harm only in the setting of infectious, inflammatory fevers, however all babies born in the setting of a maternal fever were at higher risk for seizures, low APGAR scores, and the need for cardiopulmonary resuscitation at birth.[6]

Accidental Dural Puncture and Postdural Puncture Headache or "Spinal Headache"

When the epidural needle is inserted too far and accidentally punctures the dural sac surrounding the spinal cord, small amounts of cerebrospinal fluid can leak out and a postural "spinal headache" results. This is a severe headache that tends to worsen with sitting or standing and improves with lying down, significantly limiting a new mother's ability to care for their baby. While it will ultimately go away on its own, more than 80% of women who experience this end up being treated due to the severity of the symptoms. "Spinal headaches" are treated with what is known as a "blood patch," where some of the patient's own blood is inserted into the epidural space, helping to seal the puncture site. The risk of an accidental puncture is approximately 1.5%, with 52% of those punctures developing into spinal headaches.[7]

Serious Complications: Nerve Injury, Infection, and Epidural Hematomas

One of the most common fears women express about epidurals is that it will "paralyze them" or otherwise damage their spine. Fortunately, the risk of serious neurological complications of epidurals is quite low. In a review of over 300,000 women who received epidurals, the rate of permanent nerve injury was shown to be as low as 0.6 in 100,000.[8] The risk of an epidural abscess or meningitis following an epidural is also extremely low, with each complication complicating only 0.2 to 3.7 per 100,000 obstetrical epidurals.[9] The incidence of an epidural hematoma, a blood clot forming in the epidural space causing compression and injury to the spinal cord, is even more uncommon, affecting only one patient in a review of six surveys involving more than 1 million obstetric epidural procedures.[10]

OTHER POSSIBLE CONSEQUENCES OF EPIDURALS

Lower Breastfeeding Rates

Another commonly expressed fear among laboring women regarding epidural administration is that the medication will reach the baby and result in some harm or "drugging" of the baby and negatively impact breastfeeding. This concern is often listed in natural childbirth texts as one of the reasons women should avoid an epidural. However, the medical evidence demonstrating this is lacking. An observational study of nearly 200 women in 1999 failed to show any effect of epidural analgesia on breastfeeding success.[11] A larger Italian observational study in the same year also failed to show any impact of epidurals on breastfeeding rates, which are universally high in Italian women, though it did show lower rates in women who had received general anesthesia during cesarean sections.[12] A later randomized controlled study did demonstrate that larger doses of fentanyl in epidurals were associated with negative impacts on breastfeeding, with mothers receiving the highest doses reporting more problems with breastfeeding in the first 24 hours and lower rates of breastfeeding at 6 weeks.[13] However, another larger randomized control trial by Wilson et al.[14] failed to show this association, with women showing similar rates of breastfeeding irrespective of epidural use, dosing, or type of administration. While there is certainly room for more study, it does not appear that epidurals significantly impact breastfeeding success and all current research supports that epidurals have less impact on breastfeeding than IV narcotic pain medications in labor.[15]

Chronic Back Pain

Back pain in pregnancy and after delivery is common. At least 40% of women report some degree of gestational back pain and some studies show a rate up to 90%. There are several reasons for this. During pregnancy, a hormone relaxin is secreted that results in increased mobility of the joints, which makes women more prone to strain injuries of the spine. Another causal factor is the biomechanical realities of pregnancy, where the enlarging uterus shifts the center of gravity forward, requiring pregnant women to lean backwards to maintain their balance. This puts additional strain on the muscles of the lower back, in particular, and increases the risk of injury. Postpartum backaches occur in up to two-thirds of women after delivery, though they resolve in the majority of women. Nonetheless, up to 7% of women still report significant back pain over 1 year from delivery.[16]

Chronic back pain was first linked to epidural use in 1990, when a large study was done in the United Kingdom, examining the effect of epidural on the development of back pain. Over 30,000 women were sent questionnaires inquiring about back pain and epidural use. Less than half of those sent the questionnaires responded, but the results were concerning, with women who received an epidural reporting significantly higher rates of back pain. The examiners conducted a very thorough statistical analysis, showing even that women who had planned cesareans had no difference in back pain rates whether or not they received epidural analgesia, whereas women who had epidurals and emergency cesareans during labor did demonstrate an increased rate of back pain, supporting the theory that prolonged immobility with epidural analgesia and the resultant damage was the culprit behind this association. They estimated that epidurals were associated with an 8 in 100 chance of developing chronic back pain after delivery.[17]

There was one major problem with this study, however. Given that less than half of those surveyed responded, the study likely overrepresented women with back pain, because those with pain were much more likely to return the survey than those who felt fine. Later, better designed studies have failed to show a link between epidurals and back pain and the 2011 *Cochrane Review* of the data examining this concern also determined that epidurals do not increase the risk of chronic back pain.[3]

DO EPIDURALS INCREASE THE CHANCE OF CESAREAN?

The million dollar question for most women considering an epidural is whether it will increase their chance of ending up in a cesarean section and fear of a cesarean is one of the main reasons women cite for choosing to forgo the pain relief epidurals offer. Unfortunately, for women trying to make an informed decision regarding epidurals, the evidence is extremely confusing and the interpretations of it vary widely. In the media, for every strongly supported article stating that epidurals increase the likelihood of cesarean and advocating for nonmedical management of labor pain, there is another article explicitly refuting this claim and encouraging women to utilize epidurals without concern. So, who is right?

That question is incredibly difficult to answer because labor is a complex and poorly understood process, influenced by a great number of factors, and the women going through that process are equally complicated and diverse. The initial concern about a possible link between epidurals and cesarean was raised by Thorp et al. (1989),[18] who observed a significantly higher rate of cesarean in patients who had received epidurals when compared to women who either received narcotics or had not received any pharmacological pain relief in labor. In the nearly 20 years that followed, study after study was performed trying to tease out the truth regarding the association. However, studying the subject has, in itself, been a considerable challenge and, consequently, the results and conclusions from these studies must be taken with a grain of salt. First and foremost, it is difficult to design a randomized controlled trial, the gold standard of medical evidence, because providers are unable to be blinded to the therapy they are studying and professional biases could potentially alter their management. It is also difficult to convince women to sign up for a study that may preclude them obtaining an epidural, which is the safest, most effective form of pharmacologic pain relief currently available. Furthermore, many providers feel it is unethical to even conduct a study that does not offer some form of pharmacologic pain relief and therefore all but 5 of the 38 randomized trials to date have compared epidurals to narcotics, not epidurals to nonpharmacologic pain relief methods.

To complicate things further, all of the studies have been conducted within the framework of the medically managed labor model, so it is uncertain whether women who were in the "non-epidural" groups were offered appropriate nonpharmacological pain management options, such as ambulation, hydrotherapy, or comfort positioning, what preparation, if any, they had for an unmedicated delivery, and to what degree either group were medically augmented in their labor with pitocin and artificial rupture of membranes. Hence, critics argue these studies are not adequately comparing intervention to no intervention, they are only comparing degrees of intervention and no study to date has adequately

THE NATURAL BIRTH PLAN

compared the low intervention, natural approach to the medically managed approach. Finally, some studies did not have comparable numbers of multiparous patients in each group, who are very likely to have a vaginal delivery regardless of labor interventions, and each of the studies had patients in the "epidural group" who progressed too rapidly to receive an epidural, as well as patients in the "no epidural group" who ultimately received an epidural, which makes interpretations of the results confusing.

So, keeping all these limitations in mind, what does the data show? In summary, the data shows an increased risk of many factors associated with cesarean, but not necessarily an increased risk of cesarean itself. Patients with epidurals are more likely to experience maternal fever, pitocin augmentation, continuous fetal monitoring, prolonged labor, malpositioned babies, and even cesarean specifically for fetal distress but overall rates of cesarean are not statistically comparable whether a woman has an epidural or not.[3] This is confusing. How does an increase in things that can lead to a cesarean not translate to an increased rate of cesareans themselves?

Certainly, many observational studies have shown the opposite. For example, in one study by Klein et al.,[19] which grouped patients according to their providers overall rate of epidural use, first-time mothers cared for by providers who utilized epidurals less than 40% of the time were observed to have a cesarean rate of 14.8%, while those who had a provider who utilized epidurals with over 70% of their patients had a cesarean rate of 23.4%. Providers who utilized epidurals at a higher rate were also shown to admit patients earlier in the labor process, utilize continuous fetal monitoring and pitocin augmentation at higher rates, and delivered more babies who were malpositioned and/or required NICU care. This suggests that epidural is a marker of labor management style that leads to more cesareans. Indeed, in the personal narratives of many new mothers and in the judgment of many in the natural birth community, an epidural, similar to an induction, is often the first step in a cascade of medical interventions that ultimately end in an operating room.

Another thorough observational study that attempted to minimize the effects of several confounding variables, such as noncompliance within the study groups and employment of different medical interventions like continuous monitoring, found a similar association of epidural with cesarean. Over 50,000 well-matched women were compared and even when groups were analyzed after excluding for confounding factors such as the setting where they delivered, their provider type, and the use of other medical interventions, cesarean was still two times more likely when epidurals were utilized. Investigators even performed a calculation in which they eliminated patients with occiuput posterior, or sunny-side up, babies from the analysis. This was done in order to solve the "chicken versus egg" debate concerning whether epidurals cause malpositioned babies or are simply utilized more frequently in the setting of fetal malposition. Even after patients with malpositioned babies were excluded, patients with an epidural were still shown to undergo cesarean at a higher rate.[19]

Other observational studies that have shown an increased incidence include a Danish cohort of over 2000 low-risk nulliparous women who were shown to have a higher risk of emergency cesarean with epidural use, a retrospective review of 1733 low-risk first-time mothers that demonstrated a 3.7-fold increased risk of cesarean with epidural, with higher rates observed the earlier the epidural was administered, and a multicenter study including over 2000 women which examined several risk factors for labor dystocia and found epidurals to have the highest association with protracted labor.[21-23] Several individuals have reexamined the data used in the *Cochrane Review* to try and understand the apparent disconnect between these observational studies, as well as their own clinical experience, and the randomized trials. One critic pointed out that the largest trial contributing to the results of the review was performed in an institution that already had a very low rate of cesarean, 12%, which is not indicative of national averages and suggests that factors which usually compound the effect of an epidural on the labor process may not be an issue at this particular institution. Furthermore, in most of the studies in the review, only patients in spontaneous labor, after 4 cm dilation, were randomized, perhaps merely demonstrating that epidurals in active labor do not alter the incidence of cesarean.[24]

Additional studies and a later review attempted to address this later critique, examining the timing of epidural as it related to cesarean rates. Nine studies were included in the *Cochrane Review* that attempted to determine if early epidurals were associated with more cesareans than later epidurals. Their conclusion was that timing of epidural had no impact on cesarean rate.[25] The overall quality of the review was good, however, critics have pointed out there were some limitations that should be considered. Six of the trials included in the review had significant overlap between their "early" and "late" epidurals and none of the trials used the current standard for true active labor of 6 cm, as defined by ACOG, meaning a significant portion of the "late" epidurals could actually have been administered in the latent stage of labor as we now understand it. Finally, there was also considerable variation in the overall rates of cesarean observed between what would otherwise be considered comparable groups of patients with similar risks of cesarean, which points to practice variations between the institutions that conducted the studies which could be masking the effect of epidural timing on the rate of cesarean.[26]

Ultimately, however, the question of whether a late epidural is better than an early epidural is significantly less important than whether epidurals, in general, contribute to the rising cesarean rate. Overall, the evidence suggests that epidural itself may be less important than the care philosophy in which it is provided. A recent study found that labor and delivery units with the most proactive or interventional management style and philosophy are associated with the highest rates of cesarean section, as well as postpartum hemorrhage, blood transfusions, and prolonged hospital stays.[27] Furthermore, none of the studies to date have explored what contribution, if any, the patient may have on the process. A patient planning a natural birth who prepares for a natural birth and has a plan in place to manage their discomfort nonpharmacologically is very different from a patient randomized to not receive an epidural who relies on narcotics or simply white-knuckles it through their labor. What is needed are studies comparing spontaneously laboring patients, both with and without intention for an epidural, in a low-intervention model with spontaneously laboring patients, with and without intention for an epidural, in a traditional high-intervention medical model. This could start to unravel how much effect the provider, the patient herself, and the epidural is having on cesarean rates. But in the absence of that information, the honest answer to the million dollar question is simply we do not really know. Epidural is associated with several things that have been shown to contribute to cesareans, but the degree to which those things will impact any individual woman is unable to be determined. In conclusion, women who want epidurals should be able to obtain them when they wish and both pharmacologic and nonpharmacologic alternatives to epidurals should be readily available to any woman who wishes to make an epidural her plan B.

I would like to utilize Hydrotherapy for Pain Relief

I had been in hard labor for several hours and really felt on the edge of losing it. I wasn't dilating very fast and it was becoming really difficult to concentrate on my breathing during the contractions and I could feel my body tensing up. My midwife suggested we try the labor tub and I eagerly agreed. I think I would have agreed to anything at that point. I worked through a few more contractions while they filled it up and then I waddled down the hall to the tub room. The pool was deep and warm and felt like pure bliss. I felt my tension and pain melt away. I still had the contractions and they still required my focus, but it wasn't pain in the way I was experiencing it on dry land. I am not sure how long I labored in the tub, but after what felt like a short time, I began to feel pressure. My midwife checked me and said it was time. We moved back to my room and I pushed my beautiful baby girl out a short while later.

—C. S., new mother

Hydrotherapy for pain relief in labor takes two forms, either intermittent warm showers or immersion in a warm labor tub. Both methods promote peripheral vasodilation, leading to a redistribution of blood flow and muscle relaxation. A reduction in blood pressure is observed as result of this effect.[28] Shower use also promotes muscle relaxation via the massage effect of the forced water on the skin and muscles. Both methods have demonstrated efficacy in the reduction of pain reported by women in labor, while tub immersion has also been shown to reduce the rate of epidural use and shorten the first stage of labor. Additional benefits of the tub are buoyancy, permitting more freedom of movement and better positioning, psychological benefits of relaxation with a decrease in anxiety and stress, and a greater feeling of maternal control and satisfaction with the birth process. One small randomized control trial even demonstrated that labor tubs can be an effective labor augmentation tool in the setting of a stalled labor, with patients utilizing labor tubs showing less need for pitocin augmentation or other obstetrical procedures.[29]

Neither method has shown any difference when compared with standard management in terms of cesarean rates, infection, pitocin use, or adverse neonatal effects, though many providers express concern particularly about infection with the use of tubs.[30] It is important to note that studies have been performed examining whether water enters the vagina. Back in the 1960s, when pregnant women were discouraged from bathing or swimming in the third trimester, Dr. Siegel had several women soak in iodine-stained water, with a white tampon placed vaginally. All of the women emerged from the soaking tubs with clean tampons, demonstrating that water does not enter the vagina.[31] Even when a more recent large observational study examined tub use in the setting of prolonged rupture of membranes, no difference in infection rates in either the women or their infants was observed.[32] The only evidenced-based concern about water immersion in the first stage of labor is that of maternal

THE NATURAL BIRTH PLAN

hyperthermia, with resultant fetal tachycardia, which is why care must be taken to keep tub water at body temperature and if an excessive maternal temperature or fetal tachycardia is observed, the mother should leave the tub to cool down.

Unfortunately, for those hoping to expand the use of hydrotherapy in American maternity units, the majority of studies concerning hydrotherapy have been observational in nature, as it is difficult to perform a true blinded randomized trial to a therapy that is clearly unable to be hidden from care providers and women are unlikely to willingly enter such a study if they desire the use of the tub, knowing they may be randomized in a group unable to access it. Nonetheless, the available evidence demonstrates that hydrotherapy can be an effective pain management tool, with little associated negative side effects, and should be available to mothers wishing to utilize it during labor. The American College of Obstetrics and Gynecology supports its use and in the United Kingdom it is part of standard health policy that all maternity units have water immersion therapy available to women.[33]

RECOMMENDATIONS REGARDING USE OF HYDROTHERAPY

There are no standard protocols for the use of hydrotherapy, but some general guidelines from the available evidence are:

- Temperature should be between 37°C and 38°C or 98.6°F and 100.4°F.
- Water temperature should be monitored to ensure therapeutic temperatures and prevent maternal or fetal hyperthermia.
- Fetal assessment and maternal vital signs should continue to be taken at appropriate intervals, with the utilization of mobile "mermaid" monitors or handheld Doppler devices.
- For shower therapy, intervals of at least 20 minutes should be utilized for efficacy.
- For immersion therapy, tub should be deep enough to reach the nipple line.
- All current research has been done in low-risk women, generally defined as: 37 to 41 weeks, singleton pregnancies in vertex position, with reassuring fetal heart rate tracing, absence of meconium fluid or evidence of infection, and without a history of prior cesarean, labor augmentation, or other indication for continuous monitoring. The main reason for restricting tub use in "higher risk" women centers

around monitoring issues, however, modern mobile monitors do permit continuous monitoring while utilizing hydrotherapy, so it seems reasonable to relax this restriction, though further research is needed.

I would like to use comfort positions and breathing techniques to manage my labor discomfort

The majority of women in the United States who are planning an unmedicated birth attend some form of childbirth education, where they are typically taught a range of techniques to manage their labor. Most of these classes focus on positioning and breath training to cope with labor pain. The philosophy of each class and breathing pattern taught varies, but all utilize the same general comfort positions to some degree. There is limited information about the efficacy of these methods as they relate to pharmacologic methods of pain management; however, for the woman who has already decided her goal is to birth without medications, that comparison is of little value. What is important for women is to feel prepared for labor. In the same way one would train for a marathon, unmedicated labor goes best with both physical and mental preparation. Anyone can wake up tomorrow and decide to enter a marathon, but without training for it, they are unlikely to be very successful. The same goes for a natural birth. Education provides the tools and the strategy. Obviously, a strategy does not guarantee a particular outcome any more than training can guarantee the marathon runner will not sprain their ankle in the middle of the race. Yet, the well-trained birther is much more likely to cross the finish line naturally.

COMMON CHILDBIRTH EDUCATION METHODS

Childbirth education began in the 1960s, when most women were still giving birth with the aid of forceps and systemic medications that significantly decreased their awareness and participation in the birth process. Women wanted to have more control over their birth experience and have their partners in the room, so they began to seek information. In the 1980s and 1990s, attendance of childbirth education was the norm, with over 70% of women taking some form of education. As epidural use has increased, however, many women feel childbirth education is not essential. In the most recent Listening to Mother's survey, only 34% of

THE NATURAL BIRTH PLAN

all women surveyed reported attending classes, though 59% of first-time mothers did receive formal education. Women today receive information regarding childbirth from a variety of sources, including online articles, videos, and books and only 10% of women indicated that their childbirth preparation class was the most informative source of education regarding labor and labor pain management.[34]

The true efficacy of childbirth education in achieving a natural birth is difficult to determine, given that education does not occur in a vacuum, independent of other factors that influence the childbirth process. The hospital where a woman delivers, her care provider's attitude toward natural birth and management practices, and the actual events of the woman's pregnancy and labor dramatically affect how she can apply her childbirth education. There are no well-designed studies that show whether education is associated with more natural births or decreases the likelihood of other medical interventions and there are no studies comparing the various forms of childbirth education to one another. This can make it difficult for expectant mothers planning a natural birth to decide on the "best method" of preparation and creates a challenge for hospitals and providers hoping to provide resources for mothers wanting to naturally birth. It is certainly an area that demands further research. However, some of the benefits of childbirth education that have been demonstrated include better communication between partners, improved confidence regarding the childbirth process, and a greater feeling of relaxation.[35]

There are many types of childbirth education available. Most hospital-provided classes are not geared toward natural birth per se, but offer information about the labor process, infant care, and specific practices at that particular hospital. Classes that are specifically designed to prepare patients for a natural birth are usually offered outside hospitals, provided by individuals who have been trained and credentialed by the organization representing the individual method. There is also an increasing tendency for individual birth workers, including doulas, lactation counselors, nurses, and prenatal yoga instructors, to design their own education classes for natural birth. There are many similarities between the methods. Nearly all advocate for a physiological process of labor and strongly advise against induction, epidurals, and other invasive interventions in the labor process. Generally all teach some form of breathing, relaxation, and positioning to cope with labor. However, it is useful for women to understand the ways in which the courses differ and the philosophy that informs the method in order to choose the approach that is most in line with their own philosophy and goals for her labor. It is also important for care providers to understand the method each woman has used to prepare for her labor so their care can complement that approach. For example, the Bradley Method encourages vocalization as a tool to work through contractions. If a woman's nurse or doctor was not familiar with this method, they might assume the woman was not managing her labor well and interfere with her process by encouraging her to labor quietly or take an epidural.

Lamaze Method

The Lamaze method is still the most widely recognized form of childbirth education, though it has gone through a number of reinventions over the years. It was introduced to the United States in the 1960s, when Marjorie Karmel and Elizabeth Bing founded the American Society for Psychoprophylaxis (ASPO), now known as Lamaze International, based on the work of French physician Dr. Fernand Lamaze. The method originally taught women a specific form of controlled breathing and conscious relaxation, with different patterns of breath being utilized at different points of the labor, but the most widely recognized and utilized breath was the shallow, rapid "he-he-ho-ho" breathing depicted in countless movies and TV shows. The breathing technique and tools like concentrating on a focal point sought to distract women from the discomfort of their contractions. Today, Lamaze takes a much broader approach to labor preparation, teaching women more comfort positions, massage techniques, and a less rigid breathing technique, similar to what is utilized in other methods of childbirth preparation. The breath now taught is termed conscious, controlled breathing which encourages women to use a deep, slow breath, either through the nose or mouth, without a specific number of breaths in any given time frame. They still encourage focusing on something, but now suggest this may be done with eyes closed or open, and they strongly support the use of labor balls, movement, and massage as other tools to cope with the labor process.[36] Most hospital birth classes are based on the Lamaze method, however, many still utilize the techniques in the older version of Lamaze.

The Bradley Method

The Bradley Method was started in 1947 by obstetrician gynecologist Dr. Robert Bradley and became more widespread after the publishing of his book, *Husband-Coached Childbirth*, in the 1960s. The method emphasizes deep and complete relaxation of the mother, using techniques such as deep abdominal breathing, maintenance of a dark labor environment of solitude, and closed eyes. Vocalization, when needed, is also encouraged. The other large premise of this Bradley Method is the preparation and utilization of supportive labor coach, usually the husband. Courses are typically taught in 12 installments and also focus on nutrition and the realities of labor in the hospital, including the risks of typical medical interventions. According to statistics published by the AAHCC, 86% of mothers who used the Bradley Method achieved a spontaneous, unmedicated vaginal birth, but it is unclear how this data was obtained and has not been studied in any independent trials.

HypnoBirthing: The Mongan Method

HypnoBirthing was developed in the late 1980s by Marie Mongan, based on her own childbirth experiences and the work of Dr. Grantly Dick-Read's *Childbirth Without Fear.* HypnoBirthing also emphasizes the importance of deep relaxation, but takes it a step further, teaching women the techniques of self-hypnosis, with deep breathing through the nose and into the belly, which attempts to maximize the inhalation and exhalation, as well as visualizations, and positive affirmations intended to break the fear-tension-pain cascade. The courses are typically taught over five sessions, with a home study practice component of breathing work and listening to the HypnoBirthing prescribed Rainbow Relaxation visualization for birth. The courses intentionally neglect extensive instruction about medical interventions, in an effort to not further their students concerns and fears about the birth process. The HypnoBirthing Institute conducted a survey of mothers who utilized their method from 2005 and 2010 and found that 70% of participants had an unmedicated birth and only 17% required a cesarean section, compared to the national rate of 32% during that same time interval. Two additional studies, though small in scale and not specifically using the HypnoBirthing curriculum, have been conducted examining self-hypnosis as a pain management tool in labor and found it to be moderately effective in decreasing the perception of labor pain, reducing the time spent in labor, and reducing the need for epidural and cesarean section. While more research could be done, at this time, HypnoBirthing has the most independent evidence in support of its methods. There have also been several spin-off classes based on Mongan curriculum, including HypnoBabies.

COMMON COMFORT POSITIONS

Ina Mae Gaskin, America's most famous midwife, has always taught that women need to be able to change their positions and move around freely during labor and much of the early discussions about laboring naturally and childbirth preparation advised walking rather than laboring in a supine position. As the number of resources for women desiring an unmedicated birth has expanded, more specific positioning for different labor patterns and discomfort is now suggested. There are multiple texts which touch on these positions, however, the most thorough by far is *The Labor Progress Handbook* (2011) by Penny Simkin, who began her career as a physical therapist and later founded DONA International, the largest organization involved in training and certifying doulas.[37] This section does not hope to reach the completeness of Simkin's text, but to provide a general guide to the most common positions that can be employed in a natural labor and what evidence, if any, supports their efficacy. Women planning a natural birth should practice these positions and feel comfortable moving in and out of them by the later weeks of pregnancy. Care providers should also be familiar with these positions in order to offer alternatives to a mother who may be struggling and help them get into a comfortable position. Sometimes a little variety is all a mother needs to emotionally and physically progress through a difficult point in her labor. In this way, doctors, nurses, and midwives have something to offer their patient besides medication. Positioning specifically for labor dystocia will be discussed separately.

Supported Swaying or Standing

This position is often humorously described by childbirth educators as bad junior high dancing, but there is something comforting about the idea of dancing through labor. In supported swaying, the laboring woman encircles her arms around her partner's neck and rests her head and chest against her partner's upper torso (Figure 6-1). The legs are kept wide apart, to maintain an open pelvis and aid in the descent of the baby. Generally the bottom is pushed out and hip swaying keeps the muscles loose. Figure of eight motions, in particular, facilitate a loose, open pelvis, though some women prefer to simply stand in between contractions, supported by their partner, and enter a small squat when the contractions occur. The assistance of the partner in this position is helpful from both a physical and emotional standpoint; however a raised bed or table can also be used for supported swaying or standing if a partner is unavailable or the woman feels more comfortable using a stable structure for support. The partner can also aid the laboring woman using a bed or table for support by massaging the lower back and sacrum.

Several studies have examined ambulatory and upright positioning in first-stage labor and, as previously discussed, walking and upright positioning are associated with less reported pain, lower rates of operative deliveries, labor augmentation, and cesarean delivery, and shorter

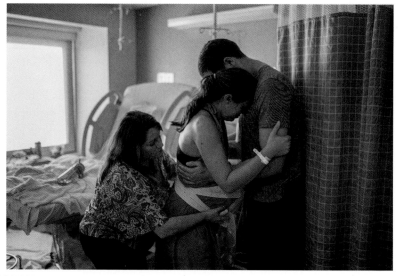

FIGURE 6-1. Supported swaying or standing.

durations of labor. Dancing, in particular, in active labor was shown to decrease pain levels and increase maternal satisfaction with labor in a small randomized control trial of 60 first-time mothers.[38]

Birth Ball Sitting

The birth ball, a large 65 cm inflatable ball, is a common tool used by naturally laboring women (Figure 6-2). When a woman's legs are tired, the birthing ball can be offered as a seat of comfort that most women prefer to hard chairs or the labor bed. As each contraction or surge begins, the laboring mother may roll the ball from side to side, the hip movement assisting in the baby's descent by helping to maintain loose muscles. When the surge ends, the mother may gently bounce, self-soothing and resting between the contractions. The mother may lean back, supported by a seated birth attendant or lean forward on a bed or the lap of her labor partner.

Recently, an interesting randomized control trial out of Taiwan demonstrated several benefits of ball use during pregnancy and labor. Women in the study were provided with an instructional book and video during pregnancy and instructed to exercise with the ball for 20 minutes three times weekly and then were provided with the ball throughout labor. They were questioned about their pain and had their labor progress tracked. Those who used the ball had a shorter first stage of labor,

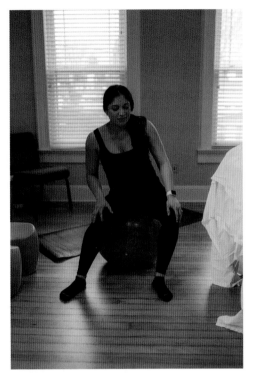

FIGURE 6-2. Ball sitting, bouncing, and circling.

reported less pain and utilized fewer epidurals, and had a lower incidence of cesarean section.[39] While this study was small in scope, it shows the promise of this inexpensive and easily utilized tool in labor.

Birthing Stool Sitting

Birthing stools, a three- or four-legged chair that supports the bottom of the laboring mother and is typically low enough to the ground to permit the woman to brace her feet on the ground for pushing leverage and stabilization, have been in use for a millennia (Figure 6-3). They were designed with an opening in front which permitted the birth attendant to access the birth canal and were intended to be sat upon in a wide-legged position, maintaining an open pelvis for delivery. They have been depicted on the walls in birthing houses of ancient Egypt and in ancient Greek art and are even mentioned in the Old Testament. In the sixteenth century, woodcut chairs became widespread and went through several modifications in the centuries that followed. They were replaced by

THE NATURAL BIRTH PLAN

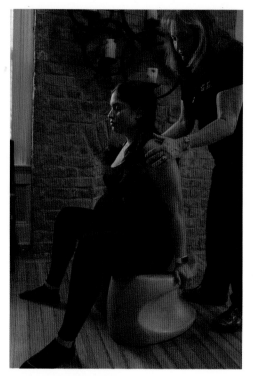

FIGURE 6-3. Birth stool or toilet sitting.

birthing beds as birth moved into the hospital in order to better position patients for forceps delivery.[40]

While intended to support the mother during the actual time of pushing and delivery, birthing stools can also be helpful in the first stage of labor, prior to full dilation. The act of sitting on an open and lower placed stool or toilet can assist a laboring mother in naturally relaxing the perineum and pelvic floor, as we are so conditioned to do while sitting on the toilet. The action is fairly instinctual. Naturally laboring mothers often have sensations of intense rectal pressure prior to full dilation, usually starting at around 7 cm dilation, which can be disconcerting for the mother and nursing staff. Many women feel more comfortable in a position and location where that sensation is "normal" and "safe," as generally people do not like to feel like they do not have control over the bowels in bed or walking down the hall. Hospital staff, however, are often fearful that a laboring woman will accidently push and deliver the baby in the toilet, so the birthing stool can be a nice alternative to the toilet in that situation. However, if a woman feels more comfortable on the toilet,

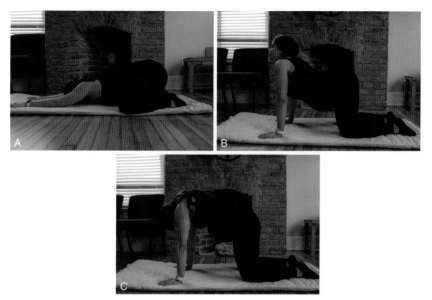

FIGURE 6-4. A little yoga in labor: (A) modified child's pose, (B) cow, and (C) cat for hand-and-knees positioning.

she should not be prohibited from laboring there. She should simply be monitored more closely for signs of being ready to deliver.

Hands-and-Knees

Hands-and-knees positioning has many benefits (Figure 6-4A–C). It helps stretch the lower back, opens the pelvis, and shifts the forces of gravity, which is theorized to assist in rotation of the descending fetal head. Simple hands and knees can be used with or without hip swaying as a comfort tool in labor or the yoga techniques of child's pose, cow, and cat may be added for additional stretching and comfort. In the cow position, the mother drops the belly down, while arching the head and neck up. The cat position is simply the opposite, the back and belly are arched up, like an angry cat, while the head and neck are dropped down. In the modified child's pose, the upper body is brought almost to the floor, with the arms outstretched, and the legs are opened wide, with the hips and knees flexed in a squatting fashion. Many women on hands and knees will instinctively drop down into this position during a contraction and sometimes sway or bounce. Labor partners can easily massage the lower back when the mother is in any of the hands-and-knees positions and all hands-and-knees positions can be done easily on a yoga mat or blanket on the floor or within the labor bed. Only a few studies have examined hands-and-knees specifically, however those that did found it was effective at relieving lower back pain and may aid in the rotation of malpositioned babies.[41-43]

Supported Squatting

Many women find squatting to be both instinctive and helpful during the labor process, however it can be difficult to balance and maintain the position free standing. Using the assistance of a labor partner, handrail, squat bar, labor ball, bed, or hanging ropes can help to both stabilize the mother and relieve fatigue (Figure 6-5). A partner can assist from behind, either sitting and allowing the mother to support her weight on her partner's thighs or standing and holding the mother under the arms, allowing the mother to grasp her partner's forearms. From the front, the partner can assist by holding the mother's hands for stabilization. When objects are used for stabilization, the mother can either hang from the objects or lean over the objects. Squatting helps open the pelvis and relax the muscles of the perineum and allows women to "lean into" any pressure sensations they may be feeling. In one small study specifically looking at squatting, women using the position in labor reported less pain when compared to simple sitting and another larger study showed a lower epidural rate and need for pitocin among patients who utilized squatting.[44,45]

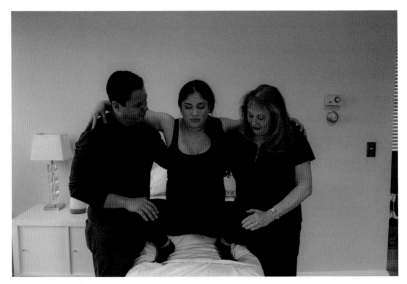

FIGURE 6-5. Supported squat.

Side-lying

While upright positions are favorable for labor, nearly all women will want and need to lay down and rest at some point in their labor. Few women find lying on their back to be comfortable or even acceptable during an unmedicated birth. Side-lying positions allow the mother to rest with less discomfort and can even aid in fetal rotation and descent (Figure 6-6). Side-lying mothers should always keep something between the legs to take pressure off the hip. Usually a pillow will suffice, though significantly raising the top leg, especially with the aid of a peanut ball as will be discussed later, can speed up the later stages of labor or help with a prolonged labor or malpositioned baby. Both knees may be bent, but assuming more of a lunge position, with the bottom leg straight and the upper leg bent at both the knee and the hip opens the pelvis to a greater degree and may be more effective. Partners can easily massage the back with the mother in this position and it is a good position if the mother requires any period of fetal monitoring. Studies have shown that women increasingly gravitate toward recumbent positions in the later stages of labor and find side-lying to be more comfortable than either sitting or lying flat on the back. Side-lying also was shown to generate more effective contractions in later labor.[46–48]

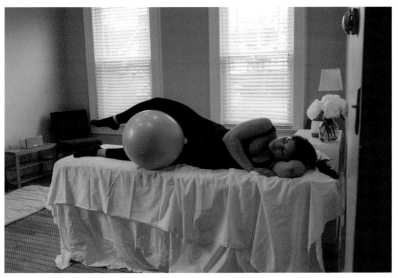

FIGURE 6-6. Side-lying.

THE NATURAL BIRTH PLAN

REFERENCES

1. Osterman MJK, Martin JA. Epidural and spinal anesthesia use during labor: 27-state reporting area, 2008. National Vital Statistics Reports, vol 59, no 5. Hyattsville, MD: National Center for Health Statistics; 2011.
2. Silva M, Halpern SH. Epidural analgesia for labor: current techniques. *Local Reg Anesth*. 2010;3:143-153. doi:10.2147/LRA.S10237.
3. Anim-Somuah M, Smyth RM, Jones L. Epidural versus non-epidural or no analgesia in labour. *Cochrane Database Syst Rev*. 2011;12(CD000331):1-127. doi:10.1002/14651858.CD000331.pub3.
4. Goer H. Epidurals: do they or don't they increase cesareans? Available at https://www.scienceandsensibility.org/p/bl/et/blogid=2&blogaid=749. Accessed January 26, 2015.
5. Greenwell EA, Wyshak G, Ringer SA, et al. Intrapartum temperature elevation, epidural use, and adverse outcome in term infants. *Pediatrics*. 2012;129(2):2010-2301.
6. Scott S. Labor epidural analgesia and maternal fever. *Anesth Analg*. 2010;111(6):1467-1475.
7. Choi PT, Galinski SE, Takeuchi L, et al. PDPH is a common complication of neuraxial blockade in parturients: a meta-analysis of obstetrical studies. *Can J Anaesth*. 2003;50(1):460-469.
8. Wong CA, Scavone BM, Dugan S, et al. Incidence of postpartum lumbosacral spine and lower extremity nerve injuries. *Obstet Gynecol*. 2003;101(1):279-288.
9. Cook TM, Counsell D, Wildsmith JA. Major complications of central neuraxial block: report on the Third National Audit Project of the Royal College of Anaesthetists. *Br J Anaesth*. 2009;102(1):179-190.
10. Chestnut DH, Wong CA, Tsen LC, et al. *Chestnut's Obstetric Anesthesia: Principles and Practice*. Philadelphia, PA: Elsevier; 2014.
11. Halpern SH, Levine T, Wilson DB, et al. Effect of labor analgesia on breastfeeding success. *Birth*. 1999;26(2):83-88.
12. Albani A, Addamo P, Renghi A, et al. The effect of breastfeeding rate of regional anesthesia technique for cesarean and vaginal childbirth. *Minerva Anestesiol*. 1999;65(9):625-630.
13. Beilin Y, Bodian CA, Weiser J, et al. Effect of labor epidural analgesia with and without fentanyl on infant breast-feeding: a prospective, randomized, double-blind study. *Anesthesiology*. 2005;103(6):1211-1217.
14. Wilson MJ, MacArthur C, Cooper GM, Bick D, Moore PA, Shennan A; COMET Study Group UK. Epidural analgesia and breastfeeding: a randomised controlled trial of epidural techniques with and without fentanyl and a non-epidural comparison group. *Anaesthesia*. 2010;65(2):145-153.
15. Akbas M, Akcan AB. Epidural analgesia and lactation. *Eurasian J Med*. 2011;43(1):45-49. doi:10.5152/eajm.2011.09.
16. Wang SM. Backaches related to pregnancy: the risk factors, etiologies, treatments and controversial issues. *Curr Opin Anaesthesiol*. 2003;16(3):269-273.
17. MacArthur C, Lewis M, Knox EG, Crawford JS. Epidural anaesthesia and long term backache after childbirth. *Br Med J*. 1990;301(6742):9-12.
18. Thorp JA, Parisi VM, Boylan PC, Johnston DA. The effect of continuous epidural analgesia on cesarean section for dystocia in nulliparous women. *Am J Obstet Gynecol*. 1989 Sep;161(3):670-5.

19. Klein MC, Grzybowski S, Harris S, et al. Epidural analgesia use as a marker for physician approach to birth: implications for maternal and newborn outcomes. *Birth.* 2001;28(4):243-248.

20. Bannister-Tyrrell M, Ford JB, Morris JM, Roberts CL. Epidural analgesia in labour and risk of caesarean delivery. *Paediatr Perinat Epidemiol.* 2014;28(5):400-411. doi:10.1111/ppe.12139.

21. Eriksen LM, Nohr EA, Kjaergaard H. Mode of delivery after epidural analgesia in a cohort of low-risk nulliparas. *Birth.* 2011;38(4):317-326. doi:10.1111/j.1523-536X.2011.00486.x.

22. Lieberman E, Lang JM, Cohen A, et al. Association of epidural analgesia with cesarean delivery in nulliparas. *Obstet Gynecol.* 1996;88(6):993-1000.

23. Kjærgaard H, Olsen J, Ottesen B, et al. Obstetric risk indicators for labour dystocia in nulliparous women: a multi-centre cohort study. *BMC Pregnancy Childbirth.* 2008;8:45. doi:10.1186/1471-2393-8-45.

24. Klein MC. Does epidural analgesia increase rate of cesarean section? *Can Fam Physician.* 2006;52(4):419-421.

25. Sng BL, Leong WL, Zeng Y, et al. Early versus late initiation of epidural analgesia for labour. *Cochrane Database Syst Rev.* 2014;10(CD00723):1-80. doi:10.1002/14651858.CD007238.pub2.

26. Goer H. Epidural anesthesia: to delay or not to delay, that is the question. Available at https://www.scienceandsensibility.org/blog/epidural-analgesia-to-delay-or-not-to-delay,-that-is-the-question. Accessed October 22, 2014.

27. Plough AC, Galvin G, Li Z, et al. Relationship between labor and delivery unit management practices and maternal outcomes. *Obstet Gynecol.* 2017;130(2):358-365. doi:10.1097/AOG.0000000000002128.

28. Cefalo RC, Andre U, Hellgers E. The effects of maternal hyperthermia on maternal and fetal cardiovascular and respiratory function. *Am J Obstet Gynecol.* 1978;131(6):687-694.

29. Cluett ER, Pickering RM, Getliffe K, Saunders NJSG. Randomised controlled trial of labouring in water compared with standard of augmentation for management of dystocia in first stage of labour. *BMJ.* 2004;328(7435):314. doi:10.1136/bmj.37963.606412.EE.

30. Cluett ER, Burns E. Immersion in water in labour and birth. *Cochrane Database Syst Rev.* 2009;(2):CD000111. Advance online publication. doi:10.1002/14651858.CD000111.pub3.

31. Siegel P. Does bath water enter the vagina? *Obstet Gynecol.* 1960;15:660-661.

32. Eriksson M, Ladfors L, Mattsson LA, Fall O. Warm tub bath during labor. A study of 1385 women with prelabor rupture of the membranes after 34 weeks of gestation. *Acta Obstet Gynecol Scand.* 1996;75(7):642-644.

33. American College of Obstetrician and Gynecologists. Immersion in water during labor and delivery. Committee Opinion No. 679. *Obstet Gynecol.* 2016;128(5): e231–e236. Available at https://www.acog.org/Resources-And-Publications/Committee-Opinions/Committee-on-Obstetric-Practice/Immersion-in-Water-During-Labor-and-Delivery. Accessed 5/2017

34. Declercq ER, Sakala C, Corry MP, Applebaum S, Herrlich A. *Listening to Mothers III: New Mothers Speak Out.* New York, NY: Childbirth Connection; 2013.

35. Koehn ML. Childbirth education outcomes: an integrative review of the literature. *J Perinat Educ.* 2002;11(3):10-19. doi:10.1624/105812402X88795.

THE NATURAL BIRTH PLAN

36. Lothian JA. Lamaze breathing: what every pregnant woman needs to know. *J Perinat Educ.* 2011;20(2):118-120. doi:10.1891/1058-1243.20.2.118.
37. Simkin P, Ancheta R. *The Labor Progress Handbook.* Ames, IA: Wiley-Blackwell; 2011.
38. Abdolahian S, Ghavi F, Abdollahifard S, Sheikhan F. Effect of dance labor on the management of active phase labor pain and clients' satisfaction: a randomized controlled trial study. *Glob J Health Sci.* 2014;6(3):219-226. doi:10.5539/gjhs.v6n3p219.
39. Gau ML, Change CY, Tian SH, Lin KC. Effects of birth ball exercise on pain and self-efficacy during childbirth: a randomised controlled trial in Taiwan. *Midwifery.* 2011;27(6):293-300.
40. Fee E, Brown TM, Beatty RL. Early modern childbirth. *Am J Public Health.* 2003;93(3):432.
41. Stremler R, Hodnett E, Petryshen P, et al. Randomized controlled trial of hands-and-knees positioning for occipitoposterior position in labor. *Birth.* 2005;32(4):243-251.
42. Andrews CM, Andrews EC. Nursing, maternal postures, and fetal position. *Nurs Res.* 1983;32(6):336-341.
43. Guittier MJ, Othenin-Girard V, de Gasquet B, et al. Maternal positioning to correct occiput posterior fetal position during the first stage of labour: a randomised controlled trial. *BJOG.* 2016;123(13):2199-2207. doi:10.1111/1471-0528.13855.
44. Valiani M, Rezaie M, Shahshahan Z. Comparative study on the influence of three delivery positions on pain intensity during the second stage of labor. *Iran J Nurs Midwifery Res.* July-August 2016;21(4):372-378. doi:10.4103/1735-9066.185578.
45. Bodner-Adler B, Bodner K, Kimberger O, Lozanov P, Husslein P, Mayerhofer K. Women's position during labour: influence on maternal and neonatal outcome. *Wien Klin Wochenschr.* October 31, 2003;115(19-20):720-723.
46. Reid AJ, Harris NL. Alternative birth positions. *Can Fam Physician.* 1988;34:1993-1998.
47. Roberts J, Malasanos L, Mendez-Bauer C. Maternal positions in labor: analysis in relation to comfort and efficiency. *Birth Defects Orig Artic Ser.* 1981;17(6):97-128.
48. Lawrence A, Lewis L, Hofmeyr GJ, Styles C. Maternal positions and mobility during first stage labour. *Cochrane Database Syst Rev.* 2013;10(CD003934):1-164. doi:10.1002/14651858.CD003934.pub4.

Delivery

CHAPTER 7

I want to birth my baby in the position that is most comfortable for me

I was really happy with my birth experience overall. I had a doula and a birth plan and the hospital staff was really supportive, but when the time came to push, they wanted me to lay on my back to deliver, which went against everything my body was telling me. Hands and knees had been the most comfortable position for me throughout the labor and I really did not want to turn around, but my doctor had never delivered a baby in that position and didn't feel like it was safe.

—D. H., new mother

The most common positions for delivery remain dorsal lithotomy (68% of vaginal deliveries) and semi-seated (23% of vaginal deliveries).[1] In the dorsal lithotomy position, the delivering woman is flat on the back with the legs widely spread, flexed at the knee and the hip, and raised with the help of labor assistants or stirrups. The semi-seated position is similar to dorsal lithotomy, except the head of the bed is raised approximately 45 degrees and legs are often not as elevated (Figure 7-1).

There are several reasons the majority of women deliver in these position, the first being that the majority of women have epidurals which simply limit their ability to deliver in alternative positions, as they are immobilized from the waist down. Second, due to this overwhelming percentage of women delivering with epidurals and the history of obstetrics that saw the majority of deliveries occurring with the aid of forceps, which necessitated a dorsal lithotomy position, most obstetricians are exclusively taught to deliver babies in a supine position and are only comfortable delivering in this manner. There is also a commonly

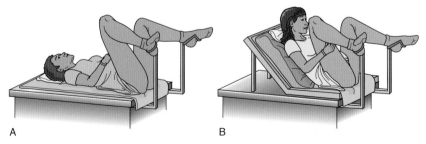

A   B

FIGURE 7-1. The most common positions for delivery remains. (A) dorsal lithotomy (68% of vaginal deliveries) and **(B)** semi-seated (23% of vaginal deliveries).

expressed concern among obstetricians that if a complication arose, such as a shoulder dystocia or an umbilical cord around the neck, it could not be easily remedied in an alternative position. Finally, supine positions for delivery facilitate continuous electronic fetal monitoring.

Unfortunately, supine positions have been shown to have several disadvantages and there are benefits associated with alternative positions, such as side-lying, squatting, and hands-and-knees positioning. There is a higher incidence of vaginal lacerations, including severe tears that injure the anal sphincter, and episiotomies in patients in lithotomy positions. Lateral, or side-lying, positions have been shown to have a decreased rate of perineal lacerations and squatting and up-right positions for delivery have been shown to shorten the second stage of labor, especially with the aid of a birth stool.[2–4] Less fetal heart rate changes have also been noted with alternative positions, which rotate the baby off the large vessels of the pelvis, maximizing blood flow to the baby. A large, randomized trial in China demonstrated a lower incidence of lacerations and episiotomies with hands-and-knees positioning as well, without any negative associations besides a longer second stage of labor, and other studies have shown less discomfort in this position as well.[5] The research to date is not considered sufficient to recommend one particular delivery position, but does demonstrate that alternative positions can be every bit as safe and efficacious as supine positions and should be used much more routinely.

The ability for women to participate in decision making regarding pushing positions is also beneficial. Women who feel they have influence on their birthing position are more likely to feel they have control over their birth experience and report a positive birth experience.[6] Doctors and midwives can best assist women in pushing by using a shared decision-making model. In this model, the provider offers instruction regarding how to best push in various positions and feedback about how each position is working, while empathetically listening and responding to how each position is feeling for the laboring mother.[7] In most natural labors, the mother and her provider will not simply choose one consistent position throughout the pushing phase, but rather alternate between them depending on the effectiveness of the pushing, the mother's comfort, and the mother's fatigue level. Flexibility and openness to trying different things or returning to a previous position are essential in helping a mother through an unmedicated second stage. Patience and positive verbal feedback are also incredibly important to help the mother psychologically through what can be a hard and frustrating process.

THE NATURAL BIRTH PLAN

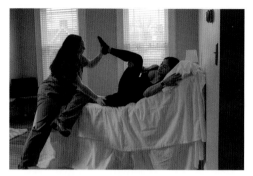

FIGURE 7-2. Alternative pushing positions: lateral or side-lying.

Side-Lying or Lateral

In the side-lying or lateral position, the mother lies on the side of her preference, bending both knees and bringing them toward her chest (Figure 7-2). During contractions, the outside leg is relaxed outwards and flexed at the hip as the mother pulls back on it by reaching under the thigh with one or both hands. This position tends to be more comfortable than supine positions, especially for mothers with malpositioned babies, and is associated with less perineal tearing. This position can also be a good option for mothers who are too fatigued to support their body weight in either an upright or hands-and-knees position. It can be combined with a pulling technique, by placing a squat bar on the bed and securing a towel or sheet to it, which the mother can then pull on during pushing while bracing her outer foot on the bar or having it held by an attendant. If delivery is performed in this position, the same maneuvers used in a supine delivery are utilized, however at a diagonal angle in keeping with the direction of the maternal pelvis. The doctor or midwife would usually deliver from the side of the bed, rather than the foot of the bed, on the same side as the outer leg.

Squatting

Many women find squatting to be an instinctual position for pushing. In this position, the legs are opened wide, with knees bent and hips fully flexed, while the weight of the woman is supported on flat feet (Figure 7-3). Most women feel the need to lean over on something to balance in this position, and a squat bar, a partner, a raised bed, or the raised back of the bed, with the woman facing inwards rather than the standard outwards, can all be utilized for this support. Squatting assists in opening the pelvis and bringing the baby to a lower station; however, it can be tiring to

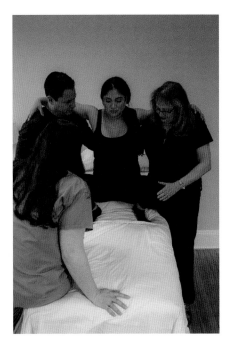

FIGURE 7-3. Squatting.

maintain for long periods of time.[8] Birthing tubs facilitate women birthing in this position due to the buoyancy of the water. Supported squatting, in which the woman is held by birth attendants on either side or within the lap of a partner, can also make the position less fatiguing. If the woman is delivering in this position, delivery can be performed either from the front, using standard delivery maneuvers, or the back, using the same maneuvers utilized in the hands-and-knees delivery, depending on which side is more easily accessible. If the woman is using a labor bed, the foot portion of the bed can be lowered to facilitate delivery. If the woman is squatting outside of the bed, the doctor or midwife can usually most easily deliver simply by sitting on the floor. Some studies have demonstrated a higher rate of tearing when mothers who have had a previous vaginal delivery utilize this position for the actual delivery, likely due to a more rapid descent and crowning of the fetal head and the direction of force on the perineum.[2]

Birth Stool

There are several types of birth stools and they provide for a supported squatting position for delivery, opening the pelvis and facilitating decent. The woman sits wide legged on the stool, either leaning back on her partner for support, grasping the back of the stool for pushing leverage, or

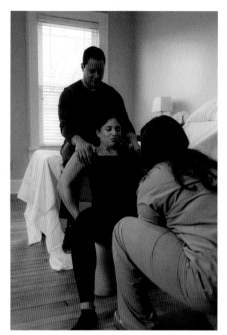

FIGURE 7-4. Birth stool.

curling forward, grasping the front of the stool or the back of her thighs for leverage (Figure 7-4). Both birth stool positions are efficacious and the woman should be encouraged to do what feels best to her. Delivery on a birth stool is less technically challenging for the doctor or midwife than a squatting position, due to the raised position of the mother and the cut out in the stool for the delivering the baby's head; however, most stools are still low enough to allow the woman to secure her feet on the ground, still requiring the practitioner to deliver kneeling or sitting on the floor. The maneuvers for a birth stool delivery are no different than in a supine delivery.

Hands-and-knees

Hands-and-knees positioning is another common position women assume when they are not guided to any specific pushing position.[9] Women using this position may assume a straight back position, with the arms straight and the hips unflexed, or they may assume more of a child's pose positioning, where the hips are flexed and the upper body is supported (Figure 7-5). Modern labor beds can easily assist women in assuming this later positioning, either by bringing the lower third section of the bed completely down

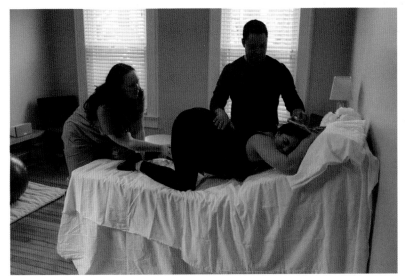

FIGURE 7-5. Hands-and-knees.

and allowing the woman to kneel on this portion facing inwards, while completely resting her upper body on the middle section of the bed, or completely raising the head of the bed, which the woman can lean over or hang from while kneeling on the middle portion facing inwards. Women report that hands-and-knees positioning is more comfortable, particularly with malpositioned babies, and possibly makes for more effective pushing and even rotation of the fetal head in women with babies in less ideal positions.[10] While studies have not demonstrated that this translates into lower rates of cesarean, the studies examining this have been plagued by small numbers and high rates of epidural, thus limiting their ability to effectively evaluate the benefits of this position for naturally laboring women.

When delivery is performed in this position, the provider must utilize a slightly different set of maneuvers. Delivery is most easily performed with the provider in a seated position behind the woman, with the entire bed raised so the woman is at the provider's arm level. Continuous fetal heart rate monitoring is challenging in this position but intermittent auscultation of the fetal heart is easily performed by the provider from underneath. It is not uncommon to feel a small anterior lip of cervix when the woman is in the hands-and-knees position, but if the woman has a strong urge to push, she most often will easily push the baby's head past this lip in one to two pushes and should not be discouraged from trying to do so. During crowning, the baby's head should be supported with an open palmed hand and attempts to stretch or support the perineum are unnecessary, as gravity is pulling the weight of the baby away from the perineum. Encouraging the woman to blow out during crowning can also help control the delivery, as often gravity can lead to a precipitous crowning process in this position. Once the head is delivered, the delivery maneuvers are then done backwards, first gently pulling up and delivering what is now the bottom shoulder (which is the traditional anterior shoulder beneath the pubic symphysis) and then gently pulling down to deliver the top shoulder (which is the traditional posterior shoulder).

Delivery complications can also be managed effectively from this position and fear of this need not be a reason to restrict a woman from birthing on all fours if she prefers it. In the event of a nuchal cord, one may simply attempt to reduce it; however, if gentle traction is applied to the cord, creating a bit of slack, most often the baby can easily be delivered through the cord, as a lesser degree of cord tension is observed on hands and knees than in the supine position. Doctors also frequently express concern about how a shoulder dystocia could be managed on hands and knees; however, much of that concern is probably unwarranted. For one, the patient only needs to completely squat down, completely flexing the hips, to achieve the standard McRobert's positioning and internal or external rotation is easily achieved in this position, as there is more often more room and flexibility when the mother is on hands and knees. The posterior shoulder is also more easily delivered, as it is on the top in this delivery position. Finally, hands-and-knees positioning, in and of itself, is also a known technique for relieving a shoulder dystocia, so while not shown in the evidence to date, it can be surmised that the incidence of shoulder dystocia in hands-and-knees deliveries may be significantly less than that observed in supine positions and, if a shoulder is unable to be reduced, the woman can simply be turned to a supine position for additional maneuvers.[11]

Pulling during Pushing

Hanging or pulling to create counter force during pushing was common in many cultures for generations.[12] Most often, a rope was tied to a tree or large pole and the mother would hang or pull against it. This motion can easily be recreated in modern maternity units with the aid of modern labor beds and a simple long sheet. The bed is put into an upright, seating position and the woman secures her feat against either the small lower handrails or the foot rests while she and an assistant engage in a game of tug-of-war with a sheet (Figure 7-6). The sheet is

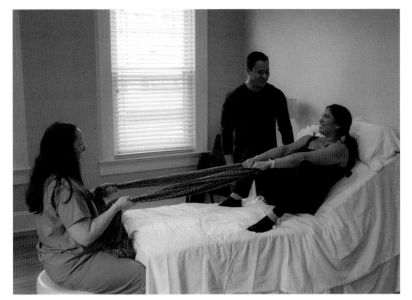

FIGURE 7-6. Tug-of-war.

generally folded in half and the woman holds the "U" side of the sheet, while the assistant holds the two ends of the sheet in each hand, leaning back and pulling with their body weight. Alternatively, the sheet can be secured to the squat bar or the back of the bed for the woman to pull against or hang from. Breathing techniques are still utilized during pushing with this method and generally the lower back of the woman rests against the bed, while the pelvis is slightly tilted forward. This technique can be helpful for women who are having a challenging time coordinating pushing efforts or who find they are "pushing in their face," as it helps the woman engage the abdominal muscles more effectively. It can even be a very helpful technique in women with epidural anesthesia.

Standing

Standing positions require little description and are also commonly utilized by women who are pushing in the position most comfortable for them. Most often, laboring women will want something to lean over, such as a bed, table, or partner and assume a wide-legged stance, often with some degree of hip flexion, similar to the squat position (Figure 7-7). Delivery is most easily facilitated from behind, using the open palm to

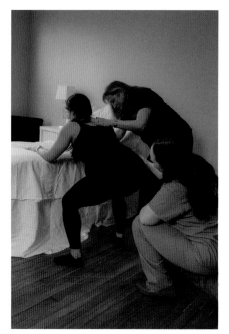

FIGURE 7-7. Standing.

support the head during crowning and control the delivery of the baby's head, followed by the same "backward" maneuvers used in hands-and-knees deliveries.

I would like to use self-directed pushing, as opposed to coached pushing

I had envisioned a calm, peaceful birth when I was pregnant with my first child. I had practiced hypnobirthing and spent a lot of time imagining that moment. I even had a specific set of music that I was planning on playing while my daughter was born. When I got to fully dilated and was ready to push, my nurse and another nurse came in and lifted my legs up. They told me to curl around my baby, hold my breath, and push for ten seconds. One of them started counting each push for me, really loudly, while the other kept saying "Push, harder, harder, harder." It was really stressful. I felt like a football coach had entered my lovely little birth room and was now screaming at me. I think it freaked my husband out too because he never even remembered to turn on my music.

—Y. N., new mother

Typically, maternal pushing is a physician- and nursing-led effort. In the most standard form of pushing, the valsalva or directed pushing technique, the laboring mother is encouraged to fill her lungs with a large breath of air, hold this breath, and bear down into her bottom for a count of 10. This effort is typically repeated three times per contraction, with each push in close succession to the last. In an alternative, spontaneous pushing, the laboring mother follows her own instincts and typically pushes three to five times per contraction. A third alternative, only studied in women with epidurals, valsalva pushing is delayed until the mother has a strong urge to push or the fetal head is on the perineum.

All of the evidence to date which compared directed to spontaneous pushing is of limited quality; however, several disadvantages to the valsalva technique have been documented. A significant decrease in fetal cerebral oxygenation has been observed, as well as lower umbilical cord pHs indicative of poor oxygenation and resultant fetal heart rate abnormalities.[13–15] In comparison, spontaneous, mother-led pushing has been associated with higher umbilical cord pHs and higher neonatal APGAR scores.[16] Maternal concerns regarding valsalva pushing include increased levels of fatigue, as well as pelvic floor damage and resultant bladder control issues. The only benefit that has been demonstrated with the traditional pushing method is a slightly shorter duration of the second stage, as compared to both spontaneous pushing and delayed pushing. However, when the bulk of the evidence is considered, it is not sufficient to recommend one form of pushing over another and, given the possible disadvantages of directed valsalva pushing, current wisdom would support allowing the laboring mother to push using the technique of her preference.[17] A woman having difficulty coordinating pushing may be guided to an alternative technique or simply given more time to labor down and develop a stronger instinct to push. Maternal wishes for a quiet, noncoached pushing stage should be respected, as cheerleading and coaching offer no documented benefit to either mother or baby, only perhaps an outlet for the provider's impatience.

I do not want an episiotomy

When I had my son, I had a nice doctor, but in the end she cut an episiotomy without really asking. She just said, "I need to make a little room here." My recovery was really rough. I sat on that stupid balloon pillow for weeks and peeing was torture. When I became pregnant with my second child, episiotomy was my number one concern. In my first visit, I told the doctor I did not want an episiotomy. I put evening primrose oil on my perineum and made my husband do the whole massage thing for weeks before I delivered. I told him if the doctor even made a move towards those scissors, he had to stop him. I think I must have said a hundred times during my labor, "Don't cut me!" My poor doctor was really reassuring and kept telling me that he had no plans to do an episiotomy. If he truly felt like one was needed, he would only do it with my permission. I tore only a little bit and had a much better recovery the second time around.

—C. W., new mother

The majority of women delivering vaginally have some degree of vaginal tearing. Tears are classified by degree, first degree to fourth degree, according to what structures they involve. Mild tears, first and second degree, involve only the vaginal mucosa or the vaginal mucosa and underlying muscles that support the perineum. Severe tears, third- and fourth-degree tears, extend further into the muscle that controls the anal sphincter or even into the anus and rectum itself. Severe tearing can lead to persistent pelvic pain, pain with intercourse, and flatulence and stool incontinence. All tearing is sutured at the time of delivery and typically require 1 to 2 weeks to heal, or longer in the case of more severe tearing. For mothers without epidurals, local injections of lidocaine are utilized for pain relief during any needed repair.

Episiotomies were introduced to the United States by Dr. Joseph DeLee in the early twentieth century as a means to shorten the second stage of labor, prevent severe perineal injury, and promote better healing, as it was hypothesized that a clean surgical cut of the perineum could be more easily repaired and heal better than an irregular tear.[18] By 1980, episiotomies were the most commonly performed obstetrical surgery, performed in 63% of births. However, there was a growing opposition to the practice, with many women feeling traumatized by the procedure, and this was expressed vocally by critics such as Sheila Kitzinger and Penny Simkin. Over the following two decades, scientific evidence against routine episiotomies mounted.[19] In the most recent *Cochrane Review* of 12 different studies, including over 12,000 women, which compared routine episiotomy to selective episiotomy, where an episiotomy is performed only for a prolonged second stage, concern for a significant tear, and/or fetal distress, routine episiotomy was found to actually be associated with more severe perineal lacerations, the very thing it was meant to avoid.[20] Furthermore, there were no benefits of routine episiotomy identified in this review to justify the higher risk of third- and fourth-degree perineal lacerations associated with episiotomies.

Newer research is even calling into question whether episiotomies should ever be performed for anything other than fetal distress and the initial study, while small in sample size, failed to demonstrate the benefit of even selective episiotomy.[21] The American College of Obstetrics and Gynecology has also issued a recent practice guideline that discourages routine episiotomy, as a means to prevent obstetric lacerations.[22]

While episiotomy rates have been decreasing steadily in response to this evidence and strong expert recommendations, it is still a common procedure. According to a recent cohort of over 2 million women who delivered in 500 different hospitals between 2006 and 2012, 15% of women received an episiotomy, though significant variation between hospitals was observed, with some institutions reporting rates as high as 34%, while others reported rates as low as 2%.[23] Few women want an episiotomy and, even more disturbingly, when they are performed, half of women surveyed indicated that they did not feel they were given a choice regarding the procedure.[1] The issue of unconsented and forced episiotomies gained national attention when a video of Kimberly Turbin's birth was made public, which clearly demonstrated an episiotomy being performed, not only without her consent, but with her explicit instruction against it. A suit alleging assault and battery was filed against her physician.[24]

An episiotomy is not just "making a little room." An episiotomy is a surgical procedure and consent for the procedure should be no less specifically and formally obtained than for any other surgery, including a thorough description of the procedure, its indications and alternatives, as well as risks and benefits. No woman should ever need to fear that an episiotomy will be performed without her being aware of it and agreeing to it. This should not even need to be included in a birth plan and the fact that it is included in so many is a testament to how much work doctors and hospitals have to do in order to regain women's trust.

I want delayed cord clamping

Since the 1950s, the routine practice in the United States was to cut the umbilical cord immediately after birth, usually within 15 to 20 seconds. There were several reasons for this practice. First, during this time period, mothers were often highly anesthetized for delivery, which resulted in possible respiratory depression in their newborns and the need for immediate resuscitation. Studies in that time period had also demonstrated that up to 90% of placental blood transfer was achieved during the first moments of delivery, so there was no need to wait to cut the umbilical cord from the standpoint of neonatal blood volume. Finally, there was concern that late clamping could increase neonatal blood counts to such a degree as to put the baby at an increased risk for newborn jaundice.[25]

In recent years, however, new research has demonstrated that a delay in umbilical cord clamping for at least 30 to 60 seconds and up to 5 minutes after birth has several benefits. Neonates demonstrate higher hemoglobin concentrations at birth and are less likely to be diagnosed with iron deficiency anemia in the first year of life when delayed clamping is performed. This is because up to 100 mL of neonatal blood is contained in the cord and placenta at the time of birth, which can represent up to a third of the total blood volume of a full-term infant. Delaying the cord clamping up to a minute allows nearly 80% of this blood volume to return to the infant, while delaying up to 3 minutes allows nearly all the blood volume to return.[26] Another benefit of delayed clamping that has not been studied is a promotion of immediate skin-to-skin contact, as the baby is simply brought to the mother's abdomen while the cord pulsates and she can immediately begin bonding with her child. This assists with the initiation of breastfeeding and respects the sanctity of the first moment between mother and child.

The research has failed to demonstrate any negative outcomes associated with delayed clamping. Rates of maternal blood loss and prolonged delivery of the placenta are the same regardless of umbilical cord clamping timing. In neonates, there was no demonstrable difference in Apgar scores, incidence of respiratory distress, NICU admissions, or polycythemia. The only difference was in the rate of jaundice requiring phototherapy, which was shown to be higher in the neonates with delayed clamping; however, only 2% higher when compared to immediate clamping.[27] One of the other concerns about delayed clamping is that it may delay needed neonatal resuscitation; however, the research has demonstrated that infants born in distress may actually benefit the most from the placental transfusion of oxygenated blood provided by delayed clamping for up to a minute. This may be considered a first step of neonatal resuscitation.[25]

As a result of this evidence, the ACOG now recommends delayed clamping in both term and preterm infants. This will hopefully go a long way toward broadening this practice, which may also have other positive effects. While not yet studied, delayed cord clamping promotes more immediate skin-to-skin, as the baby is simply brought to the mother's abdomen while the cord finishes pulsating and she can immediately begin bonding with her child. This facilitates the initiation of breastfeeding and respects the sanctity of the first moments between mother and child.

I want a water birth

A lot of people ask me why I wanted a water birth. They were amazed that I wasn't afraid the baby would drown or something like that. I was more like, "why wouldn't I have a water birth?" Water has always been soothing for me. I am most relaxed in a bath, pool, or floating in the ocean. I liked to imagine my baby relaxed in the same way, floating around in his little indoor swimming pool, happy and calm. It just seemed natural to me for him to go from water to water, that this would be a much more natural transition. My water birth was a beautiful experience. The water completely eased my contraction pain and I just began to feel the baby coming down and out. I easily pushed and pulled him up to me. I was in complete control of the process. There was no anxiety, no stress, just me and my baby making this journey.

—S. R., new mother

Giving birth in the water, rather than simply laboring within it, is judged by many to be simply one of the newest trends in natural childbirth. However, throughout history, there have been stories of women going to natural water sources to birth and in some cultures this is still common practice. Yet it was not until the 1980s that water birth entered modern maternity care with the work of Dr. Michael Odent, a French obstetrician, who is a vocal advocate for more humane birth practices and obstetrics reform. Odent published an article in *The Lancet* describing the outcomes of over 100 births that occurred within water and observed a reduction in pain and faster labors in the women who delivered this way. He also felt birth in the water offered a more peaceful transition for the neonate from the aqueous environment of his or her mother to the outside world.[28] Within 10 years, all labor units in England and Wales installed tubs for labor and half of the units offered tubs for birthing. In 1995, the first International Waterbirth Congress was held, reporting on the results of over 19,000 water births. In the United States, in 1989, Water Birth International began assisting with installation of birthing tubs within hospitals, as well as offering portable inflatable birthing tubs for out-of-hospital birth, and by 2000, water birth was widespread enough within the United States that the International Waterbirth Congress was held in Portland, Oregon.[29] However, it was not until the late 1990s and early 2000s that much of the research started emerging regarding the practice.

THE NATURAL BIRTH PLAN

POSSIBLE BENEFITS OF WATER BIRTH

Less Pain and Lower Rates of Epidural

One of the most common reason women cite for wanting a water birth is a desire for the pain relief it may provide. Multiple studies have demonstrated less or equivalent reported pain in women both laboring and delivering in the water when compared to women birthing conventionally. Interestingly, these studies have not excluded women with epidurals in the conventional groups, meaning even the studies which failed to demonstrate that water births are less painful than land births have demonstrated that water birth is comparable to pharmacological methods of pain relief, without the numerous side effects previously discussed.[30–34] The *Cochrane Review* concluded on the basis of the two small randomized trials alone that examined pain in water birth that there was no statistical benefit to water birth in regards to pain; however, they also did not acknowledge the inclusion of epidurals in the control group and did not consider the many observational studies that did demonstrate a difference in self-reported pain.

Most naturally laboring women are not seeking an option for pain relief that is better than currently available pharmacological options. Naturally laboring women are seeking options that provide a comparable alternative to pharmacologic pain relief. Many women who are planning a natural birth report a great deal of anxiety specifically about the pain associated with pushing stage of labor, as they often see this as the point of no return in regards to pharmacological options. They also know they will have no reference point for what to expect earlier in the labor, as the sensations of the second state of labor are unique to that stage. For these women, this data is reassuring and increases their desire to have water birth as an option in their delivery.

Ease of Delivery in Upright Positions

Another benefit offered by birthing tubs is the buoyancy water provides. Labor is often a long and physically demanding process and, as previously mentioned, women often find it difficult to maintain upright or kneeling positions in the second stage of labor for prolonged periods of time, even if this position is more comfortable and preferable to them. In a study which specifically examined whether water birth facilitated alternative pushing positions, it was observed that 87% of women utilizing birthing tubs delivered in an upright position.[35]

Maternal Satisfaction with Delivery

Water is frequently characterized by such words as tranquil, peaceful, serene and, not surprisingly, women often describe their water births using similar terminology. The perceived calmness of a water delivery is a common motivating factor in women seeking to birth within water. Subjective things, such as the peacefulness of a birth experience, are difficult to measure and assign value to. However, when women who have a water birth are asked to evaluate their satisfaction with their delivery, in one study, up to 92% of patients would choose to or consider delivering in the water again, whereas only 48% of the women in the conventional delivery group could say the same.[36] Nikodem et al. (1999) also demonstrated high satisfaction scores in the water birth patients, with fewer patients indicating they had difficulty managing the pushing stage of their delivery.

POSSIBLE RISKS OF WATER BIRTH

Umbilical Cord Avulsion

A snapped umbilical cord, when the umbilical cord breaks either at the umbilical or placental attachment site rather than being clamped and cut, is a serious complication observed in both conventional deliveries and water births. The rate of umbilical cord avulsion in conventional births has not been well studied, but can lead to a need for neonatal transfusion, oxygen deprivation, and possible ischemic encephalopathy. Concern about a possible association with water birth and snapped umbilical cords was generated from a British survey in 1999 examining perinatal morbidity and mortality in the setting of water birth. While the overall water birth morbidity and mortality observed in this study was no different than that of births performed out of water, five snapped umbilical cords were reported out of a total of 4032 births. The authors postulated that the possible higher rate of cord tearing could be due to the practice of rapidly bring the baby to the mother's chest in a water birth, with the cord still attached.[37] In 2012, Burns et al. directly compared the incidence of umbilical cord rupture rates in over 8000 women who delivered either in water or conventionally. Twenty snapped umbilical cords occurred and 90% of those were in the water birth group, supporting the suspicion of earlier examiners that water birth may be associated with higher rates of these cord incidents.[38]

However, it is important to note that this study did not indicate whether immediate cord clamping was performed in the conventional delivery group, which would theoretically decrease the rate of umbilical cord tears if the mechanism of tearing is to rapidly bring the baby to the maternal chest. A study examining the rate of umbilical cord avulsion in traditional deliveries with delayed cord clamping would provide more insight as to whether cord avulsion was a result of water birth or simply the practices associated with delayed cord clamping. The study also did not indicate whether nuchal cords, umbilical cords wrapped around the neck, were checked for and/or reduced at the time of delivery. A recent Italian study found that 79% of water births were "hands off" deliveries, where the delivery was not controlled in any way by the midwife or doctor.[35] This would suggest that management of nuchal cords, an event that complicates one in four deliveries, indeed is not typical in water birth and that more training in controlling the rate of fetal expulsion and reduction of nuchal cords in water births may be indicated. A review in 2014 of all incidents of umbilical cord avulsions in the literature to date estimated a rate of 3.1 per 1000 water births.[39]

Increased Rate of Perineal Lacerations

Several studies have shown higher rates of perineal lacerations in water births when compared to traditional delivery. The mechanism for this is possibly the same as the mechanism for increased umbilical cord events, less control of the rate of delivery by the provider. However, these studies have shown only an increase in the rate of first- and second-degree lacerations, as opposed to severe third- and fourth-degree lacerations that involve the anal sphincter muscles and the rectum itself.[33,34,40,41] These studies also demonstrated significantly higher episiotomy rates in conventional deliveries as compared to water births, where episiotomies rarely if ever occur. Given the known association of episiotomies with third- and fourth-degree lacerations, a lower episiotomy rate is a clear benefit of water birth which is not leading to more overall lacerations. On the contrary, water birth, by inhibiting episiotomies, is preventing mild first- and second-degree lacerations from becoming more severe third- and fourth-degree lacerations, accounting for the higher numbers of these mild lacerations seen in the water birth groups.

Aspiration, Respiratory Distress, and Infection

One of the most common and certainly most serious concerns regarding water birth, which is expressed by health care providers and the lay public alike, is that the baby could inhale contaminated tub water, resulting in drowning, respiratory distress, or pneumonia. This is an understandable concern, given that throughout history, the first cry has been the affirmation that a child made it through the birth process intact. Many people incorrectly assume that the moment the baby's head emerges, he or she must breath, not realizing that baby is still connected to a supply of oxygenated blood for as long as the umbilical cord is intact.

In a water birth, there are several mechanisms that prevent the child from taking that first breath until it emerges from the water; however, these mechanisms by no means infallibly prevent aspiration. Neonates have what is termed the "dive reflex," which theoretically prevents the baby from inhaling water. Facial skin receptors along the trigeminal nerve are stimulated by contact with water and produce apnea and a closed larynx. However, critics of water birth have argued the dive reflex is only initiated in the presence of cold water and, indeed, studies have shown that there are less, however not absent, indicators of an activated dive reflex when participants were submerged in warm versus cold water.[42,43] There are also chemoreceptors in the larynx that prevent fluid aspiration; however, interestingly, cooler water (one to two degrees below the recommended water temperature) may actually cause these same receptors to stimulate breathing rather than suppress it, emphasizing the importance of appropriate water temperature in both stage 1 and stage 2 labor. The mild hypoxia that is present in nearly all uncompromised neonates at birth is also somewhat protective, inhibiting breathing until the child is born. However, this also is not a perfect system, because if the child becomes too hypoxic, a gasping reflex may actually be stimulated, which is why appropriate monitoring is important for water birth. Any evidence of fetal distress should be considered sufficient cause to abandon a water birth plan.[44]

There have been a small number of case reports of aspiration associated with water birth, which have resulted in serious neonatal compromise and even deaths, demonstrating that aspiration is indeed a small but serious risk in water birth of which patients should be informed.[45–47] There have also been case reports of infections in babies born within birth tubs, mainly *Pseudomonas aeruginosa* and *Legionella pneumophila*; however, each of these case reports were also associated with another risk factor for infection, including improper pool disinfection, improper water temperature control, and immersion in stagnant water or water from a contaminated source.[48–51] However, because the majority of studies have been observational in nature, it is difficult to determine the exact rate of either aspiration or infection associated with water birth. Yet, with proper understanding of the reflex pathways that initiate and inhibit breathing upon birth and appropriate water sources and tub protocols, these risks should be significantly reduced. Indeed, multiple large surveys, each examining thousands of women in the United Kingdom, where water immersion for both labor and birth is widely available and regulated by standard protocols, found no increased rate of infection, neonatal mortality, or other poor neonatal or maternal outcomes.[37,52,53] Each of these surveys concluded that there was no reason to deny the option of water birth to low-risk women based on a very small sample of case reports.

Yet, the American College of Obstetrics and Gynecologists has done just that, explicitly stating that birth should occur "on land, not in water."[54] This is despite the fact that they acknowledged openly in the exact same statement that the *Cochrane Review*, which reviewed 12 different studies involving over 3000 women, found no neonatal risk associated with delivery in water and a second, more recent, meta-analysis and review confirmed this conclusion.[55,56] They explained this seemingly contradictory recommendation was based on their determination that the data to date was insufficient to completely eliminate the possibility that "an additional rare but serious adverse outcome" could occur. However, based on the thousands of women who have already been observed without poor neonatal outcomes, even if this theoretical "additional serious adverse outcome" existed, it would be such a rare event that it would seem extremely unlikely to warrant the universal banning of water birth. Yet, that fact and the fact that this risk is still a theorized possibility have not stopped many of the less than 10% of maternity units in the United States that have labor tubs from banning water birth in their institutions on the basis of the ACOG Committee Opinion.[57]

Unfortunately, this means that many women who are determined to have a water birth are again left with only extremes to choose from. Either they must give up on the idea of a water birth or birth outside of a hospital, whether that is at home or in a freestanding birth center that permits water birth. Water birth outside of the hospital is likely to be significantly more dangerous than water birth within the hospital, where protocols are more likely to be strictly adhered to and where any complications, should they occur, can be managed appropriately. The ability to have a water birth may not seem like a big deal to some, but many women rely on water immersion to manage their unmedicated birth and leaving the tub when fully dilated is both physically difficult and emotionally stressful. It is also stressful to work through the later part of labor in the tub when staff, who are instructed not to "let" women deliver in the water, are anxiously supervising the labor in an attempt to prevent an "accidental water birth" on their watch. Often this anxiety leads to women being instructed to leave the tub before they are ready to deliver, when they are at the height of their labor intensity, and still could have benefited significantly from hydrotherapy. Again, fear as policy is not good medicine and in regards to water birth, in particular, fear more than science is dominating much of the policy making and care women receive.

A balanced approach to the water birth debate would be appropriate counseling of women about the concerns about actual delivery within the water, as they compare to documented benefits, without exaggerating either. A recommendation to exit the pool for delivery can be given without prohibiting a woman from choosing not to do so. Many women, properly informed about the concerns regarding water birth, may choose to leave the tub on their own accord. However, ultimately, the autonomy of women should be the guiding principle, particularly when they are sitting in a birth tub fully dilated. Finally, alternatives should be explored that may help many women find their own balance, such as building birthing stools or access doors into the birthing tubs and simply draining the water when women reach full dilation and are ready to push. This would prevent the need to move a woman in the advanced stage of labor, but minimize any concerns about aspiration and cord tearing.

THE NATURAL BIRTH PLAN

REFERENCES

1. Declercq ER, Sakala C, Corry MP, Applebaum S, Herrlich A. Major survey findings of listening to mothers SM III: pregnancy and birth: report of the third national U.S. survey of women's childbearing experiences. *J Perinat Educ*. 2014;23(1):9-16. doi:10.1891/1058-1243.23.1.9.
2. Elvander C, Ahlberg M, Thies-Lagergren L, Cnattingius S, Stephansson O. Birth position and obstetric anal sphincter injury: a population-based study of 113,000 spontaneous births. *BMC Pregnancy Childbirth*. 2015;15:252. doi:10.1186/s12884-015-0689-7.
3. Gupta JK, Sood A, Hofmeyr GJ, et al. Position in the second stage of labour for women without epidural anaesthesia. *Cochrane Database Syst Rev*. 2017;2017(5): 1-132. CD002006. doi:10.1002/14651858.CD002006.pub4.
4. Moraloglu O, Kansu-Celik H, Tasci Y, et al. The influence of different maternal pushing positions on birth outcomes at the second stage of labor in nulliparous women. *J Maternal-Fetal and Neonatal Med*. 2016;30(2):245-249.

5. Zhang H, Huang S, Guo X, et al. A randomised controlled trial in comparing maternal and neonatal outcomes between hands-and-knees delivery position and supine position in China. *Midwifery*. 2017;50:117-124. doi:10.1016/j.midw.2017.03.022. [Epub March 31, 2017].

6. Nieuwenhuijze MJ, de Jonge A, Korstjens I, et al. Influence on birthing positions affects women's sense of control in second stage of labour. *Midwifery*. 2012;29(11): e107-e114. doi:10.1016/j.midw.2012.12.007.

7. Nieuwenhuijze M, Low LK, Korstjens I, Lagro-Janssen T. The role of maternity care providers in promoting shared decision-making regarding birthing positions during second stage labor. *J Midwifery Womens Health*. 2014;59(3):277-285. doi:10.1111/jmwh.12187.

8. Reitter A, Daviss BA, Bisits A, et al. Does pregnancy and/or shifting positions create more room in a woman's pelvis? *Am J Obstet Gynecol*. 2014;211(6):662.e1-662.e9. doi:10.1016/j.ajog.2014.06.029. [Epub June 17, 2014].

9. Rossi MA, Lindell SG. Maternal positions and pushing techniques in a nonprescriptive environment. *J Obstet Gynecol Neonatal Nurs*. 1986;15(3):203-208. PubMed PMID: 3635590.

10. Hodnett ED, Stremler R, Halpern SH, Weston J, Windrim R. Repeated hands-and-knees positioning during labour: a randomized pilot study. *Peer J*. 2013;1:e25. doi:10.7717/peerj.25.

11. Bruner JP, Drummond SB, Meenan AL, Gaskin IM. All-fours maneuver for reducing shoulder dystocia during labor. *J Reprod Med*. 1998;43(5):439-443. PubMed PMID:9610468.

12. Vireday P. Historical and traditional birthing positions. [Blog post]. Available at http://wellroundedmama.blogspot.com/2015/03/historical-and-traditional-birthing.html. Accessed March 2015.

13. Aldrich CJ, D'Antona D, Spencer JA, et al. The effect of maternal pushing on fetal cerebral oxygenation and blood volume during the second stage of labour. *Br J Obstet Gynaecol*. 1995;102(6):448-453.

14. Barnett MM, Humenic SS. Infant outcome in relation to second stage labor. *Birth*. 1982;9(4):221-229.

15. Caldeyro-Barcia R, Giussi G, Storch E. The bearing-down efforts and their effects on fetal heart rate, oxygenation and acid base balance. *J Perinat Med*. 1981;9(1):63-67.

16. Yildirim G, Beji NK. Effects of pushing techniques in birth on mother and fetus: a randomized study. *Birth*. 2008;35(1):25-30. doi:10.1111/j.1523-536X.2007.00208.x.

17. Lemos A, Amorim MMR, Dornelas de Andrade A, et al. Pushing/bearing down methods for the second stage of labour. *Cochrane Database Syst Rev*. 2017;2017(3): 1-111. CD009124. doi:10.1002/14651858.CD009124.pub3.

18. Joseph B. DeLee and the practice of preventive obstetrics. *Am J Public Health*. 1988;78(10):1353-1361.

19. Kitzinger S. *Episiotomy and the Second Stage of Labor*. Seattle, WA: Penny Press; 1984.

20. Jiang H, Qian X, Carroli G, Garner P. Selective versus routine use of episiotomy for vaginal birth. *Cochrane Database Syst Rev*. 2017;(2):CD000081. Advance online publication. doi:10.1002/14651858.CD000081.pub3.

21. Amorim M, Coutinho IC, Melo I, Katz L. Selective episiotomy vs. implementation of a non-episiotomy protocol: a randomized clinical trial. *Reprod Health*. 2017;14:55. doi:10.1186/s12978-017-0315-4.

22. American College of Obstetricians and Gynecologists. Practice bulletin No. 165: prevention and management of obstetric lacerations at vaginal delivery. *Obstet Gynecol.* 2016;128(1):e1-e15. doi:10.1097/AOG.0000000000001523.

23. Friedman AM, Ananth CV, Prendergast E, et al. Variation in and factors associated with use of episiotomy. *JAMA.* 2015;313(2):197-199. doi:10.1001/jama.2014.14774.

24. Weiner J. "Don't cut me!": discouraged by experts, episiotomies still common in some hospitals. Available at http://khn.org/news/dont-cut-me-discouraged-by-experts-episiotomies-still-common-in-some-hospitals/. Accessed July 19, 2016.

25. Raju TNK, Singal N. Optimal timing for clamping the umbilical cord after birth. *Clin Perinatol.* 2012;39(4). doi:10.1016/j.clp.2012.09.006.

26. American Congress of Obstetricians and Gynecologists, Committee on Obstetric Practice. Delayed umbilical cord clamping after birth, Committee Opinion 684. *Obstet Gynecol.* 2017;129:e5-e10.

27. McDonald SJ, Middleton P, Dowswell T, Morris PS. Effect of timing of umbilical cord clamping of term infants on maternal and neonatal outcomes. *Cochrane Database Syst Rev.* 2013;11(7):1-96. CD004074. doi:10.1002/14651858.CD004074.pub3.

28. Odent M. Birth under water. *Lancet.* 1983;2(8365-8366):1476-1477.

29. Dekker R. Evidence on water birth. Available at https://evidencebasedbirth.com/waterbirth/. Accessed July 10, 2014.

30. Nikodem C, Hofmeyr GJ, Nolte AGW, et al. The effects of water on birth: a randomized controlled trial. Proceedings of the 14th Conference on Priorities in Perinatal Care in South Africa; South Africa. March 7–10, 1995. pp. 163-166. 1999.

31. Eberhard J, Stein S, Geissbuehler V. Experience of pain and analgesia with water and land births. *J Psychosom Obstet Gynaecol.* 2005;26(2):127-133.

32. Chaichian S, Akhlaghi A, Rousta F, Safavi M. Experience of water birth delivery in Iran. *Arch Iran Med.* 2009;12(5):468-471.

33. Mollamahmutoğlu L, Moraloğlu Ö, Özyer Ş, et al. The effects of immersion in water on labor, birth and newborn and comparison with epidural analgesia and conventional vaginal delivery. *J Turk Ger Gynecol Assoc.* 2012;13(1):45-49. doi:10.5152/jtgga.2012.03.

34. Otigbah CM, Dhanjal MK, Harmsworth G, Chard T. A retrospective comparison of water births and conventional vaginal deliveries. *Eur J Obstet Gynecol Reprod Biol.* 2000;91(1):15-20.

35. Henderson J, Burns EE, Regalia AL, et al. Labouring women who used a birthing pool in obstetric units in Italy: prospective observational study. *BMC Pregnancy Childbirth.* 2014;14:17. doi:10.1186/1471-2393-14-17.

36. Torkamani SA, Kangani F, Janani F. The effects of delivery in water on duration of delivery and pain compared with normal delivery. *Pak J Med Sci.* 2010;26(3):551-555

37. Gilbert RE, Tookey PA. Perinatal mortality and morbidity among babies delivered in water: surveillance study and postal survey. *BMJ.* 1999;319(7208):483-487.

38. Burns EE, Boulton MG, Cluett E, et al. Characteristics, interventions, and outcomes of women who used a birthing pool: a prospective observational study. *Birth.* 2012;39(3):192-202. doi:10.1111/j.1523-536X.2012.00548.x.

39. Schafer R. Umbilical cord avulsion in waterbirth. *J Midwifery Womens Health.* 2014;59(1):91-94. doi:10.1111/jmwh.12157.

40. Geissbuehler V, Stein S, Eberhard J. Waterbirths compared with landbirths: an observational study of nine years. *J Perinat Med.* 2004;32(4):308-314.

41. Menakaya U, Albayati S, Vella E, et al. A retrospective comparison of water birth and conventional vaginal birth among women deemed to be low risk in a

secondary level hospital in Australia. *Women Birth.* 2013;26(2):114-118. doi:10.1016/j.wombi.2012.10.002.

42. Choate JK, Denton KM, Evans RG, Hodgson Y. Using stimulation of the diving reflex in humans to teach integrative physiology. *Adv Physiol Educ.* 2014;38(4):355-365. doi:10.1152/advan.00125.2013.

43. Jones C. An update on water immersion during labor and delivery. Available at https://sciencebasedmedicine.org/an-update-on-water-immersion-during-labor-and-delivery/. Accessed March 28, 2014.

44. Johnson P. Birth under water—to breathe or not to breathe. *Br J Obstet Gynaecol.* 1996;103(3):202-208.

45. Kassim Z, Sellars M, Greenough A. Underwater birth and neonatal respiratory distress. *BMJ.* 2005;330(7499):1071-1072.

46. Bowden K, Kessler D, Pinette M, Wilson E. Underwater birth: missing the evidence or missing the point? *Pediatrics.* 2003;112(4):972-973.

47. Nguyen S, Kuschel C, Teele R, Spooner C. Water birth—a near-drowning experience. *Pediatrics.* 2002;110(2 pt 1):411-413.

48. Rawal J, Shah A, Stirk F, Mehtar S. Water birth and infection in babies. *BMJ.* 1994;309(6953):511.

49. Byard RW, Zuccollo JM. Forensic issues in cases of water birth fatalities. *Am J Forensic Med Pathol.* 2010;31(3):258-260. doi:10.1097/PAF.0b013e3181e12eb8.

50. Collins SL, Afshar B, Walker JT, et al. Heated birthing pools as a source of Legionnaires' disease. *Epidemiol Infect.* 2016;144(4):796-802. doi:10.1017/S0950268815001983.

51. Franzin L, Cabodi D, Scolfaro C, Gioannini P. Microbiological investigations on a nosocomial case of *Legionella pneumophila* pneumonia associated with water birth and review of neonatal cases. *Infez Med.* 2004;12(1):69-75.

52. Thoeni A, Zech N, Moroder L, Ploner F. Review of 1600 water births. Does water birth increase the risk of neonatal infection? *J Matern Fetal Neonatal Med.* 2005;17(5):357-361.

53. Alderdice F, Renfrew M, Marchant S, et al. Labour and birth in water in England and Wales: survey report. *Br J Midwifery.* 1995;3(7):376-382.

54. American College of Obstetrician and Gynecologists. Immersion in water during labor and delivery. Committee Opinion No. 679. *Obstet Gynecol.* 2016;128(5):e231-e236. Available at https://www.acog.org/Resources-And-Publications/Committee-Opinions/Committee-on-Obstetric-Practice/Immersion-in-Water-During-Labor-and-Delivery. Accessed May 2017.

55. Cluett ER, Burns E. Immersion in water in labour and birth. *Cochrane Database Syst Rev.* 2009;(2):CD000111. doi:10.1002/14651858.CD000111.pub3.

56. Taylor H, Kleine I, Bewley S, Loucaides E, Sutcliffe A. Neonatal outcomes of waterbirth: a systematic review and meta-analysis. *Arch Dis Child Fetal Neonatal Ed.* 2016;101(4):F357-F365. doi:10.1136/archdischild-2015-309600.

57. Harper B. Birth, bath, and beyond: the science and safety of water immersion during labor and birth. *J Perinat Educ.* 2014;23(3):124-134. doi:10.1891/1058-1243.23.3.124.

CHAPTER 8

Post-Delivery Maternal and Infant Care

I want immediate skin-to-skin contact with my baby

After pushing hard and long to deliver my daughter, there was a moment of perfect peace when they laid her on my chest. The early morning light was just coming in through the window and there was a faint mist glowing in the air from the rain the night before. She lifted her head up, opened her eyes, blinking several times, and then stared right into me. All the fussing she had been doing quieted as she just took me in. I remember thinking that no one would ever know me like this little person who had come from me, who was half me. In that moment, she was not an infant. She held a wisdom in her eyes beyond my own, like she knew all the secrets of the universe. It was the most beautiful moment of my life.

—A. B., new mother

In busy, modern labor and delivery units, the most important thing that has been lost to technology is an appreciation and respect for the blessed moment of welcoming new life into the world. In all the medical zeal and general angst that accompanies those first minutes after a baby is born, it is rare that the team slows down long enough to honor the moment and to allow space for the parents to experience and appreciate the first precious gaze of their new child. Parents are also guilty of rushing through the moment, often too busy worrying about getting a picture or notifying family to really take it in. But in truth, there is little that "needs" to be done in those first minutes. Weighing and footprints can wait. Babies are capable of coughing and sneezing in order to expel the fluid which nurses and doctors are so quick to suction. The cord can be left alone. Family in the waiting room or a few states away is capable of pacing in anticipation for a few minutes more. The first minutes that a parent spends with their child is a time which should be remembered and staff should count themselves privileged to witness it, not inconvenienced by the few extra minutes it takes to keep it sacred.

Skin-to-skin contact refers to the practice of placing the newly born, naked infant, directly to mother's chest. The infant is placed "tummy to tummy" on the mother's abdomen or chest, with only a warm blanket placed on top of the child. The mother's body temperature maintains the baby's body temperature at a thermoneutral range and the process of breastfeeding is initiated.[1] Any necessary infant care is performed on the mother's chest, except in the event of a true emergency.

Until the twentieth century, skin-to-skin contact and limited separation of mother and child was the norm and essential for survival of the neonate in a time without formula or infant warmers. Immediate initiation of breast-feeding was also important for the mother, in order to facilitate uterine contraction post delivery and minimize uterine bleeding. However, as birth moved into the hospital and most mothers received significant amounts of anesthesia during their labors, separation became the standard. Infants were handed off to nursing staff immediately after delivery for initial resuscitation, followed by bathing, warming, and feeding. Mothers often did not see their children for several hours. It was felt that new mothers needed rest above all else and generally all infant care was performed by nurses in the hospital nursery for the mother's entire hospital stay of up to a week.

This practice, however, is not natural by any definition of the word. Minimal separation of mothers and their young is observed across all mammalian species. The importance of skin-to-skin and keeping mothers and babies together was not really appreciated by the medical community; however, until the value of breastfeeding was accepted and ways to improve breastfeeding rates were explored. It is interesting that, for the medical community, skin-to-skin contact and minimal separation of women and their infants came to be considered the "intervention" to be studied, rather than the true intervention, that of removing the infant from the mother.

Nonetheless, there are several documented benefits of immediate skin-to-skin contact in the medical literature. In mammalian physiology, close contact between the mother and her baby is necessary in order to initiate the sequence of behaviors that lead to the first breastfeeding episode. Newborns have been observed to go through nine distinct behaviors during the initiation of breastfeeding[2]:

- Birth cry
- Relaxation
- Awakening
- Activity: looking at mother and breast, rooting, hand-to-mouth movements
- Crawling: infant localizes the areola and nipple by smell and migrates toward it
- Resting
- Familiarization: touching and licking the nipple
- Suckling
- Sleeping

Separation of the mother and newborn interrupts this sequence and delays the initiation of breastfeeding. Even quickly taking the baby away for a few minutes to weigh, obtain footprints, and place identifying bands initiates a stress response that makes it less likely to achieve breastfeeding in that initial "golden hour" after birth. Babies, upon separation, will immediately offer a protest cry of distress and, while across the room from their mother, cry ten times more than babies on their mother's chest.[3] Maintenance of skin-to-skin and breastfeeding, through the release of oxytocin, lowers cortisol levels and the "fight or flight" response in both mothers and babies, making for calmer more confident mothers.[4,5] Early initiation of breastfeeding is shown to be associated with both higher breastfeeding rates upon leaving the hospital and higher rates of continued breastfeeding in the months that follow.[6,7] Other maternal benefits of skin-to-skin contact include less postpartum bleeding and anemia and quicker expulsion of the placenta.[8,9]

The most recent *Cochrane Review* on the subject acknowledged these multiple benefits of skin-to-skin contact without finding any evidence of negative associations with the practice.[10] The World Health Organization (WHO) and the United Nations Children's Fund created the Baby Friendly Hospital Initiative in order to encourage breastfeeding friendly practices within hospitals and birthing centers worldwide. The organization offers the baby friendly designation to institutions that implement the "ten steps to successful breastfeeding," one of which is helping mothers initiate breastfeeding within 1 hour and uninterrupted skin-to-skin contact is an essential part of that effort. These steps are promoted by all maternal and child health authorities including the American College of Obstetricians and Gynecologists (ACOG), the American Academy of Pediatrics, and the American College of Nurse-Midwives.[11]

I decline post-delivery pitocin

After I delivered my son, the nurse suddenly started attaching something to my IV. When I asked, she told me it was just a little pit to keep me from bleeding. I was like, "What! I just went through this whole thing naturally and NOW you are giving me drugs!" It seemed really ridiculous.

—M. G., new mother

During pregnancy, up to 40% of the maternal blood supply is directed to the uterus and the uterine vessels dilate in order to accommodate that increased blood flow. Immediately after delivery, the uterus suddenly has a lot of empty space and those enlarged vessels can quickly expel a great deal of blood unless the uterus rapidly contracts, thereby constricting the vessels and limiting vaginal bleeding. Post-delivery administration of pitocin is part of what is termed "active management" of the third stage of labor, which includes early cord clamping, traction on the umbilical cord to facilitate rapid placental delivery, and administration of pitocin to more efficiently and reliably contract the uterus. Postpartum hemorrhage is defined by the World Health Organization as a blood loss of more than 500 ml following delivery and complicates up to 4% of vaginal deliveries. Twenty percent of maternal deaths related to childbirth are a result of postpartum hemorrhage.[12,13] Postpartum hemorrhage is serious and can kill a woman within only a few hours.

A number of studies have been performed examining whether prophylactic pitocin administration, either immediately after delivery of the baby or delivery of the placenta, reduces the risk of a postpartum hemorrhage when compared to expectant management of the third stage of labor. Expectant management of the third stage is basically a hands-off approach where the cord is left uncut until it naturally ceases pulsating and the placenta spontaneously separates and is expressed from the uterus. While one aspect of expectant management of the third stage, delayed cord clamping, has not been shown to increase maternal blood loss, when it is compared to routine prophylactic pitocin augmentation, expectant management is associated with a greater risk of postpartum hemorrhage.[14] In nine different trials, including over 9000 women, routine pitocin administration after delivery was shown to decrease overall blood loss and reduce the chance of a postpartum hemorrhage, including the risk of a severe postpartum hemorrhage of over 1 L.[15] Pitocin was determined to be the most effective medication at reducing this risk and routine administration after delivery also decreased the need for any additional medications to contract the uterus.

While pitocin has a bad reputation, especially among mothers wishing to labor naturally, the objections to pitocin after delivery, when it no longer affects the labor process and cannot be transferred to the baby, are less numerous. Some mothers report anecdotally that their after-birth cramping was worse with pitocin. Some worry that synthetic oxytocin will interfere with breastfeeding efforts, though no study to date has shown this and pitocin has such a short half-life that, in theory, this should not be a concern. Other women simply feel they would rather take a "wait and see" approach, especially if they have just gone through an entire labor without receiving medications. They often do not want medications after delivery unless truly needed. However, a "wait and see" approach is actually just treatment of uterine atony and bleeding if it occurs, which is associated with higher blood losses and greater

THE NATURAL BIRTH PLAN

incidences of true hemorrhage. Ultimately, given the high frequency of hemorrhage and the rapid pace at which it can become life threatening, this is a situation where the intervention is likely the lesser of the evils. Certainly, the evidence supports that conclusion. That said, women are entitled to take their chances if they are strongly opposed to this preventative measure, but they should understand the difference between intrapartum pitocin and postpartum pitocin and the potential benefits of the treatment. Women choosing to forego routine postpartum pitocin should also be aware of the conditions that may increase their risk of a postpartum hemorrhage and they may wish to reconsider their decision if they have any of the following[16]:

- Maternal age >40
- Large baby
- Prolonged labor and/or instrumental delivery
- Labor induction or augmentation
- High maternal BMI
- Multiple gestation
- Preeclampsia, hypertension
- History of a previous postpartum hemorrhage

I decline eye ointment for my baby

In the United States, it is considered standard of care to apply erythromycin eye ointment to all newborns shortly after delivery, as prophylactic treatment for neonatal ophthalmia, conjunctivitis occurring within the first 30 days of life. Neonatal ophthalmia can be caused by a number of organisms, including *Neisseria gonorrhoeae* (<1% of US cases), *Chlamydia trachomatis* (2–40% of US cases), and other bacteria such as *Staphylococcus, Streptococcus, Haemophilus*, and other Gram-negative bacterial species (20–50% of US cases). It can also be caused by viral infections such as herpes simplex, adenovirus, and enterovirus.[17] In the majority of cases, it is a mild illness, easily treated with either topical or oral antibiotics. However, *N. gonorrhoeae* conjunctivitis, which develops in up to 50% of neonates exposed to the bacteria during delivery, can quickly progress and lead to permanent vision damage or even blindness.

Prophylaxis against *N. gonorrhoeae* was initiated in the late 1800s by Dr. Carl Siegmund Franz Credé, who discovered that application of silver nitrate to infants' eyes after birth decreased the incidence of conjunctivitis from 7% to 0.5%.[18] Throughout the twentieth century, this practice was widely adopted, though the recommended prophylaxis was changed from silver nitrate to erythromycin, which was less irritating, not associated with chemical conjunctivitis, and more effective in preventing *C. trachomatis* conjunctivitis. Many states even adopted laws that mandated prophylaxis which are still in place and enforced in several states.[19] In the last decade, however, the practice has been called into question by many within and outside the medical community. The primary reason for this is the unreliable efficacy of erythromycin. Up to 30% of *N. gonorrhoeae* is resistant to erythromycin and topical erythromycin has questionable ability to prevent *C. trachomatis* and does not prevent other, more serious, complications from the infection.[20] Routine prophylaxis has already been abandoned in several European countries without an increase in neonatal ophthalmia-related blindness.[21] Critics of prophylaxis argue that a superior form of prevention would be routine screening of all pregnant women for both *N. gonorrhoeae* and *C. trachomatis* in the first trimester of pregnancy, treatment and test of cure for all infected patients, and third trimester rescreening and appropriate treatment for all at-risk patients. Alternative prevention strategies have also been suggested including colostrum administration to the eyes, which was shown to have potential efficacy in one small randomized control trial, and povidone-iodine administration, which has demonstrated efficacy but, like silver nitrate, is associated with significant rates of chemical conjunctivitis.[22,23]

Despite the questionable effectiveness for prophylaxis, erythromycin ointment is not associated with significant side effects and supporters of prophylaxis argue that it also prevents other forms of bacterial conjunctivitis that, while less severe, are more common. This claim has not been studied, but given the current knowledge regarding bacterial sensitivities, it seems a reasonable assumption. The suggested side-effects and concerns regarding its use are mainly eye irritation, blurred vision that may impede bonding, and contribution to overall antibiotic resistance.[24] These seem to be relatively minor concerns which the benefits of prophylaxis may very well outweigh for most parents. However, the recommendation for prophylaxis is also not based on overwhelmingly strong evidence, given current antibiotic resistance, and parents should be able to weigh the benefits and side effects for themselves. Regardless of prophylaxis policies, improved screening of all women for the more serious infections appears prudent, particularly if parents are electing to forgo any prophylaxis.

I decline vitamin K injection for my baby

The growing trend of vitamin K refusal first made national headlines in 2013, when the CDC reported that five infants in Tennessee had

THE NATURAL BIRTH PLAN

developed vitamin K deficiency bleeding (VKDB) in an 8-month period, with four of the babies presenting with bleeding into the brain and one baby presenting with gastrointestinal bleeding.[25,26] An additional two babies were identified with vitamin K deficiency without bleeding. All of the infants survived; however, three had permanent neurological damage and two required emergency brain surgery. All of the parents of the affected children had refused for their babies to receive the standard vitamin K injection, which is typically administered shortly after birth.

Vitamin K deficiency bleeding, formerly known as hemorrhagic disease of the newborn, is a rare but potentially lethal condition which can develop in infants that do not have a sufficient amount of vitamin K to support the development of blood clotting factors. Placental transfer of vitamin K is limited and vitamin K does not enter breast milk to any large degree. Exclusively breast-fed infants are at significantly higher risk of deficiency. VKDB has three distinct presentations[27]:

- Early-onset VKDB: occurs within the first 24 hours after birth and is associated with cephalohematoma, bleeding between the skin and the skull, gastrointestinal bleeding, or intracranial bleeding into the brain.
- Classic VKDB: the most common (0.25–1.7% of neonates), occurs within the first 2 to 7 days of life, and usually consists of milder bleeding from the umbilicus site, gastrointestinal tract, circumcision site, or puncture sites.
- Late VKDB: occurs after the second week of life up to 6 months of age, with an incidence of 4.4 to 7.2 per 100,000 live births; however, it can occur as commonly as 1 in 15,000 to 1 in 20,000 infants who are exclusively breast-fed. Fifty percent of cases present with intracranial bleeding, with a 20% mortality.

In 1961, as a result of a large Swedish study demonstrating a five-fold reduction in the risk of newborn bleeding with administration of either oral or injected vitamin K, the American Academy of Pediatrics recommended that all infants receive a vitamin K injection at birth.[28] This practice significantly reduced the incidence of VKDB in the United States and continued unchallenged until the 1990s, when a small study (800 patients) out of the United Kingdom demonstrated an association between vitamin K injections and childhood leukemia.[29] Consequently, vitamin K injections were substituted with oral vitamin K supplementation throughout the United Kingdom and a number of follow-up studies were performed, both examining the concern about a possible association of vitamin K injections with leukemia and comparing the efficacy of oral vitamin K regimens to injectable vitamin K regimens.

The follow-up studies on the issue of a possible cancer link were extremely reassuring. Less than 2 years after the initial study of concern was published, two large trials, one involving 1.4 million children and a second involving 50,000 children, found no association between vitamin K injections and childhood cancer or any other adverse outcome, aside from mild swelling or bruising at the injection site.[30,31] Ten additional, high-quality case-controlled studies were also performed in the following years and no link between childhood cancer and injectable vitamin K was identified.[32] To date, there is simply no evidence that vitamin K has any association with childhood cancers, yet when parents who refused the vitamin K injection were asked why they declined it, this was a common explanation they offered, in addition to concerns about other "toxins" in the injection or the injection containing too much, synthetic vitamin K.[33] Why do parents believe this? Unfortunately, similar to vaccines, there are a number of "health-promoting" websites specifically encouraging parents to forgo the vitamin K injection and spreading misinformation.[34–36] Several of these sites incorrectly reassure parents that increasing the amount of maternal dietary vitamin K in the later weeks of pregnancy and during breastfeeding will provide adequate vitamin K for the newborn. They also describe and provide links to the study demonstrating an association with cancer without discussing all the evidence that disproved it. It is no wonder that parents are afraid and it is always easier to just not do something, as opposed to taking an active action. Often, when health decisions are being made, people feel less responsibility for an act of omission. If something bad happens, it is nature's fault, not their own.

Many who are opposed to or simply nervous about injectable vitamin K suggest oral vitamin K may be used as an alternative and this method of VKDB prevention is actually utilized in several countries. Oral vitamin K has been shown to be equally effective as injectable vitamin K in preventing VKDB in the first 2 weeks of life. However, in countries that rely on oral vitamin K, higher rates of late VKDB, the more serious form of the disease, are observed. In a review of data from four different countries, failure of oral vitamin K regimens occurred in 1.2 to 1.9 per 100,000 live births, as opposed to no failures observed with the injectable form. Failure rates were higher in babies that did not complete the recommended additional four doses in the weeks following birth

THE NATURAL BIRTH PLAN

(2–4 per 100,000) and noncompliance with oral regimens has been shown to be around 7%.[37] Furthermore, there is no approved oral formulation in the United States, so multiple doses of the parenteral formula must be used, which infants are likely to spit out, making for inconsistent administration even when all the proper follow-up doses are given. While the overall risk of failure is low and oral supplementation certainly is superior to no vitamin K supplementation at all, given the lack of any adverse associations with the injectable form, oral supplementation seems like more trouble for less benefit.

What about the other reasons and concerns parents raised when refusing injectable vitamin K? In respect to the dosing concern, the vitamin K in the injectable form is released in a delayed release fashion, with activity up to 2 months after the initial injection, meaning that, while the medication is administered in a single large dose, the actual medication is only entering the bloodstream in small amounts slowly over time.[38] The same dose of vitamin K is used in oral regimens and a larger quantity is absorbed at one time. With oral regimens, the child also actually ends up receiving more medication because of the multiple doses required. Another common concern is that other components in the vitamin K injection may be "toxic." Aside from the actual vitamin K, the other ingredients included in the injection are polysorbate 80, propylene glycol, sodium acetate anhydrous, and glacial acetic acid.[39] Polysorbate 80 is a plant-derived ingredient that helps the vitamin K dissolve into the liquid formulation necessary for an injection and is actually listed as a "green chemical." Sodium acetate anhydrous is a combination of salt and bicarbonate and glacial acetic acid is vinegar, all ingredients that are safe and part of routine diets. Propylene glycol is the only controversial ingredient because it is a preservative that has caused adverse reactions in preterm infants; however, those reactions occurred at much higher doses and only when the ingredient was contained in IV fluids, not a fat-soluble injection.[40,41] The small amount of propylene glycol in the vitamin K injection is not of concern. Another issue that understandably worries parents is the package insert for the medication states that deaths have occurred as a result of administration. This disclaimer was added by manufacturers for medico-legal reasons and, in fact, the extremely rare deaths from vitamin K injections have been in adults, due to anaphylactic reactions, and only a single case report of anaphylaxis in an infant has ever been reported.[42] An infant is certainly many times more likely to die as a result of not receiving vitamin K prophylaxis than as a result of a reaction to the vitamin K injection itself.

I want rooming-in with my baby

Having my baby with me in the hospital was so essential. I really learned to understand the little cues that meant she was hungry before she was screaming, which made the latching on process so much easier than when she was already starving and upset. I also spent a lot of time just cuddling with her and getting to know every part of her face, her hands, her feet...marvelling at this person I had grown inside me. It was nice to have the nurses as a backup in case I was worried about something, but I wanted to know how to take care of my baby by the time we went home. Any time she was taken to the nursery, I could feel my stress levels rise. It did not feel natural for us to be separated for any amount of time.

—J. D., new mother

Rooming-in, or non-separation of mothers and babies in the postpartum period, is the natural continuation of what begins with skin-to-skin contact after birth and is an essential part of honoring the dyad that is the mother–child unit. Again, like skin-to-skin, this is not an intervention, but given the widespread and deeply ingrained practice of keeping babies in the nursery, separated from their mothers after delivery, many studies have been done in order to demonstrate to doctors, nurses, and hospital administrators that rooming-in should be the standard of care in maternity units nationwide.

There are many documented benefits to rooming-in. Keeping mothers and babies together encourages on demand feeding and better latching, likely because feeding cues are more quickly observed and responded to, and, as a result, babies who room-in are fed more frequently and establish a better milk supply.[43–45] Mothers also report less breast engorgement and are more likely to feel confident in their parenting skills when leaving the hospital.[46] Observational studies demonstrate a higher rate of exclusive breastfeeding among babies who room-in, as well a longer duration of breastfeeding.[47,48]

Most of the concerns regarding rooming-in center on infant safety. Historically, nursery care was thought to decrease the risk of infant infections due to exposure from outside guests. However, infection outbreaks within nurseries led researchers to believe rooming-in was actually more likely to decrease the risk of neonatal infectious exposure.[49] As rooming-in has become more widespread, the more serious risk of rooming-in appears to be infant falls, most often from mothers falling asleep with their newborns in the bed. Several case reports of infant falls resulting in significant brain injury or death have been published, with the rate of in-hospital falls estimated to be 1.6 to 4.14 per 10,000 births or 600 to 1600 falls nationwide per year.[50,51] The risk appears greatest in patients who are utilizing narcotics for pain relief. Some proposals to limit this risk include parent education regarding the dangers of bedsharing, bed design changes that would make beds lower to the ground, with higher and longer bed rails, and more frequent nursing rounds in order to minimize the numbers of mothers accidently falling asleep with their babies in the bed.

The only randomized controlled trial to date that attempted to separate out the benefits of skin-to-skin and rooming-in, by randomizing patients according to skin-to-skin use and rooming-in versus nursery care, did not demonstrate that rooming-in was associated with better breastfeeding outcomes.[52] As a result of this trial, the most recent *Cochrane Review* did not conclude that postpartum rooming-in had a significant impact on breastfeeding rates, despite the observational studies that showed rooming-in promoted other practices which were associated with higher rates of breastfeeding success. However, regardless of whether rooming-in is better than nursery care, it is important to remember that separation of infants from their mothers is the intervention, not the other way around. Nursery care should be demonstrated to be superior to non-separation in order for that to become the standard of care and, to date, there is no evidence to that effect. Furthermore, even if nursery care were demonstrated to be "better" or "safer," babies belong to their parents and no hospital policy should dictate where a baby sleeps. That decision belongs to the parents alone.

I plan to keep my placenta for encapsulation

I suffered from severe postpartum depression and anxiety after my first child. In fact, it was so bad I put off having a second child for four years because I was so worried about what would happen to me and happen to my child if I were to go through the same thing again. But, as my son got older, I really wanted him to have a sibling, so I did extensive research into what might help prevent depression this time around. I worked with a counsellor and had a plan in place with my doctor, but I also found my amazing placenta encapsulator. She picked up my placenta a few hours after I had my second son and within two days delivered my pills. I would take one whenever I was feeling off and within a few moments, I felt better. It was such a different experience. I know there are those that say it is just a placebo effect, but I have taken full on antidepressants before and did not notice as quick of a response as with placenta pills. I would recommend them to anyone who suffered from postpartum depression in the past or simply wants to avoid it in the future. If I have another child, I would definitely do it again.

—T. C., new mother

Placentophagy, the act of consuming one's placenta, is observed in several mammalian species, but has occurred only rarely in human cultures and usually not post birth as in other species, but as treatment for various other maladies.[53] This changed, however, in the late 1980s when Raven Lang, an American midwife who opened California's first birthing center, learned about its use in Traditional Chinese medicine. She presented placental encapsulation, a process where the placenta is cooked, dehydrated, and placed into capsules for consumption postpartum, at the Midwives Alliance of North America's annual conference.[54] Placental encapsulation was purported by Lang to be a remedy for postpartum depression, low breast milk supply, anemia, and postpartum bleeding and, since that time, numerous organizations have been formed that promote the practice. These organizations train and certify placenta encapsulators and market placental encapsulation to new mothers. Other methods of placentophagy exist, including consuming it raw in a "placenta smoothie" or cooked by either baking or steaming; however, encapsulation is the most widespread type of placentophagy probably due to its improvement on palatability.

The majority of women who decide to encapsulate their placenta have a history of postpartum depression or anxiety.[55] The etiology of postpartum depression is multifactorial; however, one possible precipitating factor is maternal sensitivity to the acute estrogen withdrawal that occurs post delivery.[56,57] Those that promote encapsulation report that the placenta contains therapeutic levels of estrogen that may restore depleted estrogen stores and, thus, decrease maternal mood lability as a consequence of low estrogen levels. Indeed, a recent study did demonstrate the presence of 16 different hormones, including estrogen, in placenta capsules at concentrations that could potentially have physiological effects.[58] However, the hormone in greatest concentration in the samples, by several times over, was actually progesterone, which has not been shown to be beneficial for postpartum depression and actually decreases in maternal circulation in the process of proper milk production. At this time, there is an ongoing large, randomized control trial to determine what benefits, if any, placental encapsulation may offer. However, to date, there is little documented evidence beyond the anecdotal

THE NATURAL BIRTH PLAN

reports of women and encapsulators that placenta encapsulation prevents postpartum depression and anxiety disorders.

There have been a few studies, however, that actually refute some of the claims made by encapsulation proponents. In one small, randomized study, consumption of placenta capsules was not demonstrated to improve maternal iron stores and the authors cautioned against iron-deficient mother relying solely on placental encapsulation for iron replacement.[59] Another dated study examined placentophagy for milk production and reported a benefit; however, this study was not performed in accordance with currently acceptable scientific protocols, and there is no additional research that has examined the claim that placenta capsules improve milk production. Furthermore, animal studies in species that routinely consume their placentas fail to demonstrate either the hormonal or lactation effects reported by encapsulation proponents.[60]

Aside from the lack of any demonstrable benefit to placental encapsulation, there is also a growing level of concern about the safety of the practice. Placenta encapsulation is not regulated by the FDA or any other state agency. It is typically performed by unlicensed individuals, who are often also doulas, lactation counselors, or some other type of "birth worker," within their own home. While certified encapsulators are supposed to adhere to OSHA guidelines on the safe handling of placentas and follow a preparation technique designed to eliminate any bacterial or viral contamination, there is no oversight of their practices or studies demonstrating that those practices, in fact, ensure the safety of the placental preparation. Most placental encapsulators are certified after a single weekend course. The potential danger of this was brought to public awareness only recently when the CDC reported a case of late-onset group beta strep bacteremia in an 11-day-old infant whose mother was consuming placenta capsules that were later found to be colonized by the same bacteria.[61] While this was a single case report, it does emphasize the potential risks involved. Hopefully more evidence will soon be available to guide mothers as to whether there are any benefits of placental encapsulation that outweigh these potential risks, but until then, parents must realize they are choosing a therapy based only on anecdotal evidence and just because something is "natural" does not necessarily mean it is beneficial or safe.

Furthermore, perhaps more than any other practice that has made itself into the natural birth community, placental encapsulation is a business that preys upon some of the most vulnerable of women seeking natural alternatives, women who have suffered postpartum depression and are desperately seeking anything that will help them avoid a recurrence, even if it is nothing more than snake oil. Doula work is hard, time-consuming work. Most doulas are physically unable to attend more than four births per month and most attend, on average, one to two births per month, which is not enough to support someone financially and it is impossible for doulas to keep another job, given the unpredictable nature of birth. Childbirth education is also not lucrative, with educators earning, at most $300 to $400 per family for several, multi-hour sessions of education that often occur on evenings and weekends, taking educators away from their family. Private lactation counseling, like doula care, is time-consuming work that does not pay well and most counselors have a limited number of clients, as few participate with insurance and are dependent on cash pay from their clients. Placenta encapsulators charge, on average, $250 for their services and can encapsulate many placentas within a short amount of time, in the comfort of their own home. Placenta encapsulation has become an easy way for "birth workers" to supplement their income and, thus, they promote it to a greater degree than the evidence would warrant. As a cottage industry, encapsulation is not held to the professional standard that it should be, given that encapsulators are handling organ tissue and preparing it for consumption. If encapsulation is shown to have benefit for mothers, the process should become standardized and encapsulators should be regulated in order to ensure patient safety, in the same way any other medical treatment would and should be.

REFERENCES

1. Chiu SH, Anderson GC, Burkhammer MD. Newborn temperature during skin-to-skin breastfeeding in couples having breastfeeding difficulties. *Birth*. 2005;32(2): 115-121.
2. Widström AM, Lilja G, Aaltomaa-Michalias P, et al. Newborn behaviour to locate the breast when skin-to-skin: a possible method for enabling early self-regulation. *Acta Paediatr*. 2011;100(1):79-85.
3. Alberts JR. Learning as adaptation of the infant. *Acta Paediatr Suppl*. 1994;397 (83):77-85.
4. Uvänas-Moberg K, Arn I, Magnusson D. The psychobiology of emotion: the role of the oxytocinergic system. *Int J Behav Med*. 2005;12(2):59-65.
5. Winberg J. Mother and newborn baby: mutual regulation of physiology and behavior—a selective review. *Dev Psychobiol*. 2005;47(3):217-229.
6. Bernard-Bonnin AC, Stachtchenko S, Girard G, Rousseau E. Hospital practices and breastfeeding duration: a meta-analysis of controlled trials. *Birth*. 1989;16(2):64-66.
7. Pérez-Escamilla R, Pollitt E, Lönnerdal B, Dewey KG. Infant feeding policies in maternity wards and their effect on breastfeeding success: an analytical overview. *Am J Public Health*. 1994;84(1):89-97.

THE NATURAL BIRTH PLAN

8. Gabriel MA, Martín LI, López Escobar A, et al. Randomized controlled trial of early skin-to-skin contact: effects on the mother and the newborn. *Acta Paediatr.* 2010;99(11):1630-1634.

9. Dordević G, Jovanović B, Dordević M. An early contact with the baby—benefit for the mother. *Med Pregl.* 2008;61(11-12):576-579. Serbian. PubMed PMID:19368275.

10. Moore ER, Anderson GC, Bergman N, Dowswell T. Early skin-to-skin contact for mothers and their healthy newborn infants. *Cochrane Database Syst Rev.* 2012;5:CD003519. doi:10.1002/14651858.CD003519.pub3.

11. Baby-Friendly USA Inc. The ten steps to successful breastfeeding. Available at https://www.babyfriendlyusa.org/about-us/baby-friendly-hospital-initiative/the-ten-steps. Accessed 4/2017.

12. Abouzaher C. Antepartum and postpartum haemorrhage. In: Murray CJ, Lopez AD, eds. *Health Dimensions of Sex and Reproduction: The Global Burden of Sexually Transmitted Diseases, HIV, Maternal Conditions, Perinatal Disorders, and Congenital Anomalies.* Boston, MA: Harvard University Press; 1998:172-174.

13. Say L, Chou D, Gemmill A, et al. Global causes of maternal death: a WHO systematic analysis. *Lancet Global Health.* 2014;2(6):e323-e333.

14. McDonald SJ, Middleton P, Dowswell T, Morris PS. Effect of timing of umbilical cord clamping of term infants on maternal and neonatal outcomes. *Cochrane Database Syst Rev.* 2013;11(7):1-96. CD004074. doi:10.1002/14651858.CD004074.pub3.

15. Westhoff G, Cotter AM, Tolosa JE. Prophylactic oxytocin for the third stage of labour to prevent postpartum haemorrhage. *Cochrane Database Syst Rev.* 2013;10:1-93. CD001808. doi:10.1002/14651858.CD001808.pub2.

16. Sebghati M, Chandraharan E. An update on the risk factors for and management of obstetric haemorrhage. *Womens Health (Lond).* 2017;13(2):34-40. doi:10.1177/1745505717716860. [Epub ahead of print]. Available at http://journals.sagepub.com/doi/abs/10.1177/1745505717716860?url_ver=Z39.88-2003&rfr_id=ori%3Arid%3Acrossref.org&rfr_dat=cr_pub%3Dpubmed&. Accessed 5/2017.

17. American Academy of Pediatrics. Prevention of neonatal ophthalmia. In: Pickering LK, Baker CJ, Kimberlin DW, Long SS, eds. *Red Book: 2012 Report of the Committee on Infectious Diseases.* 29th ed. Elk Grove Village, IL: American Academy of Pediatrics; 2012:880-882.

18. Hoyme UB. Clinical significance of Credé's prophylaxis in Germany at present. *Infect Dis Obstet Gynecol.* 1993;1(1):32-36. doi:10.1155/S1064744993000080.

19. Standler RB. Statutory law in the USA: requiring silver nitrate in eyes of newborns. Available at http://www.rbs2.com/SilvNitr.pdf. Accessed 5/2017.

20. Moore DL, MacDonald NE; and Canadian Paediatric Society, Infectious Diseases and Immunization Committee. Preventing ophthalmia neonatorum. *Can J Infect Dis Med Microbiol.* 2015;26(3):122-125.

21. Darling EK, McDonald H. A meta-analysis of the efficacy of ocular prophylactic agents used for the prevention of gonococcal and chlamydial ophthalmia neonatorum. *J Midwifery Womens Health.* 2010;55(4):319-327.

22. Ghaemi S, Navaei P, Rahimirad S, et al. Evaluation of preventive effects of colostrum against neonatal conjunctivitis: a randomized clinical trial. *J Educ Health Promot.* 2014;3:63. doi:10.4103/2277-9531.134776.

23. Ali Z, Khadije D, Elahe A, et al. Prophylaxis of ophthalmia neonatorum comparison of betadine, erythromycin and no prophylaxis. *J Trop Pediatr.* 2007;53(6):388-392.

24. Hedberg K, Ristinen TL, Soler JT, et al. Outbreak of erythromycin-resistant staphylococcal conjunctivitis in a newborn nursery. *Pediatr Infect Dis J.* 1990;9(4):268-273.

25. Centers for Disease Control and Prevention (CDC). Notes from the field: late vitamin K deficiency bleeding in infants whose parents declined vitamin K prophylaxis—Tennessee, 2013. *Morb Mortal Wkly Rep.* 2013;62(45):901-902.

26. Schulte R, Jordan LC, Morad A, et al. Rise in late onset vitamin K deficiency bleeding in young infants because of omission or refusal of prophylaxis at birth. *Pediatr Neurol.* 2014;50(6):564-568. doi:10.1016/j.pediatrneurol.2014.02.013.

27. Block SL. Playing newborn intracranial roulette: parental refusal of vitamin K injection. *Pediatric Annals.* 2014;43(2):53-59.

28. American Academy of Pediatrics, Committee on Nutrition. Vitamin K compounds and the water-soluble analogues: use in therapy and prophylaxis in pediatrics. *Pediatrics.* 1961;28(3):501-507.

29. Golding J, Greenwood R, Birmingham K, Mott M. Childhood cancer, intramuscular vitamin K, and pethidine given during labour. *BMJ.* 1992;305(6849):341-346.

30. Ekelund H, Finnström O, Gunnarskog J, et al. Administration of vitamin K to newborn infants and childhood cancer. *BMJ.* 1993;307(6896):89-91.

31. Klebanoff MA, Read JS, Mills JL, et al. The risk of childhood cancer after neonatal exposure to vitamin K. *N Engl J Med.* 1993;329(13):905-908. doi:10.1056/NEJM199309233291301.

32. Ross JA, Davies SM. Vitamin K prophylaxis and childhood cancer. *Med Pediatr Oncol.* 2000;34(6):434-437.

33. Hamrick HJ, Gable EK, Freeman EH, et al. Reasons for refusal of newborn vitamin K prophylaxis: implications for management and education. *Hosp Pediatr.* 2016;6(1):15-21.

34. Sarah, the Healthy Home Economist. Skip that newborn vitamin k shot. Available at http://www.thehealthyhomeeconomist.com/skip-that-newborn-vitamin-k-shot/. Accessed 5/2017.

35. Rothville K. Vitamin K: controversy? What controversy? Available at http://www.vaclib.org/basic/vitamin-k.htm. Accessed 5/2017.

36. Heimer M. Synthetic vitamin k shot for my baby? No thanks. Available at http://www.livingwhole.org/synthetic-vitamin-k-shot/. Accessed 5/2017.

37. American Academy of Pediatrics: Committee on Fetus and Newborn. Controversies regarding vitamin K and the newborn. *Pediatrics.* 2003;112(1):191-192.

38. Loughnan PM, McDougall PN. Does intramuscular vitamin K1 act as an unintended depot preparation? *J Paediatr Child Health.* 1996;32(3):251-254.

39. Merck & Co. Phytonadione package insert. Available at https://www.accessdata.fda.gov/drugsatfda_docs/label/2003/012223Orig1s039Lbl.pdf. Accessed 5/2017.

40. MacDonald MG, Getson PR, Glasgow AM, et al. Propylene glycol: increased incidence of seizures in low birth weight infants. *Pediatrics.* 1987;79(4):622-625.

41. Jardine DS. Relationship of benzyl alcohol to kernicterus, intraventricular hemorrhage, and mortality in preterm infants. *Pediatrics.* 1989;83(2):153-160.

42. Koklu E, Taskale T, Koklu S, Ariguloglu EA. Anaphylactic shock due to vitamin K in a newborn and review of literature. *J Matern Fetal Neonatal Med.* 2014;27(11):1180-1181.

43. Bigelow AE, Power M, Gillis DE, et al. Breastfeeding, skin-to-skin contact, and mother-infant interactions over infants' first three months. *Infant Ment Health J.* 2014;35(1):51-62.

44. Yamauchi Y, Yamanouchi I. Breast-feeding frequency during the first 24 hours after birth in full-term neonates. *Pediatrics.* 1990;86(2):171-175.

45. Wilde CJ, Knight CH, Flint DJ. Control of milk secretion and apoptosis during mammary involution. *J Mammary Gland Biol Neoplasia.* 1999;4(2):129-136.

THE NATURAL BIRTH PLAN

46. O'Connor S, Vietze PM, Sherrod KB, et al. Reduced incidence of parenting inadequacy following rooming-in. *Pediatrics*. 1980;66(2):176-182.

47. Buranasin B. The effects of rooming-in on the success of breastfeeding and the decline in abandonment of children. *Asia Pac J Public Health*. 1991;5(3):217-220.

48. Wright A, Rice S, Wells S. Changing hospital practices to increase the duration of breastfeeding. *Pediatrics*. 1996;97(5):669-675.

49. Hillier K. Babies and bacteria: phage typing, bacteriologists, and the birth of infection control. *Bull Hist Med*. 2006;80(4):733-761.

50. Helsley L. Newborn falls/drops in the hospital setting. Available at https://www.mnhospitals.org/Portals/0/Documents/ptsafety/falls/MHA-6-20-11.pdf. Accessed June 20, 2011.

51. Thatch BT. Deaths and near deaths of healthy newborn infants while bed sharing on maternity wards. *J Perinatol*. 2014;34:275-279.

52. Jaafar SH, Ho JJ, Lee KS. Rooming-in for new mother and infant versus separate care for increasing the duration of breastfeeding. *Cochrane Database Syst Rev*. 2016;8:1-28. CD006641. doi:10.1002/14651858.CD006641.pub3.

53. Young SM, Benyshek DC. In search of human placentophagy: a cross-cultural survey of human placenta consumption, disposal practices, and cultural beliefs. *Ecol Food Nutr*. 2010;49(6):467-484.

54. IPEN Placental Network. Placental encapsulation. Available at https://placentaremediesnetwork.org/placenta-encapsulation/. Accessed 5/2017.

55. Selander J, Cantor A, Young SM, Benyshek DC. Human maternal placentophagy: a survey of self-reported motivations and experiences associated with placenta consumption. *Ecol Food Nutr*. 2013;52(2):93-115.

56. Ahokas A, Kaukoranta J, Wahlbeck K, Aito M. Estrogen deficiency in severe postpartum depression: successful treatment with sublingual physiologic 17beta-estradiol: a preliminary study. *J Clin Psychiatry*. 2001;62(5):332-336.

57. Gregoire AJ, Kumar R, Everitt B, et al. Transdermal oestrogen for treatment of severe postnatal depression. *Lancet*. 1996;347(9006):930-933.

58. Young SM, Gryder LK, Zava D, et al. Presence and concentration of 17 hormones in human placenta processed for encapsulation and consumption. *Placenta*. 2016;43:86-89.

59. Gryder LK, Young SM, Zava D, et al. Effects of human maternal placentophagy on maternal postpartum iron status: a randomized, double-blind, placebo-controlled pilot study. *J Midwifery Womens Health*. 2017;62(1):68-79.

60. Coyle CW, Hulse KE, Wisner KL, et al. Placentophagy: therapeutic miracle or myth? *Arch Womens Ment Health*. 2015;18(5):673-680. doi:10.1007/s00737-015-0538-8.

61. Buser GL, Sayonara M, Zhang AY, et al. *Notes from the field*: late-onset infant group B streptococcus infection associated with maternal consumption of capsules containing dehydrated placenta—Oregon, 2016. Centers for Disease Control and Prevention. *Morb Mortal Wkly Rep*. 66(25):677-678.

Alternative Tools for Common Challenges

We cannot solve our problems with the same thinking we used when we created them.
—Albert Einstein

CHAPTER 9

Labor Dystocia

BABY LEO'S BIRTH

Leo's mother seemed to be a naturally anxious person, so I was not surprised when she reached out to me early one evening describing contractions that were consistent with a latent labor pattern. First time mothers often need reassurance during this phase of the labor, even though they are not ready to head to the hospital and do not "need" to call. However, Leo's mother seemed more uncomfortable than most and I worried that I was missing something, but I gave her some precautions and went about my evening. She called again around 1 am, now very uncomfortable with contractions, but still without a regular pattern to the labor. I told her to try a bath or a shower to ease her discomfort and wait and see if the contractions became more regular. If so, she was to head to the hospital.

No further call came that night, but by morning my phone was ringing again and Leo's mother was now sounding desperate, though the contractions were still not regular. I instructed her to meet me in the office in a few hours when we opened. I hoped she was far enough along to be admitted, because she was obviously having a difficult time. When she arrived, I knew at once she was not really in active labor. She was exhausted and miserable, but not breathing through contractions or showing any other signs of active labor. When I examined her, she was only two centimeters and the baby was still high in the pelvis. I saw the frustration on both her and her husband's face. I sent them back home with instructions to rest.

No further calls came that day, but at 2 am my phone was ringing again and she now was having mostly regular contractions. I sent her to the hospital and tried to go back to sleep, while awaiting word of her exam. Two hours later the call came in and the laborist had examined and found her to be four centimeters dilated. I hoped she would continue to progress and gave the orders for admission. By morning she was six centimeters, but still with a strange contraction pattern, where contractions would group up together and then space out sometimes for as many as ten minutes. She felt a lot of pressure with contractions, even though the baby was still high. She described it mostly as "front pressure" versus "back pressure." She continued to work through the labor for several more hours, walking, trying different positions, and using the shower. However, nothing seemed to bring the baby down and she remained six to seven centimeters until the afternoon. We decided to try breaking her water. That seemed to increase the intensity of the contractions and improved the pattern, but the dilation did not progress. I could tell Leo's head was not positioned correctly when I examined her, but she was so uncomfortable, it was difficult to determine exactly which way the baby was facing. She finally decided to get an epidural, too exhausted at this point to keep working through her contractions. After she was comfortable, we also started pitocin to try and help improve the pattern of the contractions. Despite all our efforts, we could not get the labor to advance and we headed into the operating room for a cesarean nearly 48 hours after her first call had come in. The Leo's head was "cocked" to the side, having entered the pelvis with one side of the head uneven from the other and he just could not descend the way he needed to.

Leo's birth story followed a common pattern that I have observed in many labors over the years. It is the story of labor dystocia, or stalled labor, but more importantly, it is a story of malposition. I have learned through experience to better manage it and I do not end up in the operating room as often as I did when I first entered private practice. However, I was not taught to recognize the signs of this problem or adjust my care of patients in response to malposition when I was in residency. One of my favorite attendings, without any malice, would passionately instruct us about how labor was simply a matter of the three P's: the Passenger, the Passageway, and the Power. The passenger was the baby and, if the baby was too big, labor could not progress normally. The passageway was the woman's pelvis and, if the pelvis was too narrow, the baby could not fit through. The power was the contractions. This was the one part of the equation we had any control over. If labor was not progressing, pitocin was solution. If labor was not progressing despite pitocin, we were taught to place an internal monitor which could determine whether or not we were giving enough pitocin. If the internal monitor measured sufficient contractions, then you knew your answer. Either the baby was too big or the mother's pelvis was too small and neither were things you could do anything about, so there was no point in continuing and the correct course of action was always a cesarean. Our hospital's rate of cesarean was over forty percent. This way of thinking was obviously missing something.

SLOWLY PROGRESSING LATENT LABOR

The first step in "managing" labor dystocia is to appropriately define it. Many providers are quick to diagnose a labor dystocia before a woman has even progressed into active labor. A woman cannot be diagnosed with a labor dystocia if she has not reached active labor and at least 6 cm of dilation. Latent labor is defined as the phase of labor when the laboring mother begins perceiving contractions, but active, predictable cervical dilation is not taking place. It is generally considered prolonged if it extends past 20 hours.[1] Many patients, like Leo's mother, have long, frustrating latent labors and, while this may be an early indicator of a malposition, it is not an indication for alarm given how frequently early malpositions self-correct. Latent labor may take a few hours or it can persist for many days. When it is prolonged, providers and patients alike find themselves resisting the urge to just "do something" in response, which often equates to medical pain relief and inductions for patients who had been hoping for a natural birth. There are certainly two ways to approach a long prodromal labor: actively or passively.

Active Approach to Prolonged Latent Labor

An active approach consists of trying various things, either medical or nonmedical, to "move the labor along." *Walking* and staying physically active are generally recommended as a way to help labor progress in natural labor texts, though there is no evidence that maternal activity truly advances a latent labor.[2] *Position changes*, such as side-lying or hands-and-knees (see Chapter 6), may help a woman advance by facilitating fetal rotation, if this is an underlying cause for her drawn out latent labor. *Sexual intercourse* has also been proposed as means to advance labor because human semen is a naturally occurring prostaglandin and synthetic prostaglandins are used to medically induce labor. So far, only one study has examined intercourse as a possible induction method and did not find increased intercourse improved outcomes; however, there was not a substantial difference in the amount of intercourse between the study and control groups and neither group was already showing signs of labor.[3] *Nipple stimulation*, when examined as a tool for induction, has been shown to decrease the number of women who have not delivered in a 72-hour window, so it seems reasonable to suggest that this may be a valid tool to help a woman progress through a slow latent phase.[4] Nipple stimulation may be performed either by hand or with a breast pump and is generally recommended to be performed for 5-minute intervals, separated by 10 minute rest periods, for up to 1 hour of duration or four pump-rest sets. Nipple stimulation may be performed as frequently as every 4 hours. There have been cases of too much stimulation of the uterus during nipple stimulation and, in one study of high-risk patients, may have even been associated with fetal harm. Therefore, caution is still advised with nipple stimulation and if contractions begin coming more frequently than every 4 minutes, it should be discontinued. *Membrane sweeping*, a more invasive method of labor stimulation in which a practitioner places a finger through the cervix and separates the bag of water away from the uterine wall, may also assist women in a prolonged latent labor, as this has been shown to decrease the likelihood of not being in labor within 48 hours.[5] However, membrane sweeping is painful and carries a small risk of early membrane rupture, so many women wish to avoid it or only use it as a latter option. If these more natural methods do not have their intended effect, the final resort in an active approach to a prolonged latent phase is medical management and intervention. Some providers offer what is termed a "morphine rest," where the mother is offered a systemic narcotic such as morphine or stadol, which is intended to help the mother obtain a little relief and rest, with the hope that this will advance the labor. Other providers simply offer a medical induction, usually in combination with an epidural, if a mother is struggling through early labor.

Passive Approach to Prolonged Latent Labor

However, given that a prolonged latent phase is not a cause for concern, a passive approach is another valid and likely better alternative. While the word passive has negative connotations in our culture, what being passive really means is accepting or allowing what happens without an active response or resistance to it. In short, a passive approach goes with the flow and often in labor and life, that is just what is needed. Mothers managing a prolonged latent labor in this fashion should focus on taking time to rest, while ensuring they remain properly hydrated and nourished. Showers or long baths are often utilized to ease discomfort. Women should continue to be emotionally supported through the process by their partner, doula, or family. Too often, partners head back to work once it is determined that it is not quite "go time," isolating a tired and uncomfortable mother who is trying to work through her prolonged early labor. Partners can help by offering massage, maintaining a calm and comforting environment for the mother to labor within, preparing meals, and offering frequent hydration. Hyperfocusing on the contraction pattern should be avoided, as this only heightens anxiety and frustration. It is nearly always clear when the labor has progressed to a more active phase, so parents do not need to fear the labor will rapidly progress without them knowing it. Distraction is a key part of this more relaxed approach. Women should be encouraged to sleep if they are able and, if they are unable, to continue through their normal daily activities as much as possible. Visiting with family or friends, watching television or a movie, "nesting" behavior such as cleaning or preparing last minute things for the baby, or reading are all activities that can help keep a mother's attention off her contractions and decrease her anxiety and discomfort in response to them.

The most valuable contributions providers and hospital staff can make during this process are reassurance and help in understanding the signs that latent labor has progressed into active labor. This is particularly true for first-time mothers who do not know what to expect from the labor process and often overreact to early labor symptoms. Patients and families should be counseled that labor is both progressive and persistent. Throughout labor, contractions will become progressively stronger, longer, and more frequent. Productive contractions, contractions that actually dilate the cervix in a rapid and predictable way, persist despite position changes and rest. A good rule of thumb for a woman in the early labor process is if she can fall asleep, she is not in active labor. If contractions stop in a particular position, they are not active labor contractions. In addition to the contraction pattern, other signs that may alert women to further progress are the presence of bloody, mucousy birth show outside of a recent cervical examination, rectal pressure, nausea, shaking, or the release of membranes. Women should be comforted in the fact that they are not alone in experiencing difficulty with this stage of the labor, especially when it extends for a long period of time, and should never be made to feel foolish for coming to the hospital "too soon."

SLOWLY PROGRESSING ACTIVE LABOR OR SECOND STAGE

Once a woman reaches the active phase of labor at approximately 6-cm dilation, dilation typically proceeds at a more predictable rate. As discussed in Chapter 5, it was previously believed that women in active labor should dilate at a rate of at least 1 cm/h. However, more recent studies demonstrate that it is perfectly normal for that rate of dilation to be as slow as 0.5 cm/h, with first-time mothers typically dilating at a slower rate than mothers who have had a previous vaginal delivery.[6] A prolonged active phase, or labor dystocia, occurs when the observed rate of dilation is slower than this 0.5 cm/h and a stalled labor, or arrest of labor, is defined as no progressive dilation for more than 2 hours.

Active phase dystocia is the most commonly observed labor abnormality and reason for deviation from a natural labor plan to one that involves epidurals, pitocin use, and cesarean sections.[7] In traditional obstetrics thinking, within the active management of labor framework, labor is viewed as a simple matter of physics. Adequate force is able to move an appropriately sized object through and adequate space: the power, the passenger, and the passageway. In this case, strong and frequent contractions are able to deliver a baby, presuming the baby is not too big or the maternal pelvis too small. Hence, all recommendations in the medical literature for management of labor dystocia center around how much power, or pitocin, should be given, how sufficient contractions are demonstrated, as measured by an internal pressure catheter in Montevideo units, and for how long it is advisable to wait in the setting of appropriate contraction strength before declaring that a vaginal delivery is impossible and proceeding with a cesarean. It is a very limited view of dystocia and, unsurprisingly, it offers a narrow range of remedies for the problem.

For a woman who presents in active labor, it is actually highly unlikely that suddenly her contractions will become inadequate to continue advancing her labor, unless something else alters the course of her labor, such as bed restriction, IV fluid administration, or an epidural. Absolute cephalopelvic disproportion (CPD), where the size of the baby's head simply will not fit through the woman's pelvis, regardless of position, is a contentious diagnosis to make clinically, in that it really cannot be proven, even with radiological studies.[8] Often women are told they are likely to have CPD, prior to labor, on the basis of a pelvic examination that reveals a prominent sacrum, a narrow pelvic arch, or an android or platypelloid pelvis. Women may also be warned about CPD if they are short in stature or short waisted, have a tall partner, are obese, or simply if their baby is suspected to be large.

While short stature and more narrow pelvis types are correlated with higher rates of labor dystocia and cesarean for CPD, the majority of women can have a vaginal delivery even when one of these risk factors are present.[9] This is because the pelvis is not a static structure. The bones of the pelvis are joined with connective tissue that can relax and stretch, increasing the dimensions of the pelvis by up to 20%, depending on maternal position. The size of a baby's head is also not constant. The fetal head has the ability to mold and elongate due to the presence of unfused sutures between the bones of the skull, facilitating passage through the narrow pelvic outlet. Several studies have shown that over 60% of patients who were diagnosed as having absolute CPD in a prior pregnancy and were offered a trial of labor in their second pregnancy went on to have a successful vaginal delivery, certainly calling into question how often absolute CPD actually occurs.[10,11]

The Fourth P: Position

More often than not, when dystocia occurs in a naturally laboring woman, it is due to *relative* CPD, meaning the baby's head cannot fit through the pelvis *in the position in which it is presenting*. Malpositions are difficult to diagnose using digital examination, with digital exams having been shown to be inaccurate up to 65% of the time when assessing fetal head position, and few providers utilize more reliable ultrasound assessments of position in routine practice.[12,13] Ideally, the baby should enter the pelvis in an occiput anterior (OA) position, with its head facing the maternal back. The most common malpositions encountered in labor are occiput posterior (OP), known as a sunny-side up baby where the head is facing out toward the mother's front, or occiput transverse (OT), where the head is facing one of the mother's hips. It is not uncommon for babies to enter labor in either one of these less ideal positions and the majority will simply rotate during the labor process, leading some to theorize that persistence of these positions are not actually malpositions, but rather intrapartum malrotations. Regardless of semantics, persistence of OP or OT positions into the later part of active labor or the second pushing stage of labor inhibits the proper flexion and extension of the fetal head as it moves under the mother's pubic bone, which is necessary for proper decent. Malpositions require the maternal pelvis to accommodate a much larger diameter of the fetal head, which is unable to mold and elongate in the usual fashion.

There are a number of factors that are known to increase the likelihood of malposition in labor. First-time mothers, mothers over the age of 35, and African American mothers all have higher rates of OP babies. Larger babies (>4000 g) and induced babies are also more likely to be OP.[14] The need for an epidural was previously believed to be a symptom of malposition, but more recent research suggests that epidurals are more likely increasing the rate of OP babies. It is surmised that epidurals either lead to early pelvic relaxation that permits babies to descend into the pelvis before proper rotation has occurred or that a more relaxed pelvis actually permits previously appropriately positioned babies to rotate to an OP position during labor.[15]

Regardless of etiology, there are few documented solutions for fetal malposition resulting in labor dystocia. In the medical research, the most promising solution appears to be *manual rotation* of the fetal head, which is generally performed at the start of the second stage of labor, prior to pushing. It is generally discouraged in the first stage of labor, due to a concern that it may increase the risk of cervical lacerations. Thus, for women who are unable to actually reach 10-cm dilation in the setting of a malposition, manual rotation is not necessarily a solution and most cesareans performed for dystocia are performed in the active phase of labor, rather than the second stage. However, manual rotation at the start of the second stage is successful 74% to 93% of the time, depending on the study, and results in a significantly lower incidence of both operative vaginal delivery and cesarean section and is associated with a shorter duration of pushing.[16–18] The American College of Obstetricians and Gynecologists lists manual rotation as one method, with strong evidence, of reducing cesarean rates.[19]

There are many proposed solutions to malpositions in the first stage of labor within the midwifery literature. Not many of these solutions have been adequately studied; however, given the significantly lower rate of cesarean among midwives, it is reasonable to assume they are doing something right. Obstetricians should be open to drawing upon the midwifery skills set, particularly in situations where modern medicine has had little to offer besides an operative solution. Most of the midwifery recommendations for encouraging rotation of an OP or OT baby are positional and include the following:

- *Forward-leaning positions*
Forward leaning positions (see Chapter 6) include *modified child's pose, hands-and-knees*, and *supported swaying or standing*. The birth ball can also be used to support the upper body in a forward-leaning position either standing or kneeling. Forward-leaning positions change the gravitational forces acting on the baby, encouraging the heavier part of the occiput to rotate against the maternal front instead of the back.[20] These positions also are more comfortable for mothers with OP babies, who frequently complain of significant back pain, as the weight of the baby's head is taken off of the lower back.[21] Forward-leaning positions also aid in achieving better alignment of the baby with the maternal pelvis and can be used in either first- or second-stage labor.

- *Side-lying positions*
Side-lying positions (see Chapter 6) are another suggested way to rotate the fetal head and also serve as more comfortable resting positions which provide a good opportunity for any needed fetal monitoring.

In a *true side-lying position*, the woman rests completely laterally, on the shoulder and hip, with both knees mildly bent, ideally with a pillow or wedge for support. If the direction of the head is known, the woman should lie on the side opposite to direction the baby is facing, on the side where to occiput is resting. For example, a baby in the right OP position should lay on her right side. The correct side to direct the mother toward can also be determined by abdominal palpation. The mother should lie on the side where the back of the baby is felt or the firm, solid side of the uterus is palpated.[22]

An alternative to true side-lying is the *semiprone* or *lateral asymmetric decubitus position*. In this position, the woman also rests completely laterally, on the shoulder and hip, but the lower leg is kept completely straight and the top leg is bent at both the knee and the hip, drawn up toward the chest. This position is also referred to as the *side-lying release* in the Spinning Babies literature by midwife Gail Tully, though she recommends a more exaggerated form where the top leg is draped over the side of a raised bed and the hip is supported by a birth attendant.[23] In the more traditional version, the top leg can be supported with a pillow or a peanut ball. The peanut ball is a 45 or 55 cm ball, literally shaped like a peanut. The ball is placed between the mother's thighs and supports the top leg in an elevated position, allowing for both an open pelvis and alternative gravitational forces to act on the fetal position. Peanut balls have not been studied specifically in regards to their effect on malpositions; however, two separate randomized control trials have demonstrated significantly shorter first stages of labor with the use of a peanut ball and one of these trials demonstrated a shorter second stage as well, with a lower incidence of operative delivery and cesarean section (Figure 9-1).[24,25]

When placing a mother in this position, the side chosen should be the opposite of that chosen in a true side-lying position, toward the direction the head is facing, on the side opposite the fetal occiput. For example, now a mother with a right OP baby will be placed on the left rather than the right. Again, choosing the side can also be done with abdominal palpation. The mother should lie on the side opposite where the fetal back is felt, or opposite to the firm, solid side of the uterus.

A recent randomized control trial of the semiprone position did not demonstrate efficacy in achieving rotation of the OP position, nor benefit in terms of labor speed or cesarean section rates, though the position was only consistently utilized for 1 hour and was not performed with a peanut ball.[26] There is certainly room for more research into this position and the peanut ball, particularly as it may benefit naturally laboring mothers.

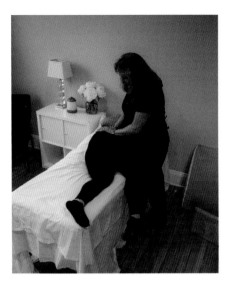

FIGURE 9-1. The semiprone or lateral asymmetric decubitus position.

- *Asymmetric positions*
  Other possible solutions to fetal malpositions that midwives tradi-tionally have employed are asymmetric positions. In these positions, the mother may either be kneeling, standing, or sitting, but raises one leg in a lunge fashion with the knee and hip bent. When sitting, the peanut ball can be used to support one leg in this fashion by placing it under the mother's knee. The suggested benefit of these positions is an increase in the dimensions of the pelvis on one side, encouraging the head to rotate into the area of more room. It is recommended that the mother lunge into the side of the occiput or where she feels the fetal back, similar to a true side-lying position. However, if the position is uncertain, she may simply alternate sides as is comfortable.

  When the position is unknown or labor dystocia occurs in the absence of an obvious malposition, a "**rollover sequence**" is recom-mended by physical therapist and childbirth educator Penny Simkin. In the rollover sequence, all of the positions that may aid in proper fetal rotation are utilized. The mother begins in a true right side-lying posi-tion, alternates to a right semiprone position, then assumes a forward-leaning position, followed by a left true side-lie and semiprone position, and finally a asymmetric sitting position.[22]

  Aside from positioning, there are other tools commonly used by mid-wives that may resolve a position-related dystocia. **Abdominal lifting** is

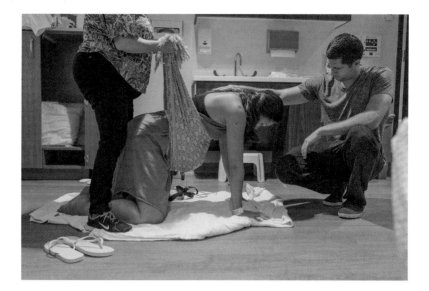

FIGURE 9-2. Abdominal lifting.

a technique that has been practiced by Mexican midwives with the aid of a rebozo, a long woven cloth approximately 45-cm wide by 150-cm long. The cloth is wrapped under the laboring mother's belly and the two ends are held by a birth attendant who applies gentle backward and upward traction (Figure 9-2).[27] This may either be done with the mother standing and the birth attendant standing behind her or with the mother in a forward-leaning position and the birth attendant standing over her. It is thought to improve upon the angle at which the baby enters the pelvis, helping to rotate the baby with contractions. It has not been studied in terms of efficacy for labor dystocia, but women who used the technique reported less pain and felt it improved their feeling of being supported by their partner and midwife.[28] The rebozo can also be used to move the mother's hips from side to side by alternating the traction applied to cloth. This can also be done with the rebozo wrapped under the woman's bottom and the birth attendant standing in front of her, moving her hips from side to side in a dance-like fashion while she leans backwards, creating a rotating asymmetric standing position that may be helpful, as well as little more fun in the labor room if some upbeat music is played. The rebozo can be substituted with a simple long hospital sheet in traditional labor and delivery units and women can also lift their belly with their hands to achieve a similar effect.

Hydrotherapy, as previously discussed, can also be considered as a noninvasive tool to remedy a prolonged labor. Apart from providing improved pain relief in a patient who is likely struggling to labor naturally at this point, one randomized controlled trial found water immersion in a labor tub to be comparable to standard labor augmentation with amniotomy and pitocin in the setting of a labor dystocia. In those that were randomized to the labor tub, there was a significantly lower rate of epidural use, no difference in the rate of operative delivery, and 29% needed no further augmentation for labor progression.[29] This study shows that there are simple, nonmedical alternatives that should be considered when labor stalls which have a high likelihood of honoring a naturally laboring woman's intention for her birth.

Inadequate Contraction Activity

While the majority of labor dystocia is due to malposition and many suggest that inadequate contraction activity is actually a symptom of malposition, even if it is not identified on examination, there are situations where contraction activity is insufficient to generate continued progression of the labor, even in active phase. Some possible cause of this are improper nourishment and hydration, prolonged immobility, and maternal exhaustion. Some of the recommendations for management of a prolonged latent labor may help augment a prolonged active labor as well such as ambulation, food and drink, nipple stimulation, and rest if needed. However, another possible cause of insufficient contractions is something referred to in midwifery texts as an "**emotional dystocia**," where fear, fatigue, and prolonged discomfort either with the labor environment or the labor itself cause the release of stress hormones which negatively impact the proper hormonal signaling necessary for proper oxytocin production. As discussed in Chapter 4, the mother's emotional state does appear to impact the labor process, though this is not often paid much attention to in traditional maternity care. If a care provider suspects that a woman's emotions are inhibiting the labor, it can be very helpful to simply talk to the woman about her thoughts and fears about the labor in an open, nonjudgmental way that acknowledges how common and normal it is for women to feel anxious during the labor process. Open dialogue will help the care providers better address what might be causing the woman distress. Prevention of "emotional dystocia" is also important. Attention to the labor environment is essential and providers need to recognize that they are part of the environment. By treating women with gentle, kind respect throughout the labor, informing them of what to expect, and obtaining their understanding and consent for any treatment, much of the maternal fear response can be avoided and hopefully, along with it, any negative consequence on the labor progress as well.

The Fifth P: Patience

On one final note, patience is crucial to the labor process and has been forgotten in our efficiency-oriented medical culture. So long as both mother and baby are doing well, everyone in the labor team should pause and consider whether they really need to do anything. Often all that is needed to resolve a labor dystocia is a little time. This was a clear message in ACOG's recommendations for avoiding cesarean.[19] In nearly every study examining labor dystocias in all stages, time was not harmful and helped a large proportion of women achieve vaginal deliveries.

REFERENCES

1. Friedman EA, Sachtleben MR. Amniotomy and the course of labor. *Obstet Gynecol.* 1963;22:755-770.
2. American College of Obstetricians and Gynecologists, Committee on Practice Bulletins-Obstetrics. Dystocia and augmentation of labor. *Int J Gynaecol Obstet.* 2004;85(3):315-324.
3. Kavanagh J, Kelly AJ, Thomas J. Sexual intercourse for cervical ripening and induction of labour. *Cochrane Database Syst Rev.* 2001;2(CD003093).
4. Kavanagh J, Kelly AJ, Thomas J. Breast stimulation for cervical ripening and induction of labour. *Cochrane Database Syst Rev.* 2005;3:1-56. CD003392.
5. Mozurkewich EL, Chilimigras JL, Berman DR, et al. Methods of induction of labour: a systematic review. *BMC Pregnancy Childbirth.* 2011;11:84. doi:10.1186/1471-2393-11-84.
6. Neal JL, Lowe NK, Patrick TE, et al. What is the slowest-yet-normal cervical dilation rate among nulliparous women with spontaneous labor onset? *J Obstet Gynecol Neonatal Nurs.* 2010;39(4):361-369.
7. Abraham W, Berhan Y. Predictors of labor abnormalities in university hospital: unmatched case control study. *BMC Pregnancy Childbirth.* 2014;4:256. doi:10.1186/1471-2393-14-256.
8. Maharaj D. Assessing cephalopelvic disproportion: back to the basics. *Obstet Gynecol Surv.* 2010;65(6):387-395. doi:10.1097/OGX.0b013e3181ecdf0c.
9. Toh-Adam R, Srisupundit K, Tongsong T. Short stature as an independent risk factor for cephalopelvic disproportion in a country of relatively small-sized mothers. *Arch Gynecol Obstet.* 2012;285(6):1513-1516. doi:10.1007/s00404-011-2168-3.
10. Impey L, O'Herlihy C. First delivery after cesarean delivery for strictly defined cephalopelvic disproportion. *Obstet Gynecol.* 1998;92(5):799-803.
11. Clark SL, Eglinton GS, Beall M, Phelan JP. Effect of indication for previous cesarean section on subsequent delivery outcome in patients undergoing a trial of labor. *J Reprod Med.* 1984;29(1):22-25.

12. Sherer DM, Miodovnik M, Bradley KS, Langer O. Intrapartum fetal head position II: comparison between transvaginal digital examination and transabdominal ultrasound assessment during the second stage of labor. *Ultrasound Obstet Gynecol.* 2002;19(3):264-268.

13. Gilboa Y, Perlman S, Karp H, et al. What do obstetricians really think about ultrasound in the delivery room? *Isr Med Assoc J.* 2017;19(4):234-236.

14. Caughey AB, Sharshiner R, Cheng YW. Fetal malposition: impact and management. *Clin Obstet Gynecol.* 2015;58(2):241-245.

15. Lieberman E, Davidson K, Lee-Parritz A, Shearer E. Changes in fetal position during labor and their association with epidural analgesia. *Obstet Gynecol.* 2005;105(5 pt 1): 974-982.

16. Shaffer BL, Cheng YW, Vargas JE, et al. Manual rotation of the fetal occiput: predictors of success and delivery. *Am J Obstet Gynecol.* 2006;194(5):e7-e9.

17. Le Ray C, Serres P, Schmitz T, et al. Manual rotation in occiput posterior or transverse position: risk factors and consequences on cesarean delivery rate. *Obstet Gynecol.* 2007;110(4):873-879.

18. Shaffer BL, Cheng YW, Vargas JE, Caughey AB. Manual rotation to reduce caesarean delivery in persistent occiput posterior or transverse position. *J Matern Fetal Neonatal Med.* 2011;24(1):65-72.

19. Caughey AB, Cahill AG, Guise JM, Rouse DJ; American College of Obstetricians and Gynecologists (College); Society for Maternal-Fetal Medicine. Safe prevention of the primary cesarean delivery. *Am J Obstet Gynecol.* 2014;210(3):179-193. doi:10.1016/j.ajog.2014.01.026.

20. Stremler R, Hodnett E, Petryshen P, et al. Randomized controlled trial of hands-and-knees positioning for occipitoposterior position in labor. *Birth.* 2005;32(4):243-251.

21. Guittier MJ, Othenin-Girard V, de Gasquet B, et al. Maternal positioning to correct occiput posterior fetal position during the first stage of labour: a randomised controlled trial. *BJOG.* 2016;123(13):2199-2207.

22. Simpkins P, Ancheta R. *The Labor Progress Handbook: Early Interventions to Prevent and Treat Dystocia.* Ames, IA: Wiley-Blackwell; 2011.

23. Tully G. Sidelying release. Available at https://spinningbabies.com/learn-more/techniques/the-fantastic-four/sidelying-release/. Accessed 6/2017.

24. Roth C, Dent SA, Parfitt SE, et al. Randomized controlled trial of use of the peanut ball during labor. *Am J Matern Child Nurs.* 2016;41(3):140-146.

25. Tussey CM, Botsios E, Gerkin RD, et al. Reducing length of labor and cesarean surgery rate using a peanut ball for women laboring with an epidural. *J Perinat Educ.* 2015;24(1):16-24.

26. Le Ray C, Lepleux F, De La Calle A, et al. Lateral asymmetric decubitus position for the rotation of occipito-posterior positions: multicenter randomized controlled trial EVADELA. *Am J Obstet Gynecol.* 2016;215(4):511.e1-511.e7.

27. Cohen SR, Thomas CR. Rebozo technique for fetal malposition in labor. *J Midwifery Womens Health.* 2015;60(4):445-451.

28. Iversen ML, Midtgaard J, Ekelin M, Hegaard HK. Danish women's experiences of the rebozo technique during labour: a qualitative explorative study. *Sex Reprod Healthc.* 2017;11:79-85.

29. Cluett ER, Pickering RM, Getliffe K, St George Saunders NJ. Randomised controlled trial of labouring in water compared with standard of augmentation for management of dystocia in first stage of labour. *BMJ.* 2004;328(7435):314.

TOOLS FOR COMMON CHALLENGES

CHAPTER 10

Fetal
Monitoring
Challenges

Every time someone comes into Labor and Delivery with a natural birth plan, I cannot help but find myself hoping they are not assigned to me. It's not for the reason you might think. I actually like taking care of naturally laboring women. I feel like I can be a much greater help to them than somebody who is just going to come in and get an epi. The reason it is so hard is because it is impossible to monitor them. Either I am running in there every fifteen minutes getting a heart rate, in the middle of everything else I have to do, or I am trying to figure out a way to keep the stupid bands in place while they are moving all over the place. I never actually get a good strip and then I have to sit there and chart that. Depending on who the doctor is, it can also be difficult. A lot of them still want the patients continuously monitored, which is nearly impossible. I had one doctor tell me they didn't give a damn if I had to sit on the floor and hold the monitor in place the entire labor. I wish my job was so easy that I could take the time to do that. I wish there was a better way to let women labor the way they want and still make sure the baby is okay. I also have to say, even though I have read the research that says it's okay for moms to be off the monitor, every time they are I still hold my breath whenever I go to put that monitor back on. It gives me angina. I guess I am just too anxious.

—S. R., Labor and Delivery Nurse

The first challenge in regards to fetal monitoring in healthy natural labors is gaining acceptance among hospitals and obstetricians that there are alternatives to continuous electronic fetal heart rate monitoring (EFM). As discussed in Chapter 5, despite the lack of evidence in support of EFM in low-risk mothers, the practice is widespread and deeply entrenched in standard obstetrics practice. Nurses, doctors, and hospital administrators need to reacquaint themselves with the evidence concerning effective fetal monitoring in order to become more open minded about options such as intermittent auscultation. However, it is unlikely that this will change anytime soon and most naturally laboring women will find their hospital and/or provider will recommend electronic monitoring for at least some portion of their labor.

Thus, practically speaking, the real challenge for women, their nurses, and their providers is to find ways to monitor that do not inhibit ambulation, positioning, and access to hydrotherapy. Mothers undergoing EFM have traditionally been restricted to the bed because monitoring was conducted via abdominal transducers, which were attached with approximately 3-feet long wires to large, bulky machines. The majority of maternity units still utilize these large monitors for some or all of their fetal monitoring. However, within the last 10 years, mobile and wireless technology has enabled a significant step in the right direction in supporting natural labor. *Mobile monitors* have become much more widespread and permit mothers to remain ambulatory, even during continuous EFM. The mechanism is the same, abdominal transducers are connected to a large, central monitor, except in the case of mobile monitors, the wires actually attach to a purse size receiver which transmits the signal wirelessly to the central machine. Newer monitors even bypass the receiver and the wires, allowing the transducers themselves to transmit the wireless signal to the central unit. Studies have demonstrated comparable quality of fetal heart rate tracings when compared to directly connected monitoring, with improvement in patient mobility and satisfaction.[1,2] Mobile monitors utilizing the purse-like receiver even allow mothers access to hydrotherapy while monitored, as the receiver can simply be kept outside of the shower or tub while the abdominal transducers, which can get wet, remain attached to the mother.

The most common frustration in mobile EFM is maintaining the proper position of the abdominal transducers, which are held in place with two separate, 1.5-inch wide elastic straps and often slide or flip as the laboring mother changes position. There are many more effective ways to attach the transducers to ambulatory mothers. All that is involved is a little creativity and patience. While no studies have been performed on these techniques, many motivated nurses, doulas, midwives, and doctors are using these techniques every day and achieving adequate fetal monitoring.

BELLY BANDS

Belly bands offer a simple, inexpensive alternative to the usual double-strapped monitoring. Belly bands are soft, fabric bands with interwoven elastic that cover the entire abdomen of the laboring mother. The transducers are held much more securely in one position on the belly as the mother changes position and the band prevents flipping of the transducer as well. The connecting wires can also be tucked into the band, reducing the risk of trips and falls (Figure 10-1).

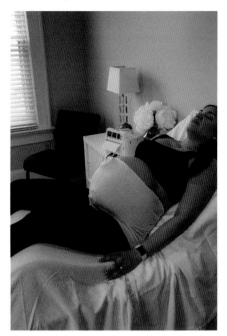

FIGURE 10-1. Belly bands.

TAPING

Another simple solution to this problem is taping the transducers in place. Kinesiology tape or wide silk surgical tape can be used. Every pregnant belly is different, but generally a long strip of tape crossing horizontally across the abdomen can be used to initially secure the transducer. Then two additional strips should be placed in an x-fashion across the transducer, again stretching from one side of the belly to the other. Vertical strips can be added on the sides of the belly for additional support and to prevent the edges of the other strips from lifting (Figure 10-2).

HYDROTHERAPY MONITORING

Securing monitors during hydrotherapy offers an even greater challenge because water rinses away the gel medium necessary for proper conduction of the Doppler fetal heart rate. Ideally, simple auscultation of the fetal heart rate every 15 minutes using a waterproof hand-held

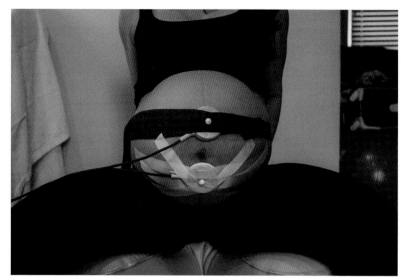

FIGURE 10-2. Taping.

Doppler should be sufficient monitoring during hydrotherapy in the low-risk mother. However, if the mother requires continuous EFM for a higher risk condition or her provider insists on it, hydrotherapy should not be withheld as a result. A large piece of tegaderm, the stretchy film-like covering used by anesthesiologists to secure epidural sites, can be placed over the Doppler transducer and then further secured by placing several strips of silk tape across the tegaderm covered transducer. This both secures the transducer in place and provides a waterproof seal that prevents loss of the transducer gel.

PATIENT-ASSISTED MONITORING

The laboring mother and her support team is an often overlooked resource in achieving adequate fetal monitoring in the ambulatory patient. After a quick, 5-minute instruction, most patients can be taught to easily adjust the transducer and find their baby's heart rate. Motivated mothers will happily assist in any way they can in order to retain freedom of movement and often take comfort in feeling in control of this part of the process. Studies have demonstrated that women are perfectly able to perform adequate EFM, even in the comfort of their own home.[3]

TOOLS FOR COMMON CHALLENGES

THE NEWEST TECHNOLOGY: ABDOMINAL SURFACE ELECTRODES

Anyone who has fought through the struggles of fetal monitoring has asked themselves or been asked by a patient, "isn't there a better way to do this?" Researchers and medical technology manufacturers are currently developing fetal monitoring via abdominal surface electrodes. These monitors stick onto the abdomen in the same fashion as EKG electrodes and are connected to a wireless transmitter that also is attached to the abdomen. Two types of peel-and-stick electrode systems are currently being marketed in the United States.[4,5]

Researchers have proposed that these systems may even be able to provide superior screening for fetal acidosis than EFM, as they are able to perform fetal electrocardiography, meaning analysis of the heart beat wave, rather than simple electrocardiotocography, meaning comparison of the heart rate to contraction pattern. However, the preliminary research indicates that the main benefit of these systems is quality, non-position dependent, mobile fetal monitoring.[6,7]

INTERMITTENT AUSCULTATION

Aside from the difficulty in getting hospitals and providers to trust intermittent auscultation, it is not without its own technical challenges in implementation. The main issue with intermittent auscultation is the time required to do it for a nursing staff that is already overburdened with patient care and documentation requirements. As one nurse told a recent patient, "you can have intermittent auscultation so long as you brought your own doppler and a nurse to do it." Typical intermittent auscultation protocols call for auscultation of the heart beat every 15 minutes in active labor, for 1- to 2-minute duration. This leaves little time for doing anything else in between and is particularly challenging with 2:1 staffing ratios, with each nurse caring for two patients. One easy administrative solution is *1:1 nursing* for naturally laboring women being monitored with intermittent auscultation. However, given the financial realities of health care today, this solution is unlikely to be implemented.

A better, simpler solution is *patient-led monitoring*. Again, easy instruction in finding the fetal heart rate can be provided when a mother presents in labor or could even be taught during outpatient prenatal visits. The mother is provided with a recording sheet to document the fetal heart rate or the heart rate check may be done with the EFM transducer so her nurse may observe the rate from outside the room. A timer should be placed in the room to remind the mother and her support team when it is time to check the heart rate and they should be instructed on the normal heart rate and when to alert their nurse with a concern. Again, this would give control of the monitoring back to the mother and allow her to conduct monitoring in comfortable positions and at times that are convenient for her in relation to her contraction pattern.

Patients have already been taught to take their own vital signs, monitor their blood sugar, inject medication, and monitor their baby's input and output. There is no reason they cannot be taught to perform this task, especially if doing so will increase the availability of intermittent auscultation as a monitoring option.

REFERENCES

1. Boatin AA, Wylie B, Goldfarb I, et al. Wireless fetal heart rate monitoring in inpatient full-term pregnant women: testing functionality and acceptability. *PLoS ONE.* 2015;10(1):e0117043. doi:10.1371/journal.pone.0117043.
2. Mugyenyi GR, Atukunda EC, Ngonzi J, et al. Functionality and acceptability of a wireless fetal heart rate monitoring device in term pregnant women in rural Southwestern Uganda. *BMC Pregnancy Childbirth.* 2017;17(1):178.
3. Kerner R, Yogev Y, Belkin A, et al. Maternal self-administered fetal heart rate monitoring and transmission from home in high-risk pregnancies. *Int J Gynaecol Obstet.* 2004;84(1):33-39.
4. OB Medical Company Press Release. OBMedical Company® announces LaborView product launch at AWHONN conference in Dallas. Available at http://www. obmedco.com/news_media.html. Accessed June 14, 2016.
5. Novii Wireless Patch System. Available at http://www.monicahealthcare.com/products/labour-and-delivery/monica-novii-wireless-patch-system. Accessed 7/2017.
6. Fuchs T, Grobelak K, Pomorski M, Zimmer M. Fetal heart rate monitoring using maternal abdominal surface electrodes in third trimester: can we obtain additional information other than CTG trace? *Adv Clin Exp Med.* 2016;25(2):309-316.
7. Martinek R, Kahankova R, Nazeran H, et al. Non-invasive fetal monitoring: a maternal surface ECG electrode placement-based novel approach for optimization of adaptive filter control parameters using the LMS and RLS algorithms. *Sensors (Basel).* 2017;17(5).pii: E1154.

TOOLS FOR COMMON CHALLENGES

CHAPTER 11

Ineffective Pain Management

The first twelve hours of my labor were easy. I had prepared well for my labor and all the tools I learned were really effective. However, at a certain point, I felt like I hit a wall and just couldn't do it anymore. I just wanted to be done. I didn't care about anything anymore, I was so tired and so uncomfortable. I told my nurse I was really having trouble and asked what else I could do and she didn't pause for a moment before saying, "get an epidural." In my state, I couldn't come up with any of my own alternatives and my husband was half-asleep on his feet by this point, so I just went with it. But it didn't feel good, it felt like I was weak or was just giving up or something. In the end, my baby was healthy and I know there are no prizes for having a natural birth, but I really did want that experience and was bummed it didn't go that way. I wish someone had been able to help me in some other way besides just: here, take the drugs.

—M. V., new mother

Ineffective pain management is usually discussed in the context of pharmacologic methods of pain relief. However, women using nonpharmacologic methods of pain management in labor can also encounter periods of time when those tools become less effective and a mother who had previously been managing her labor well finds herself having difficulty coping. The typical medical response to this situation would simply be to offer pharmacologic pain relief. However, there are many alternatives that can be tried before abandoning the plan for an unmedicated birth. An understanding of some of the common patterns of uncontrolled pain can guide care providers and laboring women toward alternatives that may be the most helpful.

COMMON PATTERNS OF PAIN OBSERVED IN NATURAL LABOR AND POSSIBLE SOLUTIONS

Significant Back Pain

"Back labor" is particularly difficult for women to manage with natural techniques. Some women predominantly feel contractions in their back, regardless of fetal position, but if a woman is complaining of strong back pain, a sunny-side up or occiput posterior baby is the usual culprit. In this position, the weight of the back of the baby's head presses against the sacrum and creates intense discomfort. **Alternative maternal positioning** can help with both fetal rotation and pain relief, particularly forward-leaning positions.[1] Most mothers find lying in the bed to be a nearly impossible position to maintain when they are suffering through a back labor. *Massage* is another option that mothers and their labor support team can try to reduce back pain. Generally, for this type of discomfort a higher pressure massage of the lower back, buttocks, and thighs is most helpful, though the pressure should always be modified for the mother's comfort. Some women may prefer *light touch or effleurage massage*, where the skin of the back and arms is gently skimmed with the fingertips instead of deeply pressing into the muscles. This also helps relax the muscles underneath and aids in calming the mother. Either technique can be easily performed with the mother in any of the forward-leaning positions and studies, while small in scope, have demonstrated less pain, shorter labors, and reduced feelings of depression and anxiety in massaged mothers.[2,3] The positive psychological effects are likely due to the touch element and more active involvement of the labor support team. Another specific hands-on technique that can be helpful for all laboring women, but particularly those with significant back pain, is counterpressure. *Counterpressure* is provided by placing the heels of both hands or fists on the woman's lower back, at the level of the sacrum, directly above the buttocks, and applying strong, steady pressure during contractions. Many women working through a back labor request counterpressure through each contraction and find that it is the only tool that enables them to continue without medical intervention (Figure 11-1).

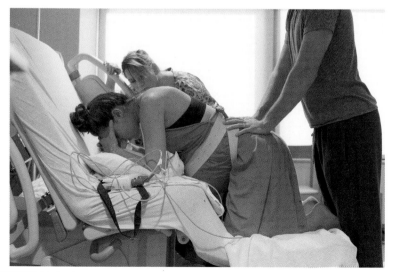

FIGURE 11-1. Counterpressure.

Hydrotherapy, as previously discussed, is one of the most effective, nonpharmacological methods of pain relief. For women struggling with significant back pain, the shower may be the most useful, as the water pressure and heat against the back aids in muscle relaxation in a manner similar to massage. Generally, however, the shower is only effective in 20-minute intervals and the mother should be encouraged to try alternatives once she finds the shower is no longer helpful. Some women go between the tub and shower, with the buoyancy of the tub relieving back pressure and the shower aiding in muscle relaxation. The best of both worlds can be a labor tub with a hand-held shower attachment which can be directed onto the lower back. On dry land, *heat packs* on the lower back can also assist a mother with poorly tolerated back pain.

Another option that may be considered is the use of a transcutaneous electrical nerve stimulation device, or *TENS unit*. The unit should be applied to the back, generally along acupressure points at the level of the sacrum and subscapular regions. TENS units have been studied widely and have not been shown to have significant benefit in labor; however, patients do report less severe pain with its use.[4] Many labor units provide access to these devices, though they can also be purchased inexpensively by individual women. If other methods are not providing relief, a TENS may take the edge off the labor discomfort to a sufficient degree to enable a naturally laboring mother to avoid pharmacologic options (Figure 11-2).

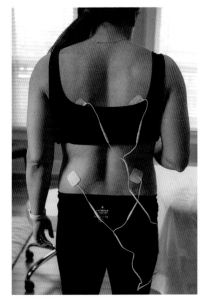

FIGURE 11-2. TENS unit.

Significant Hip Pain

Significant hip pain, like back pain, is often an indication of fetal malposition. An occiput transverse (OT) position generally creates hip pain on the side opposite to the direction the baby is facing, as the heavy back of the baby's head pushes against the hip. An acynclitic position, where the baby's head is angled against one hip or another, also creates hip pain. *Alternative maternal positioning* offers a good first step toward correcting these types of malpositions. Side-lying positions, the rollover sequence, and asymmetrical lunges and stances, as described in Chapters 6 and 9, are the best positions to try with a mother complaining of hip pain.

Another technique that may provide relief for significant hip pain is a *hip squeeze.* During the hip squeeze, which is usually performed with the mother in any of the forward-leaning positions, the woman's support partner places the full palm of each hand across the outer edge of the woman's hips and across the gluteal muscles, below the level of the iliac crests, which are the bones that can be felt at the top of buttocks, at the base of the lower back. The support partner then squeezes inwards during contractions. The exact location and intensity of the pressure applied should be modified to the mother's comfort. Alternatively, a *rebozo* or long sheet can be wrapped from front to back, across the woman's hips, then pulled tight or even tied tightly across her buttocks and lower back to provide similar pressure against the hips. While this technique has not been studied in labor, the use of pelvic support belts in pregnancy, which this technique mimics, has been shown to improve pelvic girdle pain.[5,6]

Massage of the gluteal muscles around the hip in question can also be helpful, as well as application of a *TENS* unit specifically to the muscles that are causing the most discomfort. *Heat and cold* can also be alternated on the hip joint to relieve discomfort and inflammation. *Hydrotherapy* is particularly effective for mother's struggling with hip pain, specifically immersion in a labor tub. The buoyancy of the water takes some of the weight of the malpositioned baby off the joint, aids in muscle relaxation, and can assist in rotation and better fetal positioning.

Premature Urge to Push

Many naturally laboring women experience intense rectal pressure and the urge to bear down before full dilation. This sensation can be quite distressing and confusing for the laboring mother, as well as her care providers. On the one hand, premature pushing can lead to cervical swelling, slowing of the labor process, and even cervical lacerations, which can be challenging to repair and cause significant maternal blood loss after delivery. But alternatively, sometimes the woman's urge to push is more reflective of what she needs to do than her cervical exam and "early" pushing allows the baby's head to stretch the cervix, achieve full dilation, and deliver the baby more rapidly.

Ideally, however, women should be pushing when the cervix is fully dilated and good decent of the head has occurred. A premature urge to push often accompanies an occiput posterior baby and, hence, many of the techniques that assist in rotation of this position help relieve a premature urge to push as well (see Chapter 9). Specifically, deeper, *knee-chest positions* in which the laboring mother's bottom is higher than her torso may take the weight of the baby's head off the rectum. Some women also find *toilet sitting* or sitting on a birth stool to be comforting, as this is position where women are accustomed to feeling rectal pressure and may find the sensation less stressful.

Modification of breathing technique may also assist a laboring mother who feels the need to push. Instead of the deep belly, Ujjayi breathing typically used throughout contractions, women with the urge to push may feel better vocalizing and grunting through contractions, which allows them to apply a modest amount of pushing pressure, satisfying the urge, while simultaneously releasing the breath, preventing forceful pushing and damage to the cervix. *Hydrotherapy*, specifically the immersion in the labor tub, is also very helpful for mothers with a premature urge to push, as again the buoyancy of the water relieves pelvic pressure sensations.

If the mother is at least 9 cm dilated, the other option is to simply do a *trial of pushing.* Often side-lying or hands-and-knees pushing positions are best when some cervix is still present, as this places less tension on the cervix and may aid in rotation of the fetal head. Forceful pushing should be avoided, to prevent both maternal exhaustion and cervical injury, and the cervix should be monitored for swelling during the pushing. If the cervix is soft and pliable, it can often be reduced behind the fetal head with gentle digital pressure. If significant cervical swelling occurs or the pushing does not seem effective and the mother continues to experience an uncontrollable urge to push, unrelieved with other methods, an epidural should be considered to prevent cervical injury.

Maternal Exhaustion

At times, a mother who had been previously managing her labor well may find difficulty coping due to sheer exhaustion. This is particularly true for women who experience prolonged labor, either latent or active, or a labor with a short interval between contractions. When laboring mothers become exhausted, they often find it difficult to maintain their breathing technique and stay mobile or in positions that might be more comfortable for them, but require physical strength to sustain.

The first thing that should be evaluated is the *hydration and nutrition status* of the laboring mother. Labor puts similar demands on the body as prolonged exercise. If a laboring woman is not eating and drinking properly, labor will quickly drain her energy. Women should be offered food and drink throughout labor, but especially if they are expressing extreme amounts of fatigue.

The next important step is to find a *manageable rest position*. Side-lying positions are frequently utilized and often a more comfortable way to rest than lying on the back. An alternative resting position is sitting relatively upright, with the legs in a wide-open butterfly position. Deep breathing during the contractions, with the eyes remaining closed, and the body in a loose and limp state may help maintain relaxation even while the mother is working through a contraction. Maintaining a relaxed state during contractions helps the mother rest more effectively in between contractions as well. Attention should also be given to ensuring a *calm atmosphere* in the room. Lights should be turned down or off. The room should be quiet or relaxing music played. Only the minimum number of people needed for support should remain with the mother. Aromatherapy may also be utilized. *Guided meditation*, such as that utilized in the HypnoBirthing technique, can also be used to quiet the mother's mind and help her rest, even if she is unable to sleep.

If the mother is unable to achieve a comfortable resting position, *hydrotherapy* can often provide sufficient relief to overcome maternal exhaustion. The labor tub is particularly helpful, as the laboring mother does not need to hold her own body weight and can easily maintain the most comfortable position, needing only to focus on her breathing technique during contractions. However, the shower can also be helpful for an overtired mother, as even a small amount of pain relief can provide an opportunity to rest and regroup.

OTHER CONSIDERATIONS IN THE SETTING OF INEFFECTIVE PAIN MANAGEMENT

Regardless of the pattern of ineffective pain management that is being observed, it is important for care providers to consider if any additional factors may be contributing to the mother's difficulty in coping.

TOOLS FOR COMMON CHALLENGES

Breathing Technique

When pain is not controlled well or a mother is under stress, her breathing pattern will often become shallow and hurried. This can lead to hyperventilation, which can be associated with dizziness, fetal heart rate changes, and pain exacerbation. It is very important to help the mother breathe slowly and deeply. Sometimes this requires verbally just talking to her through each contraction when pain is difficult to manage. The mother should be breathing through the nose, deeply into the belly. Counting the breath can assist the mother in maximizing her inhalation and exhalation when she is losing her focus. Ensuring she maintains relaxed shoulders and jaw will also aid in more effective breathing.

Proper Emotional Support

Working through an unmedicated labor can be lonely and isolating for many women. Hands-on support from an engaged and loving team is essential. Any criticism of the way the woman is laboring should be avoided. Comments like, "you need to calm down," or "you are making this worse for yourself," are particularly undermining of naturally laboring woman's emotional well-being and ability to continue through the process. All comments should be empathetic, encouraging, and complementary. It is tiring and difficult to support a woman through labor, but consideration of her emotional needs should supersede any personal concerns. If a member of the labor team is having difficulty maintaining proper emotional support, rest for that team member should be provided. A short break to eat something or get some fresh air can help a team member provide better support when they are in the room.

Respecting a Change in Plan

While providers and support team members should not jump to offer pharmacologic pain relief to a mother who is struggling with pain, but intends a natural birth, it is also important that if she expresses a desire for medical options, this is respected. Once a mother makes a definitive statement requesting pain relief, while alternatives can still be offered, the team should begin moving forward in providing pharmacologic relief and should not attempt to talk the laboring mother out of that decision. Specifics in managing this change in labor plan will be discussed in the following chapter; however, more often than not, a laboring mother knows what she needs and what she is capable of. Sometimes flexibility is required and can help a mother reach her overall goals. That flexibility should be encouraged and praised.

REFERENCES

1. Guittier MJ, Othenin-Girard V, de Gasquet B, et al. Maternal positioning to correct occiput posterior fetal position during the first stage of labour: a randomised controlled trial. *BJOG.* 2016;123(13):2199-2207.
2. Field T, Hernandez-Reif M, Taylor S, Quintino O, Burman I. Labor pain is reduced by massage therapy. *J Psychosom Obstet Gynaecol.* 1997;18(4):286-291.
3. Smith CA, Levett KM, Collins CT, Jones L. Massage, reflexology and other manual methods for pain management in labour. *Cochrane Database Syst Rev.* 2012;2:1-45. CD009290.
4. Dowswell T, Bedwell C, Lavender T, Neilson JP. Transcutaneous electrical nerve stimulation (TENS) for pain relief in labour. *Cochrane Database Syst Rev.* 2009;2: 1-75. CD007214.
5. Bertuit J, Van Lint CE, Rooze M, Feipel V. Pregnancy and pelvic girdle pain: analysis of pelvic belt on pain. *J Clin Nurs.* May 25, 2017. [Epub ahead of print]. doi:10.1111/jocn.13888.
6. Mens JM. Does a pelvic belt reduce hip adduction weakness in pregnancy-related posterior pelvic girdle pain? A case-control study. *Eur J Phys Rehabil Med.* March 1, 2017. [Epub ahead of print]. doi:10.23736/S1973-9087.17.04442-2. Available at https://www.minervamedica.it/en/journals/europa-medicophysica/article.php?cod=R33Y9999N00A17030101. Accessed May 2017

CHAPTER 12

Integrating Medical Intervention into a Natural Birth Plan

The expression "life is what happens while you are busy making other plans," often applies in both life and labor. Labor is frequently the initiation for parents into the reality that kids will most often do what they want, in the way they want, when they want and parental control and influence over them is limited. This recognition of the unpredictability of the labor process and a willingness to adapt one's plan for labor in response to the situation is important for all women intending to labor naturally, as it helps reduce the negative feelings of disappointment or failure that may otherwise develop if the need for medical intervention arises. However, it is equally important for medical staff to recognize that helping laboring women maintain as much control over the process as possible reduces the likelihood that the birth will be traumatic for their patients or that their patients will suffer from postpartum depression and anxiety disorders.[1] Too often, when a natural labor begins to veer off course, to borrow from another common expression, the baby is thrown out with the bath water. The decision to alter course and utilize any medical intervention in the labor process leads to a complete abandonment of all the intentions the parents had for their delivery and a uniform adoption of the traditional medical birth model. This tendency is not usually necessary and often leaves mothers feeling that they in some way failed or that their desired birth was taken from them.

THE STEPWISE MODEL FOR MEDICAL INTERVENTION

When intervention is truly indicated, a preferable management strategy is a stepwise model. In this model, medical intervention is implemented in progressive fashion, both in terms of the aggressiveness and quantity of interventions. The goal is to utilize the intervention that addresses care goals but interferes with the patient's birth plan to the least degree and to introduce only a single intervention at a time, to the degree possible given the specific indication for the modification in plans. This method is best illustrated through several real-life examples. However, prior to those examples, it is important to also explore how decision making is approached within the stepwise model. Integral to the stepwise model of intervention is a shared decision-making process, which is borne out in the medical literature as a sound method for making medical decisions that are effective in terms of outcomes and satisfying for the patient involved. This method of decision making is advocated by proponents of a true informed consent dialogue between patients and providers, rather than the typical paper form, sign on the bottom line, style of informed consent which is most commonly performed.

Shared Decision Making

Shared decision making is defined as "an approach where clinicians and patients share the best available evidence when faced with the task of making decisions, and where patients are supported to consider options, to achieve informed preferences."[2] Decisions are made both in respect to the science and the patient's values. Ideally, this approach should be utilized in all areas of medicine, but it has particular relevance to obstetrics, where there are many "preference-sensitive" situations. These are situations in which there are several reasonable options or where there is insufficient data to definitively recommend a specific course of action or significant "gray" exists because of competing maternal–fetal risks and benefits. Yet, even in these difficult situations, many providers are hesitant to employ shared decision making with their patients due to concerns that patients are either unwilling or unable to participate in these types of discussions or the process will be too time consuming. These concerns, however, have not been validated by the research. With proper education and encouragement, patients have been shown to be more than capable of discussing and making care decisions.[3]

The Informed Medical Decisions Foundation describes *six steps of shared decision making*[4]:

1. *Invite the patient to participate*: Often women do not realize that (1) a decision needs to be made, even if that decision simply is to do nothing, and (2) she is able to share in the process of reaching that decision and ultimately that decision is her's to make. The invitation to participate really should begin long before the onset of labor. Women should be educated about their care throughout pregnancy and encouraged to make decisions regarding what antepartum screening tests they desire, diet and exercise recommendations, and delivery planning. Ideally, the woman and her chosen care provider should have established a nice pattern of working together toward shared goals for her health long before they ever enter the delivery room. As a patient, if one is not invited to participate in care decisions, she should politely but firmly inform her care provider that she desires this and plans to be a part of the decision-making process. If a provider is unwilling to agree with or belittles her request, she should seek out an alternative care provider.

2. *Present the options*: Typically, women are offered an intervention which they either consent to or refuse. It is rare that more than one or two options to address a particular challenge are presented; however, in most situations there are many possible courses of action. Providers should initially discuss these options in an impartial way, without a discussion of the pros and cons involved. Providers should also ask the patient if she can think of any alternatives that were not mentioned to help foster openness and inclusion. If a laboring woman or her support team finds that all options are not being presented by their care providers, they should clarify for the provider the options presented, as they understood them, suggest any alternatives they can think of, and ask if there are any alternative options that have not been discussed.

3. *Provide information on risks and benefits:* For each option presented, information on the risks and benefits should be discussed. This sounds simple when initially considered, however, in obstetrics, this process is extremely complex. For one, given any intervention, there are two sets of risks and benefits to be considered, that of the mother and that of the baby. Often what represents a risk for one is done for the benefit of the other. For example, in response to concerning changes on the fetal heart rate tracing, a cesarean delivery may be recommended. The risks for the baby in a cesarean are relatively minimal and the risk of not performing the cesarean in this particular situation may easily outweigh those risks. However, for the mother, there is no benefit of the cesarean for her health specifically, intentionally disregarding the mental health implications of stress over her baby's well-being and coping with any potential harm that may come to her baby. For the mother, the cesarean carries significantly more risk of physical harm than waiting for a vaginal delivery. Further complicating this particular discussion is the unreliability in fetal heart rate tracings to predict fetal stress and harm. It is important that both maternal and fetal risk and benefit are given equal consideration and care should be taken by the provider to avoid prioritizing one over the other.

Another reason discussions of risk and benefit are so challenging is because the simplest way to present options is by making qualitative comparisons; however, the most informative for the patient making the decision is communication regarding the absolute risk of a course of action as it contrasts with the potential benefits. For example, one can easily say that an elective repeat cesarean section is safer for the baby than attempting a VBAC and this is technically a true statement. Many providers present this exact qualification of the risks and benefits of an elective repeat cesarean to patients who have had a previous cesarean and it very quickly ends the discussion concerning mode of delivery because who wouldn't choose what is safer for their baby? However, this is very misleading and could even be termed coercive because, as previously discussed, the absolute risk of injury to a baby during a TOLAC (trial of labor after previous cesarean) is low, approximately 1 in 1000 births, and the risk of the mother experiencing a significant complication of an elective repeat cesarean, such as a deep venous thromboembolism, hemorrhage with a need for blood transfusion, or hysterectomy, is comparable or even higher than the risk to her baby in a TOLAC.[5,6] In an interesting flip of the previous qualitative assessment, the risk of maternal mortality is also significantly higher in a repeat cesarean when compared to a TOLAC, but again the absolute risk is a much more reasonable way to discuss the frightening topic of maternal mortality. The risk of maternal mortality in a TOLAC is 3.8 per 100,000 deliveries, while the risk in an elective repeat cesarean is 13.4 per 100,000 deliveries, which is higher but to such a small degree that most would not factor this difference in absolute risk into their consideration.[7] Quoting exact numbers is not necessary in these discussions, but giving some quantitative reference to the qualitative assessments is. A better way to present this information to a patient considering either a repeat cesarean or a TOLAC would be to say that, "**while there is no risk-free option to deliver your baby, the risk of serious harm to you or your baby with either option is very low, occurring in only approximately 1 in 1000 births. In a TOLAC, that risk primarily applies to the baby, while in a repeat cesarean that risk primarily applies to the mother. The safest option for both mother and baby is a successful VBAC and, statistically, 80% of women can have a successful VBAC. However, the next safest option is a scheduled repeat cesarean and many women prefer the predictability and controlled conditions of a repeat cesarean over the unpredictability of labor. It is up to me to help you determine if you are a good candidate for a trial of labor and up to you to decide which option seems the most reasonable for you.**"

Finally, there is a tendency in discussions of the benefit and risk of various interventions to "snowball," or discuss the possible implications of that option, 10 steps down the line. An example of this would be counseling a patient desiring an early epidural that an early epidural increases her risk of a maternal fever, but rather than stopping there, going on to say that this may mean she is more likely to need pitocin or a cesarean section and her baby may need to be admitted to NICU.

TOOLS FOR COMMON CHALLENGES

If her baby goes to NICU, this may make it more difficult to breastfeed and her baby may also need antibiotics, which may cause changes in the baby's gut flora which are not yet fully understood. Two or three "risks" down the line, it is hard to remember what the initial risk even was. All the patient hears is bad piled on bad. Snowballed discussions are frightening for the patient and often manipulative, meant however unintentionally to dissuade the patient from a particular course of action. Attempts should be made to prevent patients from feeling overwhelmed by information and discussions of risk should be restricted to the intervention being discussed and its immediate known consequences. If the patient asks for elaboration on other possible outcomes if that complication occurred, it can then be explored, again with proper quantitative clarification.

Ideally, risks and benefits of common medical interventions should be explored prior to labor and delivery, during antenatal childbirth education. In this way, women and their partners can think about and consider these interventions outside of the stress of a labor complication. Decision aids, literature, or visual presentations that have been designed to educate patients about the risks and benefits of particular medical interventions and have been studied for their education efficacy are another way patients may obtain valuable information about delivery options during the antenatal period that is accurate, up-to-date, and generally unbiased. Antenatal education keeps intrapartum, in labor, conversations concerning management options and their risks and benefits manageable, as providers are able to reference and expand upon knowledge that the patient already possesses. Patients are able to ask more informed, pertinent questions, from a less fearful position.

4. *Help the patient evaluate the options based on her goals or concerns:* During these discussions of situations that have more than one reasonable option or where maternal and fetal interests conflict to some degree, it is the patient's goals and values that should direct the decision-making process and help prioritize the maternal–fetal interests. The provider should provide room for the patient to express those goals and values and offer advice that acknowledges and supports those preferences. For example, in a situation where maternal and fetal interests conflict, a mother with other children and/or her spouse may prioritize her well-being over that of the baby she carries simply for the reason that her well-being is so critical to the well-being of their other children. This does not mean the interests of the baby

are not taken into account, but only that, all else being equal, the safety of the mother is the priority. A first-time mother, on the other hand, may be quick to completely neglect her own interests in favor of her child, or a woman or her family may feel culturally or religiously obligated to consider the child first. Again, the mother is not forgotten in this situation, but recommendations may be tailored to what is safe for both yet safest for the baby, even if only to a small degree.

5. *Facilitate deliberation and decision making*: Doctors and midwives can aid in decision making by expanding on options for care to the degree the patient wishes and encouraging the patient to express her feelings about each option presented and addressing specific concerns. The care provider should provide plenty of opportunities for follow-up discussion and questions, but also provide time for independent consideration of the options by the patient and her family. In an outpatient setting, this can be done over several appointments. In labor and delivery, this is best done by offering the patient time to consider, while the provider steps out of the room with either a promise to return for further discussion after a specific time period or an indication to the patient that they should reach out when they are ready to discuss things further or have reached a decision. Patients should always feel comfortable asking additional questions and asking for time for private consideration before agreeing to any intervention.

6. *Assist with implementation:* Once the patient makes a decision, her doctor, midwife, or nurse should go about working with the other members of the health care team to bring about that action as quickly as possible or, if that decision is inaction, to communicate that preference to others so she is not further questioned about it in a way that may be interpreted as pressuring.

A helpful decision-making acronym, suggested in multiple natural birth resources, is for patients to use their *B-R-A-I-N* when considering various medical interventions:

B: Benefits—what are the benefits of this option?
R: Risks—what are the risks of this option?
A: Alternatives—what other choices do I have?
I: Intuition—how am I feeling about this option?
N: Nothing—what if I did nothing for 5 minutes, 1 hour, 5 hours, or a day?

This acronym is essentially a simplification of the shared decision-making steps, but may be a helpful way for some patients to think about problems in labor and possible solutions to them. It can also be a nonintimidating way for providers to guide their patients through shared decision making.

EXAMPLES OF THE STEPWISE MODEL WITH SHARED DECISION MAKING

Example 1: Baby Chloe's Birth, Ineffective Pain Relief and Slow Labor Progress

Chloe's mother was older and had undergone years of infertility treatment before Chloe was miraculously and spontaneously conceived. Despite this incredibly precious cargo, Chloe's mother was remarkably calm and relaxed throughout the entire pregnancy. After so many years of being poked and prodded, she very much wanted to keep Chloe's birth in the nature of how it began. She practiced yoga and prepared for an unmedicated childbirth using hypnobirthing. However, despite all this preparation, when labor hit it was hard and relentless. It began immediately with contractions every 2 to 3 minutes that were strong and painful and labor progressed very slowly. It took over 16 hours to reach 5-cm dilation and by that point, she was done. She asked for an epidural.

- *Traditional approach:* Typically this scenario would lead to IV fluid administration, epidural anesthesia, pitocin augmentation, continuous fetal heart rate monitoring, and possibly the placement of a Foley catheter and continuous monitoring of both maternal heart rate and oxygen saturation. Food and drink would almost universally be restricted as well.
- *Stepwise approach:* In this type of situation, only one problem should be addressed at a time. Ineffective pain relief is typically the more pressing concern for the patient and is usually best tackled first; however, the patient could also be offered the choice to only explore options for advancing the labor. Assuming nonmedical methods of pain relief have been exhausted (see Chapter 11) and the patient is requesting pharmacological relief, the type of pain medication offered should reflect where the mother is in her labor process and her goals. If the mother is experiencing a prolonged latent labor, often systemic

medications, such as morphine and stadol, can provide the rest and temporary comfort she needs to regroup and continue laboring in the manner she initially desired. If the problem is arising later in the labor process, epidural anesthesia is usually more appropriate, as it has a lower risk of neonatal respiratory depression close to delivery, and is more effective than systemic medications.

We discussed the epidural at length. I reviewed the benefits of the epidural, including the effective pain relief it was very likely to provide with little to no transfer of medication to the baby and the opportunity it offered for rest. We also reviewed the ways it may change her labor plan. I recommended continuous fetal monitoring with the epidural, because of the possible blood pressure changes and risk for fetal distress. I also let her know that she would need IV fluids to reduce the chance of these blood pressure changes and that once she received the epidural, she would likely be in the bed from that point forward. She asked about alternatives and I reviewed all the non pharmacological options she could try again, including the tub and different positions. I also offered IV pain medication, as she was early enough in the process that I did not worry this would affect the baby negatively at birth. She quickly rejected this suggestion and told me her number one goal was to expose the baby to as little medicine as possible and have a peaceful birth. She also really did not want a cesarean. I suggested that we could start IV fluids in anticipation of an epidural and reassess her cervix in an hour or so, try something to move the labor along faster like breaking the water or starting pitocin, or just give everything a little more time without doing anything. She worked through a few more contractions and then decidedly said she wanted the epidural. Her nurse called anesthesia and started infusing the necessary fluid as quickly as she could. She received her epidural roughly thirty minutes later and was comfortable and sleeping after about an hour.

- *Stepwise approach (continued):* While most feel continuous monitoring is indicated with an epidural and many anesthesiologists recommend continuous maternal monitoring as well, once the mother and baby have demonstrated adequate tolerance of the epidural for 1 to 2 hours, this monitoring can be relaxed, particularly for the mother. After this initial observation period, food and drink can again be offered as well, as the risk of cesarean is lower outside the initial epidural administration period and, even if surgery was required after this time, it would be very unlikely to require general anesthesia when a well-functioning epidural is on board.

TOOLS FOR COMMON CHALLENGES

After the epidural, I left her alone to rest for several hours until she began to feel pressure and asked to be checked. Somewhere along the line, her water had broken but she hadn't noticed. She was happily fully dilated and pushed well, even with the epidural. She easily delivered Chloe after an hour or so of pushing. I placed Chloe directly on her mother's chest when she was born, waited to cut her cord for a few minutes, and then her nurse helped guide breastfeeding.

- *Stepwise approach (continued):* Immediate pitocin augmentation to address the slowed labor is often not necessary, as frequently the epidural alone can relax the pelvis and bring about labor progression. Reevaluation of the mother after 2 to 4 hours of rest with the epidural is a reasonable alternative and, if necessary, discussions about augmentation can ensue at that point. If augmentation is still indicated, providers should consider and offer alternatives to pitocin augmentation, including prostaglandins, if early in the labor, or alternative positioning, amniotomy, and/or nipple stimulation, if in more advanced labor. Once full dilation is achieved, an offer can be made to reduce or discontinue the epidural and any possible pitocin augmentation in order to allow the mother enough sensation and freedom of movement to push in the position she desired. Regardless of the manner she eventually delivers in, any requests for skin-to-skin and post-baby care can still be honored even when medical intervention is necessary.

Example 2: Baby Luca's Birth, Failure of Descent and Suspected Big Baby

Luca was the second child in his family. His mother had a long and trying first labor with his older sister which had culminated in a serious shoulder dystocia, where the head delivered but the shoulder was stuck and required multiple maneuvers to reduce. Luca's sister had required emergency resuscitation at birth, which was traumatising for both of her parents, but ultimately did well and suffered no long term consequences of her dramatic entry. Luca was suspected to be of similar size and, prior to labor, we discussed the chance of a recurrent shoulder dystocia and the option of an elective cesarean in order to avoid it. Luca's mother really did not want a cesarean, especially with a toddler at home, and did not want to consider a primary elective cesarean. She wanted to see how the labor went and I reassured her that second labors were most often easier, faster, and less likely to result in a problem at delivery, though we could not guarantee she would not experience another shoulder dystocia. When she was just over 40 weeks, her water broke overnight and labor began, but rather than the fast labor I expected with a second baby, it moved very slowly throughout the night and into the next day. It took eight hours for her to progress from three centimeters to seven and even after she reached seven, it took another five hours to reach eight centimeters. The baby also remained very high in the pelvis. Throughout the day, we used non-pharmacological options for pain relief. I suspected a malposition with the slow descent of the baby and stagnated dilation, but was also worried the size of the baby could be complicating things as well. By the evening, Luca's mother was very tired and frustrated. We discussed an epidural as a means to help her rest and possibly relax the pelvis and aid in the descent of the baby. At that point, she felt that she really needed a break and had exhausted everything else she could physically do. She did not want to consider any other alternatives, so we quickly went through what she could expect and then placed the epidural. I reassessed her cervix two hours later and, disappointingly, she was still eight centimeters and her contractions had slowed to every seven minutes. We discussed options, including nipple stimulation, pitocin augmentation, or proceeding with a cesarean at this time due to the concern that a large baby was generating the abnormal labor pattern. After reviewing all the options, we all felt pitocin was her best chance of avoiding a cesarean, which was still her goal. We continued the pitocin for several more hours and finally reached 9.5 centimeters, with just a small portion of cervix remaining anteriorly. However, the baby remained very high in the pelvis and, on examination, I could tell this was not due to a malposition. I again discussed my concern that this baby was larger than we were anticipating and, while I felt confident that she could likely achieve a vaginal delivery if we proceeded, I was worried that there were several red flags that could be indicating a significant risk of a shoulder dystocia, including the slow labor and the persistently high station. She and her husband informed me that, while they did not want a cesarean, more than anything they did not want to experience another shoulder dystocia, even if it did not result in a bad outcome. We discussed the cesarean in more detail and then she and her husband took several minutes privately to consider the options. They decided they would prefer a cesarean rather than take the risk, which they now felt was high, of experiencing what they had experienced with their daughter. I performed her cesarean a short time later. Baby Luca, in all his ten pound glory, was born in the operating room to calm voices, with the music of his mother's choice playing, and, after a brief assessment of his wellbeing by the neonatologist, was handed to his mother for skin-to-skin bonding.

He immediately began nursing and stayed with his parents until the surgery was finished. He and his mother went to the recovery room together and his mother had an uncomplicated recovery. She felt very confident in the choice she had made and happy with her birth experience.

- *Traditional approach:* Most providers would have recommended Luca's mother have an elective cesarean simply based on his estimated size and her history of a previous shoulder dystocia. Some providers may not have even offered his mother a choice in this discussion and insisted on a cesarean. Other providers may have utilized a tool called the PeriCALM shoulder screen, a commercially available computer model that is said to identify women at high risk for shoulder dystocia, though its efficacy in preventing shoulder dystocia is, at this time, unproven.[8,9] Providers using this model perform a growth ultrasound in the last month of pregnancy for women determined to be at risk based on medical history and combine the estimated fetal weight with several additional parameters to determine the likelihood of a shoulder dystocia. Patients who, based on the model's calculations, are determined to be at high risk of a shoulder dystocia are typically offered a cesarean and those who decline are often asked to sign a form acknowledging that a vaginal delivery is against medical advice. Many women report feeling unduly pressured into a cesarean by this practice.

Typical care during a cesarean is also often impersonal and not reflective of the patient's birth plan for a calm atmosphere and post-delivery infant care. It is commonplace for loud extraneous conversations between caregivers to be ongoing while a cesarean is performed. Upon delivery, the infant is usually taken for an initial evaluation to a warmer across the room from the mother, where she often cannot even see the baby. Once the initial evaluation is completed, most hospitals afford only a brief period of time for the mother to see and touch her baby before both her support person and the baby are taken to the nursery for further infant assessment, leaving the mother alone for the remainder of the surgery. Few hospitals permit more than one maternal support person in the operating room and most hospitals bring the baby to the nursery for post-delivery monitoring, where the baby may spend anywhere from 1 to 4 hours away from the mother. Research suggests that this approach to cesarean delivery contributes to the lower rates of breastfeeding observed in mothers undergoing cesarean sections when compared to mothers who give birth vaginally. Mothers who deliver by cesarean take longer to achieve the first successful breastfeeding session, have lower rates of breastfeeding at discharge, and have lower rates of exclusive breastfeeding 12 weeks after delivery.[10,11]

- *Stepwise approach:* In the stepwise approach, the risk of a recurrent shoulder dystocia would be discussed during the antepartum period in a balanced way. The patient is able to consider that risk and make a decision according to her own priorities and values. In this situation, the patient made the decision to see how labor progressed, rather than proceeding with a scheduled cesarean that may or may not have been necessary. When the labor did not progress in the expected fashion, the patient was given the opportunity to explore other solutions to the failure of descent and slow progression of labor in a progressive way. First an epidural was given, followed by pitocin only when the epidural failed to achieve the intended effect and the contraction pattern slowed. Other less aggressive options were presented as well. While the pitocin was largely successful at achieving dilation, when the high station of the head did not improve, the possible implication of this was discussed with the parents and they were again presented with the option to proceed with a cesarean given their expressed concern about experiencing another traumatic shoulder dystocia. When they ultimately decided to proceed with a cesarean, the cesarean was performed, to the greatest degree possible, in a manner in keeping with their overall intention for their birth. While some might argue that Luca's birth ended in the same manner it would have if his parents had just elected for a cesarean in the first place and the labor process was a waste of time which increased both his and his mother's risk, that knowledge was truly only hindsight. The process of the labor is what demonstrated to Luca's parents that the risk of shoulder dystocia was one they were no longer willing to afford. Giving Luca's mother time and the ability to consider and make her own decisions through a difficult labor maintained her sense of autonomy and allowed her to gain confidence in the decision for a cesarean, whereas she likely would have always wondered if it was necessary had it been imposed on her.

THE GENTLE CESAREAN

Baby Luca was delivered with many components of what is termed a "gentle cesarean." This approach to a cesarean aims to improve the experience of families in the operating room and increase practices that promote breastfeeding and early maternal–child bonding. Gentle cesareans include several elements[12]:

1. Limited conversation between caregivers, with effort made to create a calm environment centered on the mother
2. Music of the mother's choice playing
3. Delayed cord clamping or cord milking at the time of delivery
4. Immediate or near-immediate skin-to-skin placement of infant, if both mother and infant are deemed stable by the pediatric, anesthesia, and obstetrics teams
5. Encouragement of early breastfeeding in the operating room
6. Avoidance of separation of mother and infant unless clinically indicated or desired by the mother

Efforts to implement gentle cesareans within hospitals have been successful, despite initial concerns expressed from physicians and staff about infant hypothermia, interference with surgical sterility, and difficulty in monitoring both mothers and babies. Gentle cesareans have been demonstrated to be safe, without an increased risk in neonatal hypothermia.[13] They are also associated with higher rates of initiation of breastfeeding, exclusive breastfeeding, and patient satisfaction.[14]

BEDSIDE MANNER

I attended medical school in Arizona and they offered this crazy elective to learn better bedside manner from horses. I could not imagine what a horse could teach me about interacting with patients, but I had always liked horses and, after spending years of my life locked inside a library, the idea of being outside was appealing. I signed up and this class quickly became my favorite part of the week and remains one of the most valuable courses I have ever taken. Standing before these intimidating but easily frightened, 1000 lb animals, I learned how my own emotions affected the way the horse would respond to me, that where I positioned my body had a direct impact on the horse, and there was a speed at which I needed to move in order to make the horse comfortable. I learned to alert the horse as I moved around it's body and where and how to first touch the horse in a way that would keep it calm. I also learned how to encourage the horse to move and that, no matter how much I wanted to, I could not move the horse. The horse had to decide to move for me. There are so many times those lessons and experiences are directly applicable to my interactions with patients and my practice of obstetrics, as I am working with women in some of their most vulnerable moments. Especially in times of stress, it is essential to slow down, be aware of your body and the tone of your speech, and work with the woman through her labor process rather than acting as an external force trying to exert control on it or her.

Bedside manner is a frequently talked about but rarely taught aspect of medical care that is critically important to provider–patient relationships, effective communication between providers and patients, and the patient's interpretation of the quality of their care. While it impacts all patient interactions, it is particularly important when working with women in labor, especially when it is necessary to incorporate medical interventions into a woman's care that she had hoped to avoid. However, patients frequently report ineffective communication with their care providers, with only one in five patients reporting satisfactory communication with their doctors.[15] When mothers were surveyed about shared decision making with their providers in labor, one in five also felt they had no ability to contribute to discussions regarding their care and that any decisions for intervention were solely made by their providers.[16]

As a first step in improving bedside manner on labor and delivery units, the doctors, midwives, and nurses working with naturally laboring women should make every effort to respect the atmosphere the patient is trying to achieve. When entering a room, care providers should always ask before making any changes to the environment, such as turning on lights, taking vital signs, or performing an exam. If the environment needs to be changed, it should only be done to the minimal degree necessary to achieve the indicated task. If the mother is laboring in quiet or with soft music playing, voices should be kept low. Care should also be taken to avoid distracting a mother in the midst of a contraction with questions or procedures.

Body language and exam style is also important. Simply moving slowly and sitting down with the patient in a relaxed manner facilitates communication and puts the laboring mother at ease. When the intention of coming into the labor room is to perform an examination, all too frequently that process of examination is initiated with little to no conversation with the patient. The provider immediately retrieves a glove upon entering the room and puts the head down on the bed, informing the patient of his or her intent as it is already being initiated. A better approach is to sit and first assess how the patient is feeling, ask if she is okay with an examination, and then perform an examination in the position most comfortable for her. Lying flat on the back for an examination, while easiest for the provider, is often difficult for women to cope with and should not be imposed on them unless necessary and with their consent for the position change.

When discussions about medical intervention are needed, in addition to the principles of shared decision making discussed previously, the patient's doctors, midwives, and nurses should also provide comfort and express empathy in their interactions with the laboring mother. There are several components of doing this effectively:

- Recognize the difficulty of making the decision: Acknowledging that these types of decisions are not easy for anyone lets the mother know that she is not alone in her struggle, nor is she wrong for having a difficult time making a choice.
- Recognize the ambiguity which is often present: There is not always a "right" choice and that can be very liberating for a woman faced with a difficult choice. A good way to phrase this is to let the mother know that there is often not a right or wrong decision, just the one that is right for her, given the set of circumstances in which she finds herself.
- Express empathy for the loss of the birth she wanted: When a mother is faced with a change in her birth plans, it is a loss of the ideal vision she had for bringing her baby in the world. It is okay for her to have sadness about that loss and she needs the space to work through those emotions. Some of the worst things care providers say to women whose births veer off the intended course are, "it doesn't matter how the baby gets out," because it matters to her or, "all that matters is the baby is healthy," because she also matters, or "don't cry, you and your baby are fine," because she can still be upset about how the labor went even if everyone is healthy at the conclusion of the process.
- Praise her decision making, hard work during the labor, and flexibility in coping with the changes: When problems in labor arise, women often feel they did something wrong. Reassuring them that they did a great job in the labor and made good choices goes a long way toward improving their feelings toward the labor experience and instilling confidence in themselves as mothers. Reinforcing that these skills are the same skills they will be using throughout their journey in parenting this child can help them keep their focus on the big picture of what their labor is all about.
- Keep yourself out of the discussion: In the stress and fatigue of caring for many women in labor, it is often easy for caregivers to forget they are not personally a factor in decisions in labor, even when those decisions are personally affecting them in terms of other

commitments, time with family, or even the ability to eat or go to the bathroom. The worse thing a care provider can do is mention other obligations outside of the patient herself as a reason for making a certain choice.

• Avoid discussions of the clock: Maintaining a ticking time clock in discussions with patients is rarely helpful and creates the impression that the provider is in a rush to just be done.

REFERENCES

1. Furuta M, Sandall J, Cooper D, Bick D. Predictors of birth-related post-traumatic stress symptoms: secondary analysis of a cohort study. *Arch Women Ment Health.* 2016;19(3):521-528.
2. Elwyn G, Laitner S, Coulter A, et al. Implementing shared decision making in the NHS. *BMJ.* 2010;341:c5146. doi:10.1136/bmj.c5146.
3. Elwyn G, Frosch D, Thomson R, et al. Shared decision making: a model for clinical practice. *J Gen Intern Med.* 2012;27(10):1361-1367. doi:10.1007/s11606-012-2077-6.
4. The Informed Medical Decisions Foundation. The six steps of shared decision making. Available at http://cdn-www.informedmedicaldecisions.org/imdfdocs/SixStepsSDM_CARD.pdf. Accessed 7/2017.
5. Galyean AM, Lagrew DC, Bush MC, Kurtzman JT. Previous cesarean section and the risk of postpartum maternal complications and adverse neonatal outcomes in future pregnancies. *J Perinatol.* 2009;29(11):726-730. doi:10.1038/jp.2009.108.
6. Menacker F, MacDorman MF, Declercq E. Neonatal mortality risk for repeat cesarean compared to vaginal birth after cesarean (VBAC) deliveries in the United States, 1998–2002 birth cohorts. *Matern Child Health J.* 2010;14(2):147-154.
7. Burrows LJ, Meyn LA, Weber AM. Maternal morbidity associated with vaginal versus cesarean delivery. *Obstet Gynecol.* 2004;103(5 pt 1):907-912.
8. Yao R, Jovanovski A. Outcomes of routine shoulder dystocia screening using a commercially available screening tool. *Am J Obstet Gynecol.* 2015;212(1):S344-S345. doi:10.1016/j.ajog.2014.10.912.
9. Daly MV, Bender C, Townsend KE, Hamilton EF. Outcomes associated with a structured prenatal counseling program for shoulder dystocia with brachial plexus injury. *Am J Obstet Gynecol.* 2012;207(2):123.e1-123.e5. doi:10.1016/j.ajog.2012.05.023.
10. Hobbs AJ, Mannion CA, McDonald SW, et al. The impact of caesarean section on breastfeeding initiation, duration and difficulties in the first four months postpartum. *BMC Pregnancy Childbirth.* 2016;16:90. doi:10.1186/s12884-016-0876-1.
11. Zanardo V, Svegliado G, Cavallin F, et al. Elective cesarean delivery: does it have a negative effect on breastfeeding? *Birth.* 2010;37(4):275-279. doi:10.1111/j.1523-536X.2010.00421.x.
12. Magee SR, Battle C, Morton J, Nothnagle M. Promotion of family-centered birth with gentle cesarean delivery. *J Am Board Fam Med.* 2014;27(5):690-693. doi:10.3122/jabfm.2014.05.140014.

13. Gouchon S, Gregori D, Picotto A, et al. Skin-to-skin contact after cesarean delivery: an experimental study. *Nurs Res.* 2010;59(2):78-84. doi:10.1097/NNR.0b013e3181d1a8bc.

14. Brady K, Bulpitt D, Chiarelli C. An interprofessional quality improvement project to implement maternal/infant skin-to-skin contact during cesarean delivery. *J Obstet Gynecol Neonatal Nurs.* 2014;43(4):488-496. doi:10.1111/1552-6909.12469.

15. Ha JF, Longnecker N. Doctor-patient communication: a review. *Ochsner J.* 2010;10(1):38-43.

16. Declercq ER, Sakala C, Corry MP, et al. Major survey findings of listening to mothers(SM) III: pregnancy and birth: report of the third national U.S. survey of women's childbearing experiences. *J Perinat Educ.* 2013;23(1):9-16. doi:10.1891/1058-1243.23.1.9.

CHAPTER 13

Special Cases: Indicated Induction, VBAC, and High-Risk Patients Wanting a Natural Birth

BABY CONNOR'S BIRTH

Connor's mother found herself in a common predicament; she was approaching 42 weeks gestation and showed no signs of labor. She had tried every natural trick and old wive's tale to bring about labor, but nothing had moved her baby along and she was getting nervous. She asked about the risks of going late and I counselled her that post-term pregnancies were at an increased risk of meconium fluid, poor fetal tolerance of labor, cesarean section, and, the most frightening of all, stillbirth, but reassured her that vast majority of post-term babies did well, that the overall risk of serious complications were low, and she was not in a substantially different place than she was just a few days before. I also counselled her that some studies had shown a possibly reduced risk of some of those complications with induction, but that induction did carry its own set of issues and she was more likely to need an epidural and possibly more likely to need a cesarean with an induction. She very much wanted a natural labor but also did not feel comfortable with the increasing risks of a post-term pregnancy. We decided on a day for induction, swept her membranes to help encourage the process along, and met at the hospital the next evening. We administered a small dose of a prostaglandin every four hours. She still was able to ambulate, with the aid of the mobile monitor, and eat as she wished. We placed a hep-lock IV just in case the baby did not tolerate the process.

Roughly ten hours later, she was nicely dilated to five centimeters and having strong, active contractions. The prostaglandin having done it's job, we now discussed the options from there. We could simply wait and see if the labor continued without any additional intervention, we could break her water to help ensure the process would continue, or we could do the more medically aggressive thing and start pitocin now that her cervix was ripened. She wanted to minimize medical interventions, but was still nervous about the labor slowing back down, so she decided to have her water broken. That really seemed to do the trick and she was eight centimeters two hours later. At this point, it had been over four hours since she had received any medication and she was uncomfortable, so we took her off the fetal monitor and she spent several hours in the labor tub with intermittent auscultation. She began to feel a lot of pressure, but when she was examined she was still only eight centimeters. She was very frustrated and, at this point, was tired and having trouble managing the labor.

We all encouraged her that she was doing really well and this was just a bump in the road. Again we discussed her options. She could get back in the tub, where she seemed to be managing her labor better, and we could just wait. Alternatively, we could attempt some different positions outside the tub. I felt she may benefit from a side-lying position because the head was a little off center when I examined her. We also reminded her that there was always the option of the epidural. She quickly expressed that she wanted the epidural and didn't feel like she had the energy to continue laboring. We told her that was fine, if that is what she wanted, but suggested she try some alternative positions while she received the necessary fluids in anticipation of the epidural, which would take thirty to forty minutes. She agreed that this was a good idea and we tried a side-lying release, with the aid of the peanut ball, while she received her fluid bolus. When the bolus was finished, she felt a strong urge to push and I suggested we examine her before she received the epidural. She agreed and was found to be fully dilated. She decided she would rather just try to push the baby out at this point, rather than get the epidural. We helped her find several comfortable pushing positions and an hour and a half later she delivered her healthy eight and half pound baby boy. The birth had not been exactly what she had planned on, but she was able to labor with most of her labor plan intact, even in the setting of an induction, and have a healthy vaginal delivery.

INDICATED INDUCTION

Indicated induction is one of the more frustrating scenarios women who wish to labor naturally find themselves in. While there is debate about what exactly constitutes an indicated induction, when truly medically necessary, it can be difficult for both women and their providers to figure out how an induction can be done in a manner conducive to a natural labor or whether an unmedicated should even be attempted.

There are certainly certain situations in which it is particularly difficult to support a natural labor. For example, in an induction performed for severe preeclampsia, it is not advisable for a woman who is extremely ill to ambulate, as she will require medications that must be closely monitored and upright positions are likely to worsen her hypertension. Furthermore, in this situation, an epidural may actually lower blood pressure and improve her chances of at least having a vaginal delivery. Given the life-threatening nature of preeclampsia, maintaining the mother's stability certainly should supersede all other concerns; however, this can and should still be done with the goal of changing as little as possible of the original intention for the patient in respect to room atmosphere and post-delivery care. Another example of a situation where supporting a natural birth plan is difficult is an induction performed for poor fetal status, such as growth restriction or oligohydramnios. These babies often have difficulty tolerating the induction process and frequently require specific positioning of the mother for stabilization of the fetal heart rate tracing, maternal oxygen and fluid supplementation, and continuous monitoring. In addition, they are at higher risk of acute distress and bradycardia requiring emergency delivery, so many providers recommend diet restriction in this circumstance.

However, most inductions are done for conditions that carry significantly less risk of complications during the labor process and the main risk to be considered is the induction itself. Some examples of these types of inductions are those performed for postdates, gestational diabetes, pre-labor release of membranes, mild gestational hypertension, maternal age, or maternal obesity. In these situations, the induction, if handled appropriately, can be completely compatible with an unmedicated delivery. Baby Conner's birth is an example of just such a birth.

Usually, for nonurgent inductions, the potential need of an induction can be anticipated several days in advance. When the need for an induction is anticipated, attempts can be made beforehand to either bring about labor nonpharmacologically or to improve upon the cervical Bishop's score prior to the induction, which makes the induction easier and more likely to succeed.[1] *Membrane sweeping* is the best studied means of bringing about labor nonpharmacologically. Studies have shown that membrane routine sweeping beginning at term reduces the likelihood of pregnancies extending to 41 and 42 weeks, which may have particular application for patients with advanced maternal age, obesity, or diabetes, in whom research suggests that postdates pregnancies are more problematic. Membrane sweeping has also been demonstrated to be effective in achieving spontaneous labor within 48 hours and reduces the need for formal induction in one out of eight women or decreases the rate of induction by 16%. The main risks associated with membrane sweeping are maternal discomfort, nonclinically significant vaginal bleeding, and pre-labor release of membranes. No differences in the rate of cesarean delivery or maternal or neonatal morbidity have been observed with membrane sweeping, making it a reasonably safe option to offer patients hoping to avoid a formal induction.[2]

Other nonpharmacological means of bringing about labor have not been thoroughly studied, but offer some promise and suggest the need for more research into alternative, nonpharmacologic means of induction. Three older observational studies examined the use of *acupuncture* as a means of induction. In these studies, induction was successful in 67% to 83% of patients and achieved a mean induction to delivery interval of 13 hours; however, there was no significant difference in cesarean rates when compared to controls.[3] More recent randomized control trials have not shown significant efficacy of acupuncture as an induction tool, though the most recent *Cochrane Review* suggests acupuncture may improve the cervical Bishop score prior to an induction.[4] Furthermore, no ill effects are associated with acupuncture so, at this time, it falls into the "may help, won't hurt" category of nonpharmacologic options that women faced with an induction may wish to pursue.

Nipple stimulation is another tool frequently recommended to bring about labor. It is known that nipple stimulation results in the release of endogenous oxytocin and generates uterine contractions. A review evaluating six randomized studies, four comparing nipple stimulation to no treatment and two comparing nipple stimulation to pitocin, found that nipple stimulation resulted in a significant decrease in the number of women not in labor within 72 hours, reduced postpartum hemorrhage rates, and was comparable to oxytocin in its efficacy in bringing about labor and achieving a vaginal delivery.[5] However, one trial performed exclusively in high-risk women, including women with post-dates pregnancies, hypertension, and intrauterine growth restriction, showed an increase in the rate of perinatal death with nipple stimulation.[6] While this study was not large in scale and provided only limited antenatal testing via a simple non-stress test prior to randomization, it does suggest caution should be used when recommending nipple stimulation in an unmonitored, outpatient setting in high-risk patients. However, in low-risk patients, it may reduce the need for pharmacological induction.

Over-the-counter agents, such as *castor oil* or *homeopathic medications*, and *sexual intercourse* are also frequently recommended in the natural childbirth community as a means to bring about labor without a formal induction. However, the limited research to date on these methods has failed to show any clear benefit to this common advice. Homeopathy has only been studied in one trial that failed to show any benefit over routine care.[7] Likewise, only one randomized study has examined sexual intercourse as a possible induction technique and did not demonstrate any benefit, though in a later observational study, couples who reported coitus at term were found to have an earlier onset of labor and reduced need for induction at 41 weeks.[8,9] Castor oil, which has demonstrated efficacy at producing uterine contractions, has also been studied only to a small degree. It was shown to be effective at producing labor in one randomized trial of 42 women; however, a larger study failed to demonstrate this benefit, though no harm was associated with its use.[10-12] Current reviews of the literature also did not find a benefit of castor oil or any other over-the-counter medications or sexual intercourse.[13]

Consequently, given the limited efficacy of nonpharmacologic options, most women who require a medically indicated induction will require an in-hospital, medical induction, with all the potential impacts on their labor plan that were previously discussed (see Chapter 5). Providers and patients must then choose the pharmacologic induction that offers the best chance of a vaginal delivery and is most conducive to nonpharmacologic methods of pain relief. The most common form of induction agents are pitocin, prostaglandin E2 dinoprostone (Cervidil), and misoprostol (Cytotec) administered orally or vaginally. Multiple trials have demonstrated a higher rate of epidural use among women induced with pitocin, compared to both women who labor spontaneously and those who are induced with prostaglandins.[14] Most women report that pitocin contractions are stronger, more frequent, and more difficult to manage with nonpharmacologic pain relief methods than spontaneous contractions. Hence, most would consider pitocin administration to be relatively noncompatible with a natural birth plan.

However, induced delivery can be achieved without pitocin. When misoprostol, administered both vaginal and orally, was compared to both oxytocin and other prostaglandin agents of induction in a large number of trials, misoprostol was associated with less epidural use, fewer failures to achieve vaginal delivery within 24 hours, and lower rates of cesarean. When misoprostol was compared to dinoprostone, misoprostol was also less likely to require pitocin augmentation. Misoprostol was associated with higher rates of uterine hyperstimulation than either oxytocin or dinoprostone, but this did not cause increased fetal distress or worse neonatal outcomes. Misoprostol was also associated with higher rates of meconium fluid, but this also was not associated with poor neonatal outcomes, suggesting that this increase may be due to an effect of misoprostol on the neonatal gastrointestinal system, rather than an indication of distress, as it is typically thought to be.[15] Studies have also compared the vaginal and oral routes of misoprostol administration and found oral administration is as effective as vaginal administration, is associated with a better neonatal condition at birth, and has less post-partum bleeding.[16] Unfortunately, despite the large quantity of evidence of its comparable safety and efficacy to other agents, misoprostol is still not FDA approved for labor induction and some providers are reluctant to use the medication "off-label." Off-label use of medications in general is common and legal, provided it is supported by quality evidence, but off-label use carries a higher medical–legal risk, especially in obstetrics. It is also unlikely that misoprostol will ever be FDA approved for induc-tion because it is an inexpensive medication that is already being widely used for this purpose, thus there is no incentive, in terms of increased revenue, for the manufacturer to go through the lengthy and expen-sive process to acquire FDA approval. Hence, many patients wishing to labor naturally may not have access to this medication which is more likely to help them achieve an unmedicated vaginal delivery than other medications.

Yet, beyond the induction agent used, there are other important ways an unmedicated delivery can be supported in induction setting. Provided the mother and baby are stable, the key to enabling an unmedi-cated delivery is maintaining ambulation and freedom of movement during the induction. This is frequently challenging, given the need to continuously monitor most patients undergoing an induction, but can be achieved by utilizing the mobile monitoring techniques and solu-tions explored in Chapter 10. Placing a hep-lock IV, as opposed to con-tinuous IV fluids, and permitting oral intake, at least for hydration, also encourages freedom of movement. However, inductions are frequently long and, in most inductions, the mother and baby are stable enough to permit eating, as well as drinking. Restricting diet contributes to both physical and emotional fatigue in all laboring women, but is par-ticularly difficult for those trying to work through their labor without medical pain relief. If signs of distress or complications develop, diet may need to be restricted in anticipation of a cesarean delivery, but this should be approached on an individualized basis rather than a blanket policy.

Maintaining access to hydrotherapy is also incredibly valuable for women undergoing induction. Often the shower or tub can be just enough of a comfort to help a mother who would otherwise have given up on her plan. However, continuous monitoring during hydrotherapy is particularly difficult and is the component of care that most frequently restricts shower and tub access in the induction setting. In order to offer induced women easier access to hydrotherapy, care providers should consider whether relaxing monitoring guidelines is possible for their patient, given the individual circumstances of the induction. This is dependent on the indication for induction, where the mother is in her labor process, and how long it has been since she has received an induction agent. For example, often with a misoprostol induction, the mother's labor progresses to the point that no additional doses of medication are necessary or a simple amniotomy will be sufficient to continue the labor. The half-life of misoprostol varies according to mode of administration, with vaginal use associated with a longer half-life than oral use; however, for both modes of administration, within 4 hours, the serum concentration of the medication is low enough to render the effect on the fetus negligible.[17] Provided fetal monitoring has been reassuring to that point, it is reasonable for a woman induced for a lower risk indication to labor in the same manner she would have if her labor had begun spontaneously, once she is out of the window where the induction agent is likely to have a fetal effect.

If the laboring mother is not outside that window or there is a medical indication for continued monitoring, hydrotherapy can still be attempted utilizing previously discussed alternative monitoring techniques, specifically using taping as a seal against the water. More frequent intermittent auscultation of the heart rate could also be considered in this setting; however, alternative regimes of intermittent auscultation in higher risk patients have not been studied and most providers are unlikely to feel comfortable utilizing intermittent auscultation methods during an induction. Yet, even in higher risk settings, providers should ask themselves how likely it is that anything is going to change in regards to the fetal status in 5, 10, 15, or even 30 minutes. Furthermore, even if a change occurred, how likely is it that this would alter management or require emergency delivery, especially if the fetal monitoring had been reassuring up to that point.

Patience is also incredibly important during all inductions, but particularly so for inductions in naturally laboring mothers. Inductions, no matter how they are performed, are long, taking, on average, 8 more hours than a spontaneous labor.[18] In a typical, medically managed induction, the goal is to safely achieve delivery, as efficiently as possible. However, a less efficient mode of induction or management style, in keeping with the stepwise model for medical intervention, may be the one that enables a woman to have an unmedicated delivery and maintain her sense of control over the process. Unless there is a more urgent need for delivery, there is no rule that says inductions must be completed in 24 hours.

VBAC

I do a lot of VBACs and I have found a common pattern over the years. The more I try and control it, the more often it fails. All the checking, nervous flustering around, obsessive fetal heart rate strip checking…it just doesn't work. I think it is because, in those situations, I make the mother so tense her body can't do what it needs to do. If I just leave the woman alone, interfering with her process to the least degree necessary to ensure the baby is safe, the better she does. Certainly, the more medical intervention that enters into the labor process, the worse it seems to go. In my experience, the less you mess with a VBAC, the less it messes with you.

Many patients desiring a natural birth are patients with a history of a previous cesarean delivery. These patients, often having personally experienced the conclusion of medicalized birth within an operating room, are highly motivated to avoid any of part of the sequence of events that may have contributed to their surgical birth. Obviously, the initial step in offering these women a natural birth is simply giving them the opportunity to have a trial of labor after cesarean (TOLAC) in the first place. Many providers give lip service to "allowing" women a TOLAC, but put policies in place that significantly restrict their ability to have a vaginal delivery. For example, many providers

- insist on delivery by the due date or 41 weeks.
- place time limits on the labor that would not apply to women who had not had a previous cesarean.
- recommend or insist on an epidural for all TOLACs, in order to have quicker access to an emergency cesarean, or restrict epidural use, in order to be able to better predict uterine rupture.
- prohibit TOLAC when the previous cesarean was performed for labor dystocia or failure of descent.
- prohibit TOLAC in the setting of suspected macrosomia.
- prohibit TOLAC in the setting of any other complication of pregnancy.
- refuse to induce or augment patients with a previous cesarean.

TOOLS FOR COMMON CHALLENGES

- prohibit TOLAC without an operative report indicating a prior low-transverse cesarean, with a two-layer closure of the uterus.
- limit TOLAC to patients with one previous cesarean.

The main risk of labor for patients with a previous cesarean when compared to patients without a previous uterine incision is the risk of uterine rupture; however, this risk is quite low. The relative safety of VBAC has been well established and it is supported by the American College of Obstetricians and Gynecologists (ACOG). Most of the restrictions listed above are, in fact, specifically addressed and refuted in the most recent practice bulletin concerning VBAC.[19] To summarize the practice bulletin in regards to these concerns, while a trial of labor attempted after the due date is less likely to result in a successful vaginal delivery, it is no more likely to result in a uterine rupture or other complication of pregnancy than in a TOLAC attempted prior to the due date. Likewise, if a pregnancy complication exists, such as preeclampsia, diabetes, or advanced maternal age, or the prior previous delivery was performed for labor dystocia and the current estimated fetal weight is greater than the prior baby's delivery weight, the trial of labor is less likely to succeed, but it is not more likely to result in uterine rupture. Epidural use or lack of use, as an independent factor, also does not alter TOLAC success or the ability to recognize uterine rupture, as the most reliable indicator of uterine rupture is a change in the fetal heart rate tracing.[20,21] Induction or augmentation of labor utilizing pitocin has been shown to be associated with an increased chance of a uterine rupture and decreased likelihood of vaginal delivery; however, the risk of uterine rupture is still less than 1% and comparable to the rate of rupture with a spontaneous labor. Hence, a medical indication for delivery prior to labor need not preclude a patient from a VBAC; however, the way in which induction would alter the risks and likelihood of success should be discussed with the patient. Similarly, suspected macrosomia has also been associated with a lower rate of successful VBAC and potentially a higher risk of uterine rupture. However, given the way suspected macrosomia impacts the vaginal delivery rate of all women, this statistic may be more reflective of provider practices when babies are suspected to be big in general, rather than something that is specific to VBAC, and the study showing a higher rate of uterine rupture was based on birth weights rather than estimated fetal weights, limiting its application to decision making in the antenatal period. Finally, VBAC success rates of patients with more than one previous cesarean section or an unknown type of surgical incision are similar to patients with one prior, low-transverse incision. There is some evidence that the risk of uterine rupture may be higher in patients with more than one previous cesarean; however, the largest studies examining the rate of rupture in this setting did not show difference in rupture rate. An unknown surgical scar, a low vertical incision, or lack of a two-layer or double closure is also not associated with an increased rate of uterine rupture.[22] However, a history of a classical cesarean or previous uterine rupture was associated with a significantly higher rate of uterine rupture, anywhere from 6% to 13%, and current evidence supports recommendations for an elective repeat cesarean in these women.

Beyond adopting less restrictive VBAC policies, providers also need be more open to nonpharmacologic coping strategies for their VBAC. Providers should be happy when a mother desiring VBAC wants to labor naturally, because the less potentially compounding variables that enter into the labor process the better. While studies may not demonstrate lower vaginal delivery rates with epidurals, given the established increased need for pitocin augmentation with epidurals, which most providers want to avoid in a trial of labor due to its association with VBAC complications, it would seem to behoove providers to make it as easy as possible for TOLAC patients to labor unmedicated.[23] Again, the main respect in which a TOLAC differs from any other labor is in the risk of uterine rupture and, given the most reliable means of predicting and responding to a potential uterine rupture is via fetal monitoring, the principal challenge for doctors, midwives, and nurses in truly supporting these patients is achieving continuous monitoring in an ambulatory woman. All too often, women with a previous cesarean are told they must stay in bed in order to properly monitor their baby. Monitoring is incredibly important in a TOLAC and continuously monitoring an ambulatory patient is frequently difficult and frustrating, but it is doable with the aid of alternative monitoring techniques and a motivated care provider. As with inductions, freedom of movement is essential to unmedicated mothers during a TOLAC, even if it takes some work to achieve.

The concern about monitoring is also the most commonly cited reason for keeping VBACs from accessing hydrotherapy. However, as previously emphasized, monitoring is possible even with hydrotherapy. Regardless of this possibility, most hospitals have specific policies prohibiting labor tub use if the patient has had a previous cesarean. Administrators frequently express concern that a uterine rupture could occur while the woman is using the labor tub, which would impede staff from being able to quickly move the patient to the operating room for an emergency cesarean. While this concern is understandable, it is a highly unlikely scenario. Given a risk of uterine rupture of 0.5% throughout the duration of a TOLAC and an average labor length of 12 hours, the risk of a uterine rupture in any 30-minute time interval is estimated to be as low as 0.02%. If one also considers that the incidence of uterine rupture without any recognizable changes in the fetal heart rate tracing is only 30%, the risk of a spontaneous rupture in a patient with a normal fetal heart rate tracing while in the labor tub for any 30-minute interval decreases even further to a mere 0.006%. This hardly seems a risk worthy of restricting all VBACs from hydrotherapy for the entirety of their labor, especially when hydrotherapy can be so helpful in minimizing the need for pharmacological pain relief.

Providers and women planning a VBAC should also be aware that TOLACs may differ from other labors in terms of length. While some evidence has shown rates of dilation in TOLAC patients are similar to patients without a uterine scar, other studies have demonstrated significantly slower dilation, especially in the setting of induction.[24,25] In anecdotal observations among providers who commonly support VBACs, rate of dilation most often reflects the extent to which the woman's labor progressed in her previous birth. Mothers who reached an advanced stage of dilation will often labor in a fashion similar to other multiparous women, while women who either did not labor or only reached an early cervical dilation in their previous labor will usually labor more slowly, often slower than even a typical nulliparous patient. Patience and reassurance are essential to helping mothers through these labors which are always more anxiety provoking for everyone involved.

Women who are planning to have a VBAC should be encouraged to prepare well for labor and have the healthiest pregnancy possible. Proper childbirth education is an essential part of minimizing medical interventions, especially early in the labor when they are more likely to cause problems in the labor. Regular exercise and careful attention to diet can help minimize excess weight gain and prevent macrosomia, which both contribute to a higher likelihood of cesarean delivery. This is particularly important if the last cesarean was performed for a labor dystocia or failure of descent. Women should work to enter into their labors with every physical advantage possible in order to improve their chances of success. A positive mental attitude is also paramount. Women often enter a

TOLAC with a significant amount of baggage from their previous delivery. It is incredibly valuable for women desiring a VBAC to work through any fear and anxiety from the previous delivery and enter labor with a clean emotional slate, to the greatest degree possible. Counseling and support groups can aid in this process, as can childbirth education methods, such as HypnoBirthing, which incorporate some element of fear release into the curriculum. Women should also discuss their previous birth with their care provider and inform him or her of the areas in which they felt well supported in their previous delivery, as well as the areas in which they felt their care was lacking and may have contributed to their cesarean. It is important for providers to understand what transpired in the previous delivery, both to help avoid a similar sequence of events and understand what may make their patient nervous or distrustful. A lack of confidence in medical care providers is a common characteristic in women desiring a VBAC and having an open, honest dialogue about care plans and management styles is essential to creating an effective provider–patient relationship, able to effectively utilize shared decision making. If a woman desires something her care provider is not comfortable with, this should be discussed long before the labor and, if it is unable to be resolved with appropriate counseling, it may be more appropriate for the patient to seek care with a different provider rather than have a significant area of contention which may lead to a combative interaction in the delivery room. Professional doula support can also be incredibly helpful to women undergoing a trial of labor, as this provides the continuous physical and emotional support which is so essential for these patients.

HIGH-RISK PATIENTS DESIRING A NATURAL BIRTH

I was 41 when I became pregnant with my first child. We had tried infertility treatments for many years without success and, just when we had reconciled ourselves to a future without children, I was suddenly late. I went to my first doctor appointment, happy and in disbelief, never for a moment considering that this miracle could be anything but that: a miracle. Unfortunately, my doctor saw it differently. Before I had even seen my baby's heartbeat, my doctor had barraged me with concerns about miscarriage, diabetes, preeclampsia, down syndrome, cesarean, and stillbirth. I was told I would need an amniocentesis, would be considered high risk and need to see a specialist, and that I would be induced on my due date. I hadn't given a whole lot of thought to my birth at that point, but suddenly I knew this wasn't the way I wanted to birth my miracle...surrounded by all this fear instead of joy.

I ended up changing to another doctor who treated my age in a much more measured way. She reassured me that, while my age was a risk factor for certain things that I could not "good health" my way out of, the fact that I was healthy and had a spontaneous pregnancy was a very good thing and this baby would just need a little closer watching. She told me as long as my pregnancy progressed normally, which was the MOST LIKELY thing, I could deliver my baby in any way I desired. She did not insist on any invasive testing and counselled me about all my choices for screening for chromosomal abnormalities, including not testing at all, which is what I chose to do because this was my miracle and I knew in my heart that nothing was wrong and even if it was, I would take the blessing I was given. My pregnancy progressed without incident and as I approached my due date, we discussed the recommendation to deliver by forty weeks. She explained the increased risk of stillbirth and the risks and benefits of induction. Ultimately, we decided I would deliver by 41 weeks but luckily I went into labor at 40 weeks and two days and had a beautiful and easy delivery. I felt so grateful to have a doctor that did not ignore my risk, but did not let it completely take over every aspect of my care and worked with me to make the choices that felt right to me.

—A. F., new mother

Many women fear that if they are given a "high-risk" label, they will be unable to have a low-intervention, nonpharmacologic delivery. Depending on the condition, this may indeed be the case. Medical intervention is certainly appropriate and lifesaving in many high-risk conditions of pregnancy. However, the "high-risk" label has come to be applied rather broadly and not all that is "high risk" is incompatible with a natural birth. Risk is typically defined in very black and white terms; a woman is either high or low risk. There is also no indication in terminology of whether that risk applies to pregnancy and labor, pregnancy alone, or labor alone. For patients and providers considering whether a natural birth or even low-intervention approach is appropriate, it is more helpful to think of risk as low, moderate, or high and define the timing of the risk.

For example, a patient with a history of premature birth or fetal loss may be high risk during the antepartum period, but if her pregnancy progresses normally to term and she enters spontaneous labor without complication, her labor and delivery is actually a low-risk event and should be treated as such. Alternatively, a patient may have a low-risk pregnancy until she suddenly goes into premature labor or develops severe preeclampsia, at which point both the remainder of her pregnancy and her delivery are significantly high risk and her care and her expectations in regards to that care must be adjusted to reflect this.

Thinking of risk in this less static way helps both providers and patients maintain flexibility in regards to labor plans. It also aids in assigning appropriate care providers to the patient and choosing the appropriate location for delivery. In general patients who are at low risk for pregnancy, labor, and delivery (AP1, IP1) may receive care from either a doctor or midwife, have a low-intervention, natural labor, and may be appropriate for either a birth center or hospital delivery. Patients in the moderate risk category for pregnancy (AP2) may also be cared for by either a doctor or midwife; however, depending on the condition, greater physician collaboration may be appropriate. For those in the moderate risk category for delivery (IP2), care may also be provided by a doctor or midwife, but with readily available physician backup, and delivery in a hospital is most appropriate. Natural labor may be possible for these patients, but they may require induction, continuous fetal monitoring, and other medical care which may make an unmedicated delivery more challenging. For those in high-risk category for either pregnancy or delivery, obstetrician-led care, with specialist collaboration of maternal–fetal medicine, is most appropriate. Delivery undoubtedly should be performed in a Level 2 or Level 3 hospital, depending on the condition, and most often a limited-intervention or natural approach is not recommended, due to the level of care necessary to ensure maternal and fetal safety. Often, high-risk patients for labor and delivery will require a cesarean delivery.

However, regardless of the risk stratification a patient finds herself within, the principles of the stepwise model and shared decision making should apply. Providers and patients should work together to achieve the healthiest pregnancy possible, especially when significant risk factors are present, with the hope that this may decrease her risk during the actual labor and delivery. Preserving as many components of the mother's initial intention for her labor and delivery, even in a high-risk setting, aids in creating a satisfying birth experience (Table 13-1).

TOOLS FOR COMMON CHALLENGES

TABLE 13-1: RISK STRATIFICATION FOR PREGNANCY, LABOR, AND DELIVERY[26,27]

Antepartum Risk	Intrapartum Risk
Low (1) Singleton pregnancy Age <40 (or 35 according to some guidelines) BMI <30 History of previous cesarean Singleton malposition: breech	**Low (1)** Singleton pregnancy Age <40 Teen pregnancy BMI <30 Diet-controlled diabetic History of fetal loss History of preterm labor
Moderate (2) Advanced maternal age Teen pregnancy Obesity Diet-controlled diabetic Well-controlled maternal medical conditions	**Moderate (2)** Advanced maternal age Obesity Insulin-controlled diabetic with good control Moderate hypertension Well-controlled maternal medical conditions History of previous cesarean Moderate placental deficiency with growth restriction, oligohydramnios
High (3) History of preterm labor History of fetal loss Coagulation defect or history of blood clot Hypertension, preeclampsia Insulin-controlled diabetic Fetal growth restriction Placental insufficiency, oligohydramnios Multiple gestation Poorly controlled maternal medical conditions Congenital abnormality in fetus Placental abnormalities: previa, accreta, percreta	**High (3)** Preterm labor Severe hypertension, preeclampsia Poorly controlled diabetic Coagulation defect, history of blood clot Severe placental deficiency with growth restriction, oligohydramnios Multiple gestation Singleton malposition: breech Poorly controlled maternal medical conditions Congenital abnormality in fetus Placental abnormalities: previa, accreta, percreta

REFERENCES

1. Davey M, King J. Caesarean section following induction of labour in uncomplicated first births—a population-based cross-sectional analysis of 42,950 births. *BMC Pregnancy Childbirth*. 2016;16(1):1. doi:1186/s12884-016-0869-0.
2. Boulvain M, Stan C, Irion O. Membrane sweeping for induction of labour. *Cochrane Database Syst Rev*. 2005;(1):1-95.

3. Smith CA, Crowther CA, Grant SJ. Acupuncture for induction of labour. *Cochrane Database Syst Rev.* 2013;(8):1-73. doi:10.1002/14651858.

4. Smith CA, Crowther CA, Collins CT, Coyle ME. Acupuncture to induce labor: a randomized controlled trial. *Obstet Gynecol.* 2008;112(5):1067-1074. doi:10.1097/AOG.0b013e31818b46bb.

5. Kavanagh J, Kelly AJ, Thomas J. Breast stimulation for cervical ripening and induction of labour. *Cochrane Database Syst Rev.* 2005;(3):1-56.

6. Damania KK, Natu U, Mhatre PN. Evaluation of two methods employed for cervical ripening. *J Postgrad Med.* 1992;38(2):58-59.

7. Beer AM, Heiliger F. Randomized, double-blind trial of Caulophyllum D4 for induction of labor after premature rupture of the membranes at term. *Geburtsh Frauenheilk.* 1999;59(9):431-435.

8. Bendvold E. Coitus and induction of labour [Samleie og induksjon av fodsel]. *Tidsskrift for Jordmodre.* 1990;96:6-8.

9. Tan PC, Andi A, Azmi N, Noraihan MN. Effect of coitus at term on length of gestation, induction of labour, and mode of delivery. *Obstet Gynecol.* 2006;108(1):134-140.

10. Azhari S, Pirdadeh S, Lotfalizadeh M, Shakeri MT. Evaluation of the effect of castor oil on initiating labor in term pregnancy. *Saudi Med J.* 2006;27(7):1011-1014.

11. Tunaru S, Althoff TF, Nüsing RM, et al. Castor oil induces laxation and uterus contraction via ricinoleic acid activating prostaglandin EP3receptors. *Proc Natl Acad Sci USA.* 2012;109(23):9179-9184. doi:10.1073/pnas.1201627109.

12. Boel ME, Lee SJ, Rijken MJ, et al. Castor oil for induction of labour: not harmful, not helpful. *Aust N Z J Obstet Gynaecol.* 2009;49(5):499-503. doi:10.1111/j.1479-828X.2009.01055.x.

13. National Collaborating Centre for Women's and Children's Health (UK). Induction of Labour: NICE Clinical Guidelines, No. 70. London, England: RCOG Press. Available at https://www.ncbi.nlm.nih.gov/books/NBK53608/. Accessed July 2017.

14. Alfirevic Z, Kelly AJ, Dowswell T. Intravenous oxytocin alone for cervical ripening and induction of labour. *Cochrane Database Syst Rev.* 2009;(4):1-322.

15. Hofmeyr GJ, Gülmezoglu AM, Pileggi C. Vaginal misoprostol for cervical ripening and induction of labour. *Cochrane Database Syst Rev.* 2010;(10):1-528. CD000941. doi:10.1002/14651858.

16. Alfirevic Z, Aflaifel N, Weeks A. Oral misoprostol for induction of labour. *Cochrane Database Syst Rev.* 2014;(6):1-342. doi:10.1002/14651858.CD001338.pub3.

17. Tang OS, Gemzell-Danielsson K, Ho PC. Misoprostol: pharmacokinetic profiles, effects on the uterus and side-effects. *Int J Gynaecol Obstet.* 2007;99(2):S160-S167. [Epub October 26, 2007]. Available at http://www.misoprostol.org/downloads/misoprostol-journals/IJGO_pharm_Tang.pdf. Accessed July 2017.

18. Glantz JC. Elective induction vs. spontaneous labor associations and outcomes. *J Reprod Med.* 2005;50(4):235-240.

19. American College of Obstetricians and Gynecologists. ACOG Practice Bulletin No. 115: vaginal birth after previous cesarean delivery. *Obstet Gynecol.* 2010;116(2 pt 1):450-463. doi:10.1097/AOG.0b013e3181eeb251.

20. Ridgeway JJ, Weyrich DL, Benedetti TJ. Fetal heart rate changes associated with uterine rupture. *Obstet Gynecol.* 2004;103(3):506-512.

21. Kieser KE, Baskett TF. A 10-year population-based study of uterine rupture. *Obstet Gynecol.* 2002;100(4):749-753.

22. Hesselman S, Högberg U, Ekholm-Selling K, et al. The risk of uterine rupture is not increased with single- compared with double-layer closure: a Swedish cohort study. *BJOG.* 2015;122(11):1535-1541.

TOOLS FOR COMMON CHALLENGES

23. Anim-Somuah M, Smyth RM, Jones L. Epidural versus non-epidural or no analgesia in labour. *Cochrane Database Syst Rev.* 2011;(12):1-127. doi:10.1002/14651858. CD000331.

24. Graseck AS, Odibo AO, Tuuli M, et al. Normal first stage of labor in women undergoing trial of labor after cesarean delivery. *Obstet Gynecol.* 2012;119(4):732-736.

25. Grantz KL, Gonzalez-Quintero V, Troendle J, et al. Labor patterns in women attempting vaginal birth after cesarean with normal neonatal outcomes. *Am J Obstet Gynecol.* 2015;213(2):226.e1-226.e6.

26. American College of Obstetricians and Gynecologists and Society for Maternal-Fetal Medicine. Levels of maternal care. Obstetric Care Consensus No. 2. *Am J Obstet Gynecol.* 2015;212(3):259-271.

27. What are the factors that put a pregnancy at risk. [Web log post]. Available at https://www.nichd.nih.gov/health/topics/high-risk/conditioninfo/pages/factors. aspx. Accessed August 15, 2017.

The Bookends of Holistic Maternity Care: The Antepartum and Postpartum Periods

The greatest medicine of all is teaching people how not to need it.

—Hippocrates

CHAPTER 14

Holistic Antepartum Care: The Foundation of a Natural Birth

At each new pregnancy consultation, I ask my patient if they have any ideas about the way they would like to birth their baby. Most new mothers indicate a preference for a vaginal delivery and a labor process that is as natural as possible, though most are not willing to take an epidural off the table. I always counsel my patient that they certainly are capable of having an unmedicated delivery. If this were not the case, we would not all be sitting here today. Women have been delivering their babies without pain relief for all of time. However, I also counsel my patients that without proper physical and mental conditioning, ultimately they are unlikely to choose to have an unmedicated delivery because labor is very hard work and if they are unprepared for it, they will most likely want an epidural. But beyond the consideration of an epidural, taking good care of their bodies with proper diet and exercise helps reduce their need for all medical interventions and makes a vaginal delivery more likely. There is nothing I can do as a physician to help a woman have a natural birth which is more important than her taking good care of herself throughout the pregnancy and preparing well for working through an unmedicated delivery. When it comes to natural birth, a woman cannot just try, she must do.

Proper self-care in pregnancy forms the foundation of a natural birth. Unfortunately, in modern time-starved obstetrics practices, few women receive counseling about the importance of proper diet and exercise unless a problem, such as gestational diabetes or excessive weight gain, has already developed. Few women are encouraged to attend childbirth preparation and the western medical viewpoint acknowledges the mind–body connections only to a limited extent, so an even smaller number of women receive any instruction in stress-reduction techniques or emotional preparation for either childbirth or parenthood. There are three hurdles to overcome in order for women to begin receiving this type of counseling in pregnancy and apply it to their pregnancy. First, as with all lifestyle modification initiatives, health care providers must begin to appreciate its value and believe it is something they can influence. Second, outpatient care structures must be modified to accommodate the time required to address these issues. Most physicians and midwives have 15 minutes or less to spend at each antenatal visit. This leaves barely enough time to perform a quick check up and address any immediate questions or concerns. Finally, women themselves must be willing to devote time to both receiving the education and committing themselves to making recommended changes in their own lifestyle. This should be a priority for all women, but for women hoping to have a natural birth, it is an essential part of making their plan a reality.

CRITICAL LIFESTYLE MODIFICATIONS FOR A NATURAL BIRTH

Proper Diet

Eating right, in general, seems like such a simple concept; however, the sheer volume of contradictory advice on proper diet and the numbers of individuals struggling with excess weight are a testament to just how difficult this is to achieve in our modern society. This difficulty in maintaining a healthy diet has a multifactorial etiology and pregnant women are not exempt from the problem, despite usually having a strong motivation to do what is best for their baby. Nearly 50% of women exceed their weight gain recommendations and women who start off pregnancy overweight or obese are even more likely to do so.[1] One reason for the challenge is that access to quality produce and fresh, unprocessed, whole foods is limited for many individuals on the basis of income and/or geographical location. Food preparation is also incredibly time consuming and with the majority of pregnant women working full time, as well as carrying an uneven burden of the household responsibilities, it is understandable that fast and easy is often prioritized over healthy in the hectic day-to-day schedule of most pregnant women. Furthermore, food consumption is tied to both cultural and emotional patterns that are deeply ingrained and challenging to modify even when one knows what they should be doing differently.

In regards to pregnancy specifically, there is a plethora of information regarding what one should or should not eat. Countless articles addressing diet are published in both online and print publications geared toward pregnancy. A simple Google search for books about diet in pregnancy yields over 15 separate results, which are in addition to the individual chapters that are devoted to diet in nearly every general pregnancy book. Family members and friends often take unique liberties with pregnant women in telling what they should and should not be eating. Many women, inundated with this unlimited supply of "helpful" diet advice, find themselves tuning out, skipping over the nutrition chapters in their pregnancy books, and frustrated by their inability to forego the cupcake in the cafeteria or the ice cream in the freezer. Yet, the voice that is often remarkably quiet in this steady stream of information is the woman's own health care provider and, interestingly, most obstetricians actually receive little to no instruction on proper diet guidelines in pregnancy, which may explain their reluctance to discuss the topic. Midwifery care is more likely to include dietary counseling, but time constraints are often limiting.

However, studies have shown that health care providers are able to bring about positive changes in their patient's diets and accomplish what all the books, magazines, and mother-in-law nagging often cannot.[2] These diet conversations do not have to be complicated or overwhelming for either the patient or the provider. Women should be provided with some general guidelines about choosing healthy foods, which can be summarized in *four simple "rules" of pregnancy eating*:

1. *Maximize protein intake*: A pregnant woman should eat at least 65 g. of protein daily. This means she should be eating protein at every meal and one or two protein-rich snacks, such as nuts, yogurt, or cheese.
2. *Maximize vegetable and fruit intake*: Women in pregnancy should eat fruit or vegetables at every meal, of varied types and colors, and incorporate produce into their snacks as well. Eating a rainbow maximizes nutritional intake. Smoothies can be an easy way to get extra fruit and vegetables, but should not be made with fruit juice or other sources of excess sugar.
3. *Limit carbohydrate intake*: Carbohydrates should be limited to roughly a cup per meal and should be brown versus white, whole grain versus white, starchy, and processed. True sweets and treats should be kept to a true once or twice a week treat.
4. *Maximize water intake*: Water should be the beverage of choice and pregnant women should have at least 2 L of water per day, with increased amounts during exercise or heat exposure. Fruit juices or sodas should be considered sweets and treats, not a daily beverage.

Women should be provided with these guidelines at their first pregnancy appointment, but informed that the first trimester is a grace period when it comes to proper eating, as most women have some degree of nausea and food aversions, which make following these guidelines challenging. The most important thing in regards to diet in the first trimester is simply staying hydrated and keeping something down, which for most women is simple carbohydrates. However, once the second trimester arrives and nausea and vomiting of pregnancy is resolving, these recommendations should be revisited and the mother reminded that second trimester is the time to begin focusing on a healthy diet. At each following visit, she should be questioned about what she is eating in a typical day and suggestions for improvement should be made.

Women should also be counseled about typical weight gain expectations and goals for pregnancy, in respect to their pre-pregnancy weight. Excessive weight gain in pregnancy is associated with an increased risk of gestational diabetes, hypertension and preeclampsia, induction, longer labors, and cesarean delivery.[3] Weight gain should be reviewed at each visit. Generally, women should not expect to gain a significant amount of weight in the first half of the pregnancy and weight gain should be limited to approximately one pound per week for the second half of the pregnancy. If a woman is exceeding or not meeting these recommendations, a more thorough assessment of her diet should be performed with a *food diary* and reviewed at the next visit. Consult with a dietician may also be considered. Research, while mixed, has indicated that dietary counseling, in and of itself, helps reduce the incidence of excessive weight gain in pregnancy.[4] However, stronger evidence exists supporting the combination of both diet and exercise in preventing women from gaining too much weight in pregnancy.[5,6]

Exercise

Like eating a proper diet, exercising in pregnancy is something most women know they should do, but many women find it difficult to accomplish. Barriers to exercise in pregnancy are numerous. Often, despite recommendations to exercise, women are afraid that it will harm their baby or they may be told by friends or family members that it is not safe. Even some doctors still give the outdated advice that women should not exercise in the first trimester and should avoid it altogether if they did not exercise prior to pregnancy. Other women simply fall out of the habit during the first trimester, when nausea and fatigue may prevent them for exercising, and never put it back into their routine. For women who did not regularly exercise prior to pregnancy, time constraints and lack of motivation are common barriers that continue to contribute to a sedentary lifestyle. Pregnancy is also a challenging time to begin an exercise regimen, as women are frequently more fatigued, with a greater amount of musculoskeletal discomfort.

However, despite these hurdles, providers should actively encourage their patients, especially those desiring a natural birth, to exercise and inquire about exercise during their routine prenatal visits. The safety of exercise in pregnancy has been well established in medical literature, for both women who were active prior to pregnancy and those that were not. Some common concerns about exercise are that it may lead to premature birth, cause fetal growth restriction, contribute to maternal hyperthermia, or result in episodes of fetal hypoxia. These concerns have been specifically examined and no association with either premature delivery or premature growth restriction has been demonstrated, except in small studies of women who maintained vigorous exercise throughout their pregnancies without appropriate accommodating caloric intake.[7] Exercise in high temperatures is not recommended; however, studies have not demonstrated increased maternal temperatures even in these conditions nor fetal anomalies as a result. The only concerns regarding exercise in healthy pregnancies that are documented in the research are an increased risk of falls and abdominal trauma, maternal sprains and strains, and maternal hypoglycemia. Pregnant women should make modifications in their exercise routine to minimize these risks; however, these concerns should not prevent women from exercising.[8]

Contraindications to exercise are few, but include[9]:

- Severe cardiovascular, respiratory, or systemic disease
- Uncontrolled hypertension or diabetes
- Placenta previa
- Ruptured membranes or premature labor
- Persistent bleeding after first trimester
- Incompetent cervix
- Preeclampsia
- Higher order multiple gestations
- Poor fetal growth

On the other hand, there are numerous *benefits of exercise in pregnancy*[9-11]:

- Maintenance and improvement in physical fitness, which aids in both stamina during labor and delivery and improved maternal condition after pregnancy
- Decreased rates of cesarean delivery and operative vaginal delivery
- Decreased risk of gestational diabetes
- Decreased incidence of preeclampsia and hypertension

These benefits have a particular relevance for women who wish to minimize technological interventions during their labor and delivery, as exercise reduces their likelihood of developing conditions that considerably restrict their ability to have an unmedicated birth.

Current recommendations are for pregnant women to exercise at least three times weekly, for a minimum of 30 consecutive minutes. Many women confuse being active during the day with adequate exercise; however, this does not have the same benefit as true, dedicated exercise in which the woman has consistent, maintained physical exertion. Women should also be encouraged to vary their exercise, incorporating cardiovascular exercise with light strengthening routines, as well as activities that help open and strengthen the pelvic floor, such as yoga and pilates. Yoga, specifically, has been shown to reduce pain during labor, shorten the total duration of labor, and improve quality of life and interpersonal relationships during pregnancy.[12]

Specific *physical activities that are suitable in pregnancy* include:

- Walking, running, and jogging
- Swimming
- Stationary cycling
- Yoga and pilates, modified for pregnancy
- Aerobics
- Strength training, modified for pregnancy

However, there are certain *activities that should be avoided in pregnancy* including:

- Activities with a high risk of falling or trauma: skiing, surfing, horseback riding, ice skating, or off-road cycling
- High impact or contact sports
- Scuba diving
- Sky diving

However, despite the clear benefits and specific recommendations from the American College of Obstetrician and Gynecologists about exercise in pregnancy, only 52% of obstetricians routinely discuss exercise and among those that do, a large portion do not counsel their patients in accordance with current guidelines. For example, despite evidence to the contrary, many obstetricians advise women not to exceed a certain heart rate, recommend reducing exercise load in the third trimester, and do not recommend sedentary women initiate exercise in pregnancy.[13] Reeducation of health care providers is an important component of women receiving the appropriate information regarding prenatal physical activity. For health care providers looking for guidance in how to encourage their pregnant patients to incorporate exercise into their routines, methods for encouraging lifestyle modification have been studied and can be applied to their practice. A tool which has demonstrated efficacy in smoking cessation, *the five A's*, has also shown to be beneficial in weight reduction and exercise promotion.[14,15] The five A's stand for *ask, advise, assess, assist,* and *arrange.* Doctors and midwives should ask about exercise at each visit, make recommendations regarding the information the patient reports, assess progress by both monitoring weight gain and reviewing food diaries, assist patients who are having challenges by exploring their individual barriers to change and suggesting solutions, and arrange specialist care with dieticians or physical therapists if indicated.

Women, for their part, must be willing to listen to their care providers and make exercise a priority. Many sedentary women are able to make a long list of why they cannot exercise; however, the truth is there are very few people who cannot exercise. It is usually simply a question of what is taking precedence in their lives. When women schedule exercise into their week and consider it a commitment that they are unable to break, they are more likely to be consistent with an exercise routine. Women should also know that exercise does not have to occur in the gym. This may be especially helpful for women that have other young children at home or work long hours. A dance party in the living room can be great exercise. Starting the day off with a yoga stretching routine is an easy modification that only requires waking 15 minutes earlier. Light hand weights and simple squats are strengthening activities that can be done while watching an evening television show. Women should be looking for all the ways they can incorporate physical activity into their day, rather than focusing on all the things that are keeping them from getting to a gym.

Stress Reduction and Mental Preparation for Birth

In addition to proper nutrition and physical activity, the emotional well-being of the mother should also be cared for in the antenatal period as part of a holistic model of care and preparation for an unmedicated delivery. While pregnancy is a happy and exciting time for most women, it also represents a major life-changing event, which is stress producing. Up to 12% of women experience depression at some point in pregnancy and one in five pregnant women meet diagnostic criteria for an anxiety disorder.[16–18] Women experiencing mood disorders in pregnancy may be more likely to desire natural birth options, as they may have a stronger desire to maintain control over their birth process than women who are not experiencing anxiety.

Treating the symptoms of depression and anxiety and reducing stress in pregnancy is important for both mother and baby. Women with mood disorders in pregnancy are more likely to have those symptoms carry on after pregnancy and affect their ability to care for their children and enjoy motherhood.[19] Studies have also shown an association between maternal stress and mood disorders and complications of pregnancy such as premature birth and fetal growth restriction.[20,21] During labor, preventing the flight or fight cascade of stress hormones is also important for proper labor progression.[22]

All women should be screened for mood disorders throughout the pregnancy and women should know that relaying any emotional concerns is as important as reporting on any other area of their health. Certainly, a history of mood disorders prior to pregnancy warrants close follow-up and referral with a mental health professional is often appropriate. Some examples of general questions which both providers and women can consider exploring are:

- *How are you feeling about this pregnancy?*
- *How are you feeling in general?*
- *What in your life is causing you stress or anxiety?*
- *How are you sleeping?*
- *How are you and your partner getting along?*
- *What is your support like in this pregnancy and what do you expect your support will be like after you have the baby?*
- *How are you feeling about the process of giving birth?*
- *What are you most nervous about in terms of labor or being a mother?*

When women are reporting depression or anxiety symptoms, a simple *daily rating system* can be helpful for both women and their providers to gage the severity of the symptoms. At the end of the day, women should give the day a 1, 2, or 3, where a 1 indicates a day with little to no symptoms, a 2 indicates a moderate amount of symptoms, and a 3 indicates a day with significant symptoms. If a woman is mainly having 1's or 2's, both she and provider can be reassured and focus on stress-reduction strategies and perhaps cognitive therapy or counseling. If a woman is reporting mainly 2's or 3's, this indicates that symptoms are at a level that likely requires specialist referral.

Stress-reduction strategies are helpful for all women, but are particularly important when women are having symptoms of anxiety or depression. Stress-reduction strategies also have particular application to an unmedicated, natural labor process, where women endure long periods of physical discomfort, in addition to considerable fear and anxiety about the process, their baby, and their level of discomfort. Formal methods of teaching stress reduction or relaxation training generally focus on *mindfulness, meditation, positive affirmations,* and *breathwork.* Mindfulness is defined as a mental state in which one focuses on the present moment, openly accepting and acknowledging all sensations, emotions, and thoughts without judging them or making an attempt to modify them. Meditation is generally described as dedicated time spent in quiet mindfulness or visualization, where the deep, Ujjayi breath is utilized to promote deep relaxation and quieting of the mind. Positive affirmations are statements spoken as a fact or truth, in the present tense with only positive language, that affirm the speaker. The intention of repeating these statements is to build the self-confidence needed to make the statements a reality. Studies have shown that both chronic and acute stress impair performance and positive self-affirmation is a valuable tool to reverse this effect.[23] Pregnant women who are provided with relaxation training during the course of their routine prenatal care demonstrate lower levels of anxiety and perceived stress when compared to women who only receive routine prenatal care.[24] This training is also effective in reducing anxiety in patients who enter pregnancy with anxiety disorders or acquire anxiety during pregnancy.[25]

These techniques have been extended into labor preparation, as well. Conscious birthing methods, such as HypnoBirthing, HypnoBabies, and Mindfulness-Based Childbirth and Parenting Education (MBCP), teach parents to use meditation and breathing in order to cope with childbirth discomfort and maintain a low-stress, relaxed mental state throughout the process. These methods help mothers-to-be learn to focus on periods of ease and rest between contractions, rather than focusing on and anticipating the more intense sensations which occur during a contraction. These courses also provide space for mothers and their partners to express their anxieties about the labor process and receive support from their partners, instructors, and classmates. By bringing those fears into the open, parents are better able to process them and release them, so they do not impact their labor process and emotional well-being. These methods have been shown to help women better cope with unmedicated birth, as well as improve their emotional response to stressful situations both during labor and in the postpartum period.[26,27]

ANTENATAL EDUCATION

Childbirth Preparation

As previously discussed, childbirth preparation utilizing a structured method should be considered essential for any mother wishing to labor without medication. This is something that should be discussed early in prenatal care and women should be encouraged to learn about the various methods and return to their care providers with any questions. While no one method of childbirth education is right for all women, methods that thoroughly inform women about the labor process, explore typical medical management and interventions, provide hands-on instruction in natural coping strategies, and address the psychological impacts of the labor process, as well as teaching stress-reduction techniques, are most effective in preparing women for their natural birth goals. To be able to cover these areas sufficiently generally requires several sessions of education and patients should be prepared to make this time commitment. Support partners should make every effort to attend childbirth education, to offer moral support, be an active participant in the process, and understand the tools which are being utilized. Care providers should also gain a firm understanding of the benefits and downsides of each method of childbirth instruction, beyond the two-line description on a website or information pamphlet, and be able to discuss the methods which may be best for their patient. Ideally, doctors and midwives should attend the various childbirth classes themselves or read their associated texts so they may work with their patients in the style of education they received. By the 28-week visit, women should have chosen and registered for their childbirth class and they should have completed their education by the 36-week visit, so they may discuss their labor plan with their doctor or midwife from an educated viewpoint.

Breastfeeding Preparation

Most mothers who plan to labor naturally also plan to breastfeed their babies. In fact, 80% of new mothers surveyed reported an intention to breastfeed. However, 60% of mothers report that they stopped breastfeeding earlier than they originally intended.[28] There have been many studies examining why so many women have difficulty achieving their breastfeeding goals and the most commonly cited reasons are lactation difficulties, concerns about the adequacy of breast milk alone to meet their child's nutritional needs and demands, complications of maternal and infants illness, and the time constraints of outside work combined with pumping demands.[29] Breastfeeding confidence is also correlated with breastfeeding duration and success and breastfeeding knowledge is strongly associated with confidence in breastfeeding.[30] Therefore, there are many individuals who encourage women to attend antenatal breastfeeding education to better prepare for and prevent breastfeeding challenges. The data on the benefits of antenatal breastfeeding education is mixed. Some studies have demonstrated improvement in both initiation of breastfeeding and duration of breastfeeding among women who receive antenatal breastfeeding education.[31,32] However, larger reviews have failed to demonstrate a clear benefit to antenatal breastfeeding education, though given the multifactorial nature of breastfeeding barriers and challenges, it is not surprising that a single intervention fails to demonstrate significant benefit.[33] When antenatal breastfeeding is included as part of a comprehensive program of intervention to promote breastfeeding in multiple settings, including outpatient antepartum care, inpatient postpartum care, and outpatient postpartum care, both in clinics and the home, it has been seen as more beneficial.[34] Thus, in the same way that natural childbirth education cannot be effective if it occurs in a vacuum, without any other support structure for natural labor, breastfeeding education is not likely to help women achieve their breastfeeding goals if there is no support in place to help women through the number of breastfeeding challenges they may face. Education in the antepartum period is simply the first step in a system of support for holistic maternity practices.

Parenting Preparation

When I was pregnant with my first baby, I did EVERYTHING to prepare for a natural labor! We attended a Bradley class for twelve entire weeks. I read at least fifteen different books, watched the Business of Being Born, and viewed every natural birth YouTube video I could find. I went to yoga twice per week. We hired a doula, used a midwife, and had a two page birth plan. When the day finally came, it felt like a final exam that I passed with flying colors. I bounced and vocalized, swayed and groaned, and rocked my birth of my nine pound baby boy. I felt so incredibly powerful and vindicated, getting to tell all those people who had told me it would never happen that I had exactly what I wanted, that I did it. But after that initial high wore off and I settled into the days and weeks to follow, I came to realize, in all my preparation, I had forgot one crucial thing. At three in the morning, after days of no sleep, laundry piled to the ceiling, and no food in the fridge, I discovered that I hadn't planned for the baby! I hadn't taken the time to figure out what we were going to do with this loud, demanding, little human being who we were now completely responsible for. I had arranged all the help I needed to birth him, but none of the help I needed to actually take care of him...and me. I didn't know how to nurse him. I didn't know how to bathe him. I didn't know how to get him to sleep anywhere but in my arms. I couldn't cook a meal or take a shower. I had passed my final exam but forgotten to register for the next course. Now, when my friends ask me about laboring and having a baby, I tell them to certainly prepare for their labor, but prepare for the whole motherhood part too.

—B. N., new mother

Very few childbirth preparation courses provide information about how to approach the first weeks and months of new parenthood. While no class or book can prepare one for the experience of new parenthood, many parents report feeling in the dark, with little support to navigate those early, challenging days. A frequent critique of antenatal education is that it inadequately prepares new parents for parenthood.[35] Parents who have previously had a child have less difficulty, as they have their previous experience to fall back on and are more confident in their infant care skills. However, even experienced parents may have challenges integrating a new baby into their family structure or experience unique difficulties with their new or existing child. Ideally, parenting courses should teach necessary infant care skills, inform parents about child development, provide instruction on child safety and warning signs of illness, and help parents begin to dialogue about child care, feeding decisions, sleep schedules, and discipline. Courses should also help new parents prepare for the changes they can expect in their personal relationship and encourage relationship building and communication skills. Parents should also be encouraged to develop a plan of support for the initial weeks after the baby comes home that addresses time for each individual to obtain rest, meal preparation, household chores, and transportation to necessary doctor visits. Parents should be provided with resources for lactation counseling and a listing of support groups and mental health professionals, should symptoms of postpartum depression or anxiety arise.

MODIFICATIONS TO THE ANTEPARTUM CARE STRUCTURE

In order for expecting women and their partners to receive the proper counseling and education to promote holistic maternity goals, the issue of time restriction in traditional antepartum care must be addressed. In the current insurance structure, women are afforded an initial confirmation of pregnancy visit, which is intended only to confirm the viability of the pregnancy and address an immediate concern. No general pregnancy counseling, information on testing options, or lifestyle recommendations are meant to be addressed at this visit. Once the pregnancy is confirmed, the patient is supposed to return for a longer initial prenatal appointment, in which all this information is discussed, in addition to a complete physical exam and typically an ultrasound to again confirm viability. Most practices only have 30 minutes available for this appointment and some only allot 15 minutes for this visit because it is not separately reimbursed. All additional appointments are 15 minutes. There is simply no way to accomplish the needs of new parents in this care structure.

Many alternatives have been suggested and studied to a limited degree. One simple solution would be to increase reimbursements for antepartum care to reflect the time necessary to deliver this level of care. With higher reimbursements, practices could afford to accept fewer patients and spend more time with the women under their care. However, given the shortage of obstetricians in the United States, this strategy, in the absence of other efforts to expand maternity services, would restrict access to care to an even larger extent.[36] Another option is a broader adoption of the Integrated Collaborative Care model, which would utilize midwifery care for improved counseling and more efficient time management within obstetrics practices (see Chapter 3). This model offers an individual approach to counseling and education, which is preferred by patients when surveyed, and allows advice to be tailored to each woman's risk stratification.[2] A third alternative is group prenatal care, most notably the Centering Pregnancy model. In this model, the physical assessment, including fetal heart rate checks, vital signs, and fundal height measurements, education, and peer support are all conducted in one group space according to the routine prenatal visit calendar. Patients are placed in Centering groups after the initial pregnancy confirmation. The model offers more time for counseling and education by delivering the information once in a group setting, rather than repetitively to each individual. Question time is also less time consuming, because there is less repetition of questions, and patients benefit from hearing concerns from their peers which they may not have considered. Group prenatal care also builds camaraderie and provides improved social and emotional support. Studies examining this method have demonstrated higher levels of patient and provider satisfaction, improved breastfeeding rates, and improved birth outcomes with group care.[37] However, this model may have logistical limitations in a busy practice, without a large meeting space, and some women may not feel comfortable in a group setting or be less likely to reveal personal concerns.

A fourth option is to design a care structure that incorporates each of these solutions, to some degree. Limiting patient numbers can be done without limiting the number of obstetric patients, but by segregating entire practices into obstetrics-focused practices, which are limited to obstetrics care and gynecology for women who are in the active childbearing years, and gynecology-focused practices, which are limited to gynecology for adolescents, pre-childbearing young women, and post-childbearing older women. In this way, obstetrics practices can design their services around providing optimal care for pregnant patients, rather than dividing their time and energy between obstetrics and gynecology needs. While this may seem to fly in the face of the longstanding tradition of OB/GYNs caring for women through all their life cycle transitions, in reality, most OB/GYNs follow a career pattern where they predominantly practice obstetrics in their early years out of residency and later transition into providing mainly gynecologic care. This would simply be designing practices around that transition. Obstetrics-based practices could more easily incorporate midwifery care and develop collaborative practice models. With less need for procedure space and pelvic exam rooms, practices could create larger group spaces and offer classes and group care. Group care, with its expanded education, counseling, and peer support could be offered monthly, each trimester, or at specific points within the pregnancy that were determined to be most beneficial. Childbirth, breastfeeding, and parenting education could all be offered within these maternity centers, which could even incorporate prenatal yoga and doula services into their prenatal centers.

This "one-stop shopping" would increase the number of patients receiving education, as they would not have to research courses in their individual communities and their classes could be scheduled well ahead of time when each patient establishes care. Offering these services, which are typically cash pay, also helps increase sources of revenue for individual practices, even without increased insurance reimbursements, and limits some of the financial barriers to natural birth support. Centralization of services is also likely to reduce costs for individual patients and increase the number of women who are able to take advantage of these important aspects of prenatal care and natural labor support, which are not currently covered by insurance companies.

REFERENCES

1. Kominiarek MA, Peaceman AM. Gestational weight gain. *Am J Obstet Gynecol.* 2017;217(6):642-651. doi:10.1016/j.ajog.2017.05.040.

2. National Collaborating Centre for Women's and Children's Health (UK). *Antenatal Care: Routine Care for the Healthy Pregnant Woman.* (NICE Clinical Guidelines, No. 62). 3: Woman-centered care and informed decision making. London: RCOG Press; 2008. Available at https://www.ncbi.nlm.nih.gov/books/NBK51901/. Accessed July 2017.

3. Institute of Medicine (US) and National Research Council (US) Committee to Reexamine IOM Pregnancy Weight Guidelines; Rasmussen KM, Yaktine AL, eds. *Weight Gain During Pregnancy: Reexamining the Guidelines.* Washington, DC: National Academies Press; 2009. Available at https://www.ncbi.nlm.nih.gov/books/NBK32818/.

4. Tieu J, Shepherd E, Middleton P, Crowther CA. Dietary advice interventions in pregnancy for preventing gestational diabetes mellitus. *Cochrane Database Syst Rev.* 2017;1:1-134. doi:10.1002/14651858.CD006674.

5. Muktabhant B, Lawrie TA, Lumbiganon P, Laopaiboon M. Diet or exercise, or both, for preventing excessive weight gain in pregnancy. *Cochrane Database Syst Rev.* 2015;(6):1-260. doi:10.1002/14651858.

6. The International Weight Management in Pregnancy (i-WIP) Collaborative Group. Effect of diet and physical activity based interventions in pregnancy on gestational weight gain and pregnancy outcomes: meta-analysis of individual participant data from randomised trials. *BMJ.* 2017;358:j3991. doi:10.1136/bmj.j3991. Available at http://www.bmj.com/content/358/bmj.j3119.

7. Tinloy J, Chuang CH, Zhu J, et al. Exercise during pregnancy and risk of late preterm birth, cesarean delivery, and hospitalizations. *Womens Health Issues.* 2014;24(1): e99-e104.

8. Hammer RL, Perkins J, Parr R. Exercise during the childbearing year. *J Perinat Educ.* 2009;9(1):1-14. doi:10.1624/105812400X87455.

9. American College of Obstetricians and Gynecologists. ACOG Committee Opinion No. 650: physical activity and exercise during pregnancy and the postpartum period. *Obstet Gynecol.* 2015;126(6):e135-e142. doi:10.1097/AOG.0000000000001214.

10. Wang C, Wei Y, Zhang X, et al. A randomized clinical trial of exercise during pregnancy to prevent gestational diabetes mellitus and improve pregnancy outcome in overweight and obese pregnant women. *Am J Obstet Gynecol.* 2017;216(4):340-351.

11. Di Mascio D, Magro-Malosso ER, Saccone G, et al. Exercise during pregnancy in normal-weight women and risk of preterm birth: a systematic review and meta-analysis of randomized controlled trials. *Am J Obstet Gynecol.* 2016;215(5):561-571.

12. Curtis K, Weinrib A, Katz J. Systematic review of yoga for pregnant women: current status and future directions. *Evid Based Complement Alternat Med.* 2012;2012(715942):1-13. doi:10.1155/2012/715942. Available at https://www.ncbi.nlm.nih.gov/pmc/articles/PMC3424788/pdf/ECAM2012-715942.pdf.

13. Entin PL, Munhall KM. Recommendations regarding exercise during pregnancy made by private/small group practice obstetricians in the USA. *J Sports Sci Med.* 2006;5(3):449-458.

14. Alexander SC, Cox ME, Boling Turer CL. Do the five A's work when physicians counsel about weight loss? *Fam Med.* 2011;43(3):179-184.

15. Serdula MK, Khan LK, Dietz WH. Weight loss counseling revisited. *JAMA.* 2003;289(14):1747-1750.

16. Gavin NI, Gaynes BN, Lohr KN, et al. Perinatal depression: a systematic review of prevalence and incidence. *Obstet Gynecol.* 2005;106(5 pt 1):1071-1083.

17. Vesga-López O, Blanco C, Keyes K, et al. Psychiatric disorders in pregnant and postpartum women in the United States. *Arch Gen Psychiatry.* 2008;65(7):805-815. doi:10.1001/archpsyc.65.7.805.

18. Grant KA, McMahon C, Austin MP. Maternal anxiety during the transition to parenthood: a prospective study. *J Affect Disord.* 2008;108(1-2):101-111.

19. Martini J, Knappe S, Beesdo-Baum K, et al. Anxiety disorders before birth and self-perceived distress during pregnancy: associations with maternal depression and obstetric, neonatal and early childhood outcomes. *Early Hum Dev.* 2010;86(5):305-310. doi:10.1016/j.earlhumdev.2010.04.004.

20. Wadhwa PD, Entringer S, Buss C, Lu MC. The contribution of maternal stress to preterm birth: issues and considerations. *Clin Perinatol.* 2011;38(3):351-384. doi:10.1016/j.clp.2011.06.007.

21. Staneva A, Bogossian F, Pritchard M, Wittkowski A. The effects of maternal depression, anxiety, and perceived stress during pregnancy on preterm birth: a systematic review. *Women Birth.* 2015;28(3):179-193. doi:10.1016/j.wombi.2015.02.003.

22. Foureur M. Creating birth space to enable an undisturbed birth. In *Birth Territory and Midwifery Guardianship: Theory for Practice, Education, and Research.* London: Elsevier Limited; 2008.

23. Creswell JD, Dutcher JM, Klein WM, et al. Self-affirmation improves problem-solving under stress. *PLoS ONE.* 2013;8(5):e62593. Available at http://journals.plos.org/plosone/article?id=10.1371/journal.pone.0062593.

24. Bastani F, Hidarnia A, Kazemnejad A, et al. A randomized controlled trial of the effects of applied relaxation training on reducing anxiety and perceived stress in pregnant women. *J Midwifery Womens Health.* 2005;50(4):e36-e40.

25. Goodman JH, Guarino A, Chenausky K, et al. CALM Pregnancy: results of a pilot study of mindfulness-based cognitive therapy for perinatal anxiety. *Arch Womens Ment Health.* 2014;17(5):373-387. doi:10.1007/s00737-013-0402-7.

26. Duncan LG, Bardacke N. Mindfulness-based childbirth and parenting education: promoting family mindfulness during the perinatal period. *J Child Fam Stud.* 2010;19(2):190-202. doi:10.1007/s10826-009-9313-7.

27. Marc I, Toureche N, Ernst E. Mind-body interventions during pregnancy for preventing or treating women's anxiety. *Cochrane Database Syst Rev.* 2011;(7):1-65. CD007559. doi:10.1002/14651858.CD007559.pub2.

28. Odom EC, Li R, Scanlon KS, et al. Reasons for earlier than desired cessation of breastfeeding. *Pediatrics.* 2013;131(3):e726-e732. doi:10.1542/peds.2012-1295.

29. Li R, Fein SB, Chen J, Grummer-Strawn LM. Why mothers stop breastfeeding: mothers' self-reported reasons for stopping during the first year. *Pediatrics.* 2008;122(suppl 2):69-76. doi:10.1542/peds.2008-1315i.

30. Chezem J, Friesen C, Boettcher J. Breastfeeding knowledge, breastfeeding confidence, and infant feeding plans: effects on actual feeding practices. *J Obstet Gynecol Neonatal Nurs.* 2003;32(1):40-47.

31. Haroon S, Das JK, Salam RA, Imdad A, Bhutta ZA. Breastfeeding promotion interventions and breastfeeding practices: a systematic review. *BMC Public Health.* 2013;13(suppl 3):S20. doi:10.1186/1471-2458-13-S3-S20.

32. Artieta-Pinedo I, Paz-Pascual C, Grandes G, et al. Antenatal education and breastfeeding in a cohort of primiparas. *J Adv Nurs.* 2013;69(7):1607-1617. doi:10.1111/jan.12022.

33. Lumbiganon P, Martis R, Laopaiboon M, et al. Antenatal breastfeeding education for increasing breastfeeding duration. *Cochrane Database Syst Rev.* 2016;(12):CD006425. doi:10.1002/14651858.CD006425.pub4.

34. Sinha B, Chowdhury R, Sankar MJ, et al. Interventions to improve breastfeeding outcomes: a systematic review and meta-analysis. *Acta Paediatrica.* 2015;104(S467):114-134.

35. Entsieh AA, Hallström IK. First-time parents' prenatal needs for early parenthood preparation—a systematic review and meta-synthesis of qualitative literature. *Midwifery.* 2016;39(Aug):1-11. doi:10.1016/j.midw.2016.04.006.

36. Rayburn W. The Obstetrician-Gynecologist Workforce in the United States: facts, figures, and implications, 2017. American Congress of Obstetrician Gynecologists. Available at https://www.acog.org/Resources-And-Publications/The-Ob-Gyn-Workforce/The-Obstetrician-Gynecologist-Workforce-in-the-United-States. Accessed July 2017.

37. Rotundo G. Centering pregnancy: the benefits of group prenatal care. *Nurs Womens Health.* 2011;15(6):508-517. doi:10.1111/j.1751-486X.2011.01678.x.

CHAPTER 15

Holistic Postpartum Care: Recognizing the Fourth Trimester

When I got home from the hospital, my wife and I felt like we had been dropped on a desert island. The first few days everyone was really excited to see the baby and brought food and company, but after that initial rush, we were alone. Neither of us had babysat much, so we were awkward even holding the kid for a while. I was afraid all the time. I would just sit up staring at her, so terrified that she would stop breathing in her sleep. I didn't have enough of a milk supply and after two weeks of crying...usually all of us crying together...we finally caved and just went to formula. I felt like the worst mother on the planet. I couldn't even figure out how to feed my baby. I wished there was someone who could help, but I didn't even have the energy to look and, even if I did, I wouldn't have known where to start. It got better in its own time, I think mainly just from the baby getting older and us gaining some experience, but I think I missed out on something... that sort of new mothering bliss I always imagined I would have. I hardly even remember what my daughter was like as a newborn, I was so stressed and sleep deprived. I was probably a bit depressed too, though I was never diagnosed or anything. I would definitely do a lot of things differently if I knew then what I know now.

—E. L., new mother

In medicine, mommy blogs, and most pregnancy books, including this one, much time and energy is spent on improving the labor and delivery process and outcomes. For the most part, the postpartum period is an afterthought and there is little planning for this time or support for the mothers navigating an entirely new set of challenges, while still physically recuperating from pregnancy and delivery. Most parents spend more time on their baby registry than on preparing for the actual realities of new parenthood. While some would argue that no book or class can adequately prepare expectant mothers and fathers for what is to come, most new parents express the desire for more than just on-the-job training and feel they would benefit from more parenting information prior to delivery and increased help after the baby arrives.[1]

With increasing awareness about the importance of breastfeeding and the resultant public health campaign to expand breastfeeding in the United States and throughout the world, some positive developments have occurred in postpartum care, but most of those improvements have been limited to the hospital, with little to no continuity with care providers following discharge. In the traditional postpartum care model, mothers who have an in-hospital vaginal delivery spend 1 to 2 days in the hospital after the birth of their child and do not see their obstetrician or midwife until well after delivery. If they are struggling with laceration healing, sleep deprivation, breastfeeding, infant care, or postpartum depression and anxiety, they are frequently isolated and left floundering at home, trying to solve the problem themselves or searching independently for resources in the community. While pediatricians see new infants frequently during this time period, these visits do not necessarily address the needs of new mothers. All too often, it is only discovered at a woman's routine postpartum visit, a full 6 to 8 weeks after delivery, that she is experiencing significant depression or anxiety, she abandoned breastfeeding due to considerable challenges, or her perineal laceration is not healing in the way it should be. Her relationship may also be strained to the breaking point as she and her partner struggle to parent together.

It is important for both women and their care providers to be better informed about the common challenges women face in the postpartum period, as well as the commonly suggested remedies to these problems. In the absence of proper or timely medical feedback, women receive a plethora of advice of varied quality from a multitude of sources. Women are often desperate to try anything that may improve their situation, but much of what is recommended to new mothers in regards to breastfeeding or infant care struggles has not necessarily been shown to be effective and women can expend a great deal of energy and money trying treatments that are not likely to solve their problem. Providers need to be familiar with these difficulties and the advice women are likely to receive so they can have an intelligent dialogue and direct their patients to those remedies that are most likely to be helpful.

BREASTFEEDING

I thought delivering my son was going to be the hard part. Boy, was I wrong. Breastfeeding was hard, like really hard. But looking at it now, I guess if breastfeeding was as easy as I thought it would be, everyone would do it.

—C. W., new mother

IMPROVED BREASTFEEDING SUPPORT

The World Health Organization recommends all infants be exclusively breastfed for at least 6 months after birth and partial breastfeeding continue until 2 years of age.[2] This recommendation is supported by multiple studies demonstrating decreased infant morbidity with this duration of exclusive breastfeeding.[3] However, most countries observe low rates of exclusive breastfeeding and shorter than recommended breastfeeding durations. This is observed even in countries where the rate of breast-feeding initiation is high, suggesting this problem is not a result of moth-ers being unwilling or unmotivated to breastfeed. Rather, it is a result of mothers being unable to achieve successful breastfeeding and over-come breastfeeding challenges. Most of the available research regard-ing breastfeeding focuses on modifications in antepartum care and in-hospital intrapartum and postpartum care. While antepartum edu-cation regarding breastfeeding has been shown to improve the rates of women initiating breastfeeding, as well as reduce the number of women not breastfeeding at all, education alone has not been shown to sig-nificantly impact exclusive breastfeeding rates later in the postpartum period.[4–6] Antenatal breastfeeding education is better thought of as an initiating step in a process of breastfeeding support. The most effec-tive intervention demonstrated by the literature, shown to improve all parameters including breastfeeding initiation, duration of any breast-feeding, and exclusive breastfeeding rates, is the combination of prac-tices included within the 10 steps of the Baby-Friendly Initiative.

In-Hospital Support: The Baby-Friendly Initiative

The Baby-Friendly Initiative was launched in 1991 as a joint effort by the World Health Organization and the United Nations Children's Fund (UNICEF) to promote global breastfeeding through broad implementa-tion of the Ten Steps to Successful Breastfeeding and the International Code of Marketing of Breast-milk Substitutes.[7] The goal of the Ten Steps is to help hospitals adopt evidence-based practices which promote breastfeeding, while the International Code aims to reduce the negative influence of formula marketing on breastfeeding within the hospital.[8]

There are multiple studies supporting each of the steps promoted by the Baby-Friendly Initiative. Since the broader adoption of the Baby-Friendly Initiative and subsequent certification of Baby-Friendly hospitals, there have also been a number of studies evaluating the imple-mentation of these steps collectively. The first of these was a large ran-domized control study of over 17,000 mother–infant pairs in Belarus, which demonstrated significant improvement in duration of breastfeed-ing with adherence to the Baby-Friendly Initiative, as well as a significant increases in the rates of predominant and exclusive breastfeeding.[9] Fol-low-up studies in Brazil, Switzerland, Taiwan, the United States, as well as other countries have supported these findings; however, the majority

The Baby-Friendly Initiative[10]	
The Ten Steps to Successful Breastfeeding	**The International Code of Marketing of Breast-milk Substitutes**
1. Have a written breastfeeding policy that is routinely communicated to all health care staff.	1. No advertising of breast-milk substitutes to families.
2. Train all health care staff in the skills necessary to implement this policy.	2. No free samples or supplies in the health care system.
3. Inform all pregnant women about the benefits and management of breastfeeding.	3. No promotion of products through health care facilities, including no free or low-cost formula.
4. Help mothers initiate breastfeeding within 1 hour of birth.	4. No contact between marketing personnel and mothers.
5. Show mothers how to breastfeed and how to maintain lactation, even if they are separated from their infants.	5. No gifts or personal samples to health workers.
6. Give infants no food or drink other than breast milk, unless medically indicated.	6. No words or pictures idealizing artificial feeding, including pictures of infants, on the labels or product.
7. Practice rooming in—allow mothers and infants to remain together 24 hours a day.	7. Information to health workers should be scientific and factual only.
8. Encourage breastfeeding on demand.	8. All information on artificial feeding, including labels, should explain the benefits of breastfeeding and the costs and hazards associated with artificial feeding.
9. Give no pacifiers or artificial nipples to breastfeeding infants.	9. Unsuitable products should not be promoted for babies.
10. Foster the establishment of breastfeeding support groups and refer mothers to them on discharge from the hospital or birth center.	10. All products should be of high quality and take account of the climate and storage conditions of the country.

of the evidence in support of the Baby-Friendly Initiative is based on research performed outside the United States.[11-15] Research has also shown, perhaps unsurprisingly, that the greater the number of steps which are actually implemented, the more positive the effect on breastfeeding outcomes, again demonstrating the importance of a comprehensive approach to breastfeeding support and promotion.[16]

Outpatient Support

However, even with full implementation of the Baby-Friendly Initiative, the rates of exclusive breastfeeding and breastfeeding duration still fall short of the goals of World Health Organization, American Academy of

Pediatrics, and other health organizations. Continuation of breastfeeding support in the outpatient setting and appropriate management of breastfeeding complications is equally important as the establishment of a strong breastfeeding foundation during the antepartum and immediate postpartum periods.

There are many approaches to outpatient breastfeeding support. Mothers may receive *individual breastfeeding counseling* sessions with a certified lactation consultant (IBCLC) or lactation counselor (CLC). Lactation consultants and counselors offer similar services, though lactation consultants have significantly more training than lactation counselors and are generally considered preferable when a significant breastfeeding challenge arises. Individual sessions with a certified lactation provider have been shown to improve rates of breastfeeding initiation, any breastfeeding, and exclusive breastfeeding.[17,18] Research has also demonstrated an association between access to breastfeeding specialists and overall breastfeeding prevalence.[19] Breastfeeding support and counseling may also be provided in group setting, either through professionally led *breastfeeding support groups*, or peer-led groups. These groups may be affiliated with the hospital, birthing center, or medical office that provided care during pregnancy and delivery or exist privately within a woman's local community. La Leche League is the most well-known peer-led breastfeeding support group and offers online resources as well. Both professional and peer-led group support has been shown to be helpful.[20] Mothers may also receive professional telephone or online support; however, face-to-face counseling and evaluation of the mother–infant dyad is the most beneficial.

Family support, particularly partner support, is also incredibly important for breastfeeding mothers. Lack of partner support is associated with early cessation of exclusive breastfeeding and less maternal confidence, while mothers who describe better partner support are more likely to report higher confidence with breastfeeding in general.[21,22] Research is ongoing to examine whether breastfeeding promotional interventions specifically geared toward fathers may aid in increasing breastfeeding rates.[23] However, from questionnaires of mothers and their partners about their experiences with breastfeeding, it appears partners play an integral role in helping women breastfeed and that breastfeeding should be something parents approach as a team.[24] Professionals should also be mindful of involving both parents when breastfeeding challenges arise. Sharing in the burden of breastfeeding with their partner may also help prevent the negative emotional effects that often accompany breastfeeding struggles.

COMMON BREASTFEEDING CHALLENGES

Low Milk Supply

Low milk supply is a common concern in the first few weeks of breast-feeding and one of the most commonly cited reasons for early weaning. For approximately 35% of all mothers who wean prior to 6 months of age, inadequacy of milk production is their primary reason for doing so.[25] In those mothers who wean the earliest, in the first week of breastfeeding, the rate of concern regarding milk supply appears even higher, with up to 65% of mothers in one study listing poor supply as their reason for breast-feeding discontinuation.[26] However, in studies that examined actual milk production via 24-hour testing and weighing, an imperfect but generally accepted method of estimating breast-milk production, mothers' perception of insufficient milk supply was not found to be associated with true insufficient supply.[27,28] Mothers most frequently rely upon their perception of their infant's satiety when making the determination regarding the sufficiency of their supply, though most mothers receive little instruction in interpreting infant satiety cues.[29–31] Mothers who feel their babies are fussy or unsettled or feed too frequently are more likely to feel their milk supply is low and begin supplementing or stop breastfeeding altogether. Alternatively, more confident mothers are less likely to perceive a low supply and are less likely to wean early. Helping mothers understand true indicators of poor milk supply and gain breastfeeding confidence is one simple way to help more mothers reach their breastfeeding goals.

Common Misperceptions of Insufficient Milk Supply	Reliable Indications of Insufficient Milk Supply
• Baby wants to feed frequently, every 1 to 2 hours • Baby suddenly wants to feed more often • Baby is fussy or difficult to soothe • Breasts feel soft • Feeding duration begins to shorten • Baby willing to take a bottle after nursing • Not a lot of production with pumping	• Poor weight gain, less than 500 g per month or 150 g per week • Baby has not regained birth weight by 2 weeks of age • Baby appears sleepy, lethargic, and has weak cry • Small amount of urine production, less than 6 wet diapers per day, with concentrated urine • Infrequent passage of hard, dry stools • Dry skin or mucous membranes • Poor muscle tone

Lactogenesis II is the process whereby breast milk begins to be produced in copious amounts, sufficient to supply the long-term nutritional needs of the baby. The timing of lactogenesis varies, occurring anywhere from 32 to 96 hours after birth, though it is considered delayed when it is more than 72 hours after birth. Lactogenesis begins when the placenta delivers and there is an immediate and rapid decrease in maternal progesterone levels and an increase in circulating levels of prolactin. Milk production is inhibited by peptides within breast milk so frequent emptying of the breast is an important part of ensuring an adequate supply.

Delayed lactogenesis is a common problem and has a significant impact on overall breastfeeding rates. As many as one in four women experience delayed onset of lactogenesis and delayed lactogenesis is a risk factor for formula supplementation, low supply long term, lack of breastfeeding exclusivity, and early discontinuation of breastfeeding.[32] Mothers who are more likely to experience delayed lactogenesis include those with diabetes, obesity, premature delivery, polycystic ovarian syndrome, and depression or anxiety treated with SSRIs.[33] Events during labor and delivery also increase the risk, including long and stressful labors, cesarean section, postpartum hemorrhage, and retained placenta. First-time mothers are also more likely to have delayed lactogenesis, with lactation occurring 10 to 35 hours later in primiparous patients when compared to multiparous patients.[34]

Fortunately, while delayed lactogenesis is common, failed lactogenesis is not. Failed lactogenesis is defined as a condition in which a mother is never able to achieve full lactation with a sufficient milk supply. There is insufficient data to precisely quantify the prevalence of failed lactogenesis, but is estimated to affect around 5% of women, though some report that the number may be as high as 15%.[35] It may be a result of either a primary inability of the mother to generate a sufficient milk supply or secondary factors, such as improper breastfeeding management or infant conditions, such as tongue tie, prematurity, or congenital heart disease. Many of the risk factors for delayed lactogenesis are also risk factors for failed lactogenesis, both due to the conditions themselves and mismanagement of delayed lactogenesis.

While many risk factors associated with failed lactation cannot be changed, it is important for mothers and their care providers to be aware of the risk factors for both delayed and failed lactation. Mothers who wish to breastfeed and are at risk of lactation failure should receive early and increased breastfeeding support from qualified lactation consultants and their obstetrics providers. Early recognition of those mothers with an inability to achieve sufficient lactation is essential, as negative early

Risk Factors for Low Milk Supply[34-36]	
Primary	**Secondary**
• Impaired maternal glucose tolerance/ decreased insulin responsiveness: diabetes, PCOS • Maternal obesity • Thyroid disorders • Anatomic breast abnormalities, insufficient mammary glandular tissue • History of breast augmentation, reduction • Significant postpartum hemorrhage, Sheehan's syndrome • Retained placental tissue	• Delayed initiation of breastfeeding • Restriction of frequency or duration of feeds • Formula supplementation • Infant tongue tie or poor latch • Prematurity • Infant medical condition • Maternal anemia • Medications: antihistamines, Decongestants, hormonal contraception, antidepressants • Maternal smoking

breastfeeding experiences, often centered around a prolonged process in vain to achieve lactation, are associated with depressive symptoms at 2 months postpartum.[37] In fact, in a survey of over 10,000 women in the United Kingdom, among those mothers who wanted to breastfeed and were unable, a twofold increase in the risk of postpartum depression was observed.[38] In other words, helping mothers breastfeed is not just good for babies, it is important for mothers too. However, equally essential is adequately supporting mothers when it is not going well and providing reassurance that an inability to breastfeed does not make someone less of a mother or negatively impact their baby. There is a delicate balance between breastfeeding promotion and promotion of maternal well-being. A formula-fed baby with a happy mother is always better than a breastfed baby with a guilt-ridden and depressed mother.

That said, there are many possible solutions to poor supply that may help mothers achieve their breastfeeding goals; however, the first step is to determine if there is a modifiable health condition which is impairing production. Initially, a complete examination of the mother should be performed, ruling out an anatomic or surgical breast abnormality, mastitis, retained placenta, or hormonal abnormality. Blood work should be obtained, examining thyroid and testosterone levels, as well as a blood count to look for anemia. The infant should also be examined for signs of malnutrition, dehydration, or structural abnormalities of the mouth, including tongue tie, which is the most common. The infant's latch should be observed for adequacy. If the mother has a history of any condition with impaired glucose control, such as diabetes, obesity, or PCOS, *metformin* may also be considered. It has been suggested through improving insulin sensitivity, metformin may improve lactogenesis, as modulation of insulin receptors is observed in the transition of colostrum to breast milk and aids in the increase in fat and protein synthesis observed in the later stages of lactogenesis.[39] The safety of metformin in lactation has been well established, with no increases in the risk of neonatal hypoglycemia having been observed.[40] Studies are ongoing examining the efficacy of metformin in treating impaired lactation.

If examination fails to demonstrate an underlying medical or latch-related cause for impaired milk supply, the first treatment usually recommended is increased stimulation of the breast and expression of breast milk. This can be done by shortening the interval between feedings, offering both breasts at each feeding, and pumping in between or immediately after feeds. Interestingly, there is limited data demonstrating the efficacy of this practice in improving milk supply, though there is some evidence that complete emptying of the breast increases the rate of lactogenesis, providing support for the advice to pump following feeds to ensure the breast is empty.[41] Yet, many mothers drive themselves to exhaustion, in an endless cycles of nursing and pumping, often advised to pump up to 15 or 20 minutes following each feeding, even when no milk is being expressed. This schedule is difficult if not impossible to maintain. A more reasonable approach would be a trial of a short duration of pumping following daytime feedings, with the priority given to achieving effective and frequent nursing sessions and adequate maternal rest. Breast massage during nursing and pumping may help increase the amount of milk expressed.[42] Newborns, especially in the setting of low milk supply, should be nursing at least every 2 to 3 hours. If the baby is going longer stretches without nursing, an additional pumping session could be considered to encourage supply. This is particularly important if the baby is receiving formula supplementation and, when supplementing, formula should always be offered after the infant has nursed from both breasts, not as a replacement for a nursing session.

Another proposed solution to low supply is increased maternal hydration and caloric intake, but there have only been a few studies examining these recommendations. The few studies on increased hydration failed to show that hydration had an impact on breast-milk production, though proper hydration is generally regarded as important for nursing mothers.[43] One older, small study examining the caloric intake of mothers with and without insufficient milk supply demonstrated that mothers with sufficient supply were eating 50% more than their counterparts with insufficient supply and that increasing calories did improve milk supply.[44] While small in scope, it does support the current recommendations that nursing mothers maintain a caloric intake of at least 500 kcal above non-lactating women. Other studies have examined whether specific nutrient supplementation may increase milk supply; however, this practice has not been shown to be beneficial.[45]

Galactogogues are also commonly recommended to lactating mothers who are struggling with supply. Galactogogues are substances believed to augment maternal milk synthesis.

Oral Galactogogues[46]	
Pharmacologic	**Botanical/Herbal**
• Domperidone • Metoclopramide • Sulpiride	• Fenugreek • Blessed thistle • Milk thistle • Torbangun leaves • Goat's rue • Barley • Anise or aniseed • Shatavari

Most of the studies on both pharmacologic and botanical galacto-gogues are limited by size, inconsistency in alternative breastfeeding support provided, and lack of randomization, controls, or blinding and, consequently, most experts are reluctant to recommend the routine use of galactogogues for low milk supply.[47] However, some agents may be beneficial and providers should consider them if alternative methods of improving milk supply have been ineffective. The most promising phar-macologic agent appears to be domperidone, which was associated with increased milk production in two well-conducted randomized trials and is the only galactogogue supported by this level of evidence. It is usually administered in doses of 10 to 20 mg, three to four times per day, for up to 8 weeks. This medication is not FDA approved for this purpose and is, in fact, strongly discouraged by the FDA due to concerns about cardiac arrhythmias associated with its use, though these cases were rare and in a different patient population.[48] The existing evidence does not seem to support the FDA's level of concern and domperidone is widely available for the purpose of increasing milk supply outside of the United States. Metoclopramide, brand name Reglan, has also been well studied as a galactogogue and demonstrated some efficacy in observational studies; however, the one randomized trial performed failed to show a benefit. It is usually administered at a dose of 30 to 45 mg per day, divided into three or four separate administrations, for 1 to 2 weeks, followed by a weeklong taper. Metoclopramide is associated with more maternal side effects than domperidone, including restlessness, drowsiness, fatigue, diarrhea, depression, and even acute dystonic reactions in a very small number of women (<0.05%). However, metoclopramide is the most easily accessible pharmacologic galactogogue in the United States and may be the only option some women and their providers have. Sulpiride, an antipsychotic medication that has been observed to cause galactorrhea in both men and women, is another suggested pharmacologic galactogogue; however, it is also associated with neurological side effects, in addition to weight gain, so it is less commonly used.[47]

As for biologic galactogogues, shatavari, torbangun, fenugreek, and milk thistle have all demonstrated some efficacy in increasing milk production in a small number of flawed studies. The extensive historical use of biologic galactogogues among many cultures also certainly suggests some benefit, as ineffective remedies tend to fall out of favor with time.[49] However, at this time and in terms of actual evidence, most of the "natural" remedies fall into the "may help, unlikely to hurt" category. Given the large percentage of women who experience low-supply concerns, there is definitely a need for more research into the potential application of galactogogues within the broader treatment of impaired lactogenesis.

Persistent Sore/Cracked Nipples

Nipple pain is another common cause of breastfeeding discontinuation. There are many possible causes for nipple pain including:

- Suboptimal positioning and poor infant latch
- Infant ankyloglossia (tongue tie)
- Nipple friction and fissures
- Infections
- Milk blisters or blebs
- Raynaud's phenomenon

The first recommendation for persistent nipple pain is an evaluation of *positioning and latch*. The nursing mother should be encouraged to assume a comfortable seated or side-lying position. When sitting, she should be semi-reclining, with a supported back, relaxed shoulders, and feet on the ground. The baby should be lying across the mother's body, supported by a nursing pillow if needed in order for the infant's nose to be in line with the mother's nipple and head slightly tilted back.

The baby's head and neck should be supported, but not gripped and the chin should be brought to the nipple, waiting for the baby to open their mouth wide and take the breast from the base of the areola, over the nipple, toward the top of the areola. A baby with a good latch should have a mouthful of breast, not just the nipple. The chin should be touching the breast and the nose should be tilted upward, allowing the baby to breathe without difficulty. Many lactation counselors and consultants encourage women to manually grasp their breast with their hand in a "C" fashion, creating a "breast sandwich" for the baby to latch onto, which can also be helpful. If the latch is uncomfortable, a finger can be inserted into the baby's mouth to break the suction and position the baby again. Helping mothers achieve proper breastfeeding positioning and latch has been shown to promote longer breastfeeding durations and decrease the incidence of breastfeeding problems.[50] Furthermore, correction of improper positioning and latch has been shown to improve nipple pain in up to 65% of patients.[51]

Flat or inverted nipples can create a particular challenge in achieving a proper latch. Often, this condition will self-correct through the process of infant suckling. Alternatively, a simple device, referred to as a Latch Assist, that applies a small amount of suction to the nipple prior to nursing can help draw out the nipple prior to infant latching and decrease related nipple pain issues. *Nipple shields* can also assist in achieving a latch in the setting of flat or inverted nipples, as well as assisting mothers with generalized nipple pain. Nipple shields have a mixed reputation in the literature and among lactation consultants, due to concerns that they prevent complete emptying of the breast, impairing the development of proper milk supply, and prevent babies from being able to independently latch, thus interfering with long-term breastfeeding success. However, they are generally regarded positively by the mothers utilizing them for pain or latch issues and are often credited by mothers for preventing their discontinuation of breastfeeding.[52] While some studies have shown issues with supply surrounding shield use, the majority of studies have not shown this and nipple shields may offer a short-term solution to nipple-related breastfeeding concerns. The majority of women do not utilize shields for more than 6 weeks.

Infant tongue tie is another possible cause of persistent nipple pain. There is much controversy in the literature regarding the definition of infant ankyloglossia, characteristics of the varying classes of the condition, its clinical significance, and appropriateness of surgical intervention. The incidence ranges from 0.02% to 5%, depending on the definition applied, though in babies with breastfeeding challenges the incidence may be as high as 13%.[53] *Frenotomy*, a simple "snipping" of the tongue tie is frequently proposed for infants with tongue tie who have latch-related issues or mothers reporting significant nipple pain with breastfeeding. It has been shown in some studies, including randomized controlled trials, to reduce nipple pain and improve breastfeeding efficacy by maternal self-report; however, the total body of evidence in support of the procedure is generally regarded as low or insufficient.[54–57]

Milk blebs or blisters are small, raised white bumps that appear on the surface of the nipple and are usually associated with pain. This may or may not be associated with a blocked duct higher up in the breast and is thought to be a result of epithelial overgrowth of the distal portion of the duct or an accumulation of particulate or fatty material in the area. Sometimes they develop early in breastfeeding due to a poor latch, but they can also develop in isolation later in breastfeeding when no latch issue or other breastfeeding complaint is present. There is little research in regards to effective treatments of milk blebs; however, it is generally recommended that an attempt be made to open the bleb by warm compresses to the nipple, rubbing the area with a towel, or piercing the bleb with a sterile needle if needed and manually draining it. *Epson salt soaks* may also help soothe blebs or other cracks or fissures of the nipple, as well as promote healing and prevent further infection of the nipple. *Topical antibiotics*, such as mupirocin ointment, can also be considered in the setting of blebs and nipple fissures, as an underlying infectious etiology is possible and the opening in the nipple may serve as an entry point for bacteria and increase the risk of mastitis. Research has shown that mothers who applied mupirocin to nipple cracks and openings reported significantly improved resolution of these complaints.[58]

Raynaud's phenomenon is a less common, but commonly misdiagnosed cause of a nipple pain. It is caused by vasoconstriction of the arterioles supplying the nipple and can result in severe pain. It is most commonly mistaken for candidiasis or thrush and many mothers and their babies are inappropriately treated with multiple rounds of antifungal medication prior to Raynaud's being properly identified. Hallmarks of the condition are significant nipple pain, blanching of the nipple, followed by blue or red discoloration, and symptoms occurring outside of feeding episodes as well, particularly with cold exposure. The bulk of the literature concerning the phenomenon consists of case reports and series. What evidence does exist suggests autoimmune disease and a history of breast surgery may be predisposing factors. Conservative treatment includes avoiding cold exposure, breastfeeding in warm environments or under a blanket, applying warm compresses to the breast, avoiding caffeine and nicotine, and the addition of oral supplements including calcium, magnesium, fish oil, and evening primrose. However, medical management is commonly needed to improve symptoms and consists of oral nifedipine, a calcium channel blocker, which is typically given for a 2-week course at a dose of 5 mg, three times daily, or one 30 mg delayed-release tablet daily. Treatment beyond 2 weeks is usually unnecessary. Nifedipine is safe in both pregnancy and breastfeeding and has demonstrated efficacy in treating Raynaud's symptoms.[59]

Other nonspecific treatments for breastfeeding-associated nipple pain include *glycerin gel dressings, lanolin cream,* and *all-purpose nipple ointment (APNO).* As with other breastfeeding remedies, there is limited research into these specific treatments and the research that does exist does not conclusively recommend their use. However, interestingly, the research does show that most women report significant improvement in their nipple pain symptoms after approximately 10 days, regardless of the remedy they utilize. The reassurance of the apparently self-limited nature of nipple pain may be enough to help women continue breastfeeding during the critical first weeks during which most women discontinue breastfeeding.[60]

Mastitis, Plugged Ducts, Engorgement

Mastitis, or inflammation and infection of the breast, is another common breastfeeding complication and is often part of a continuum of breast-feeding symptoms including breast engorgement and plugged ducts. Nipple disrupture and cracking may also be a precursor to mastitis. Symptoms of mastitis include maternal fever, decreased milk production from one or both breasts, extreme breast tenderness, and redness of the skin. The breast is also typically firm and warm to the touch. It affects up to 18% of women and half of cases occur in the first month of breastfeeding.[61]

Milk stasis creates a reservoir for bacterial growth. Therefore, the best prevention of mastitis appears to be frequent emptying of the breast, confirmation of a proper latch to permit adequate emptying from all areas of the breast, and avoidance of external compression of the breast with ill-fitting bras or prone sleeping.[62] Oral *lecithin* supplementation, at a dose of 1200 mg, three to four times daily, is another commonly recommended way to prevent engorgement, blockages, and subsequent infection; however, no studies to date have confirmed this recommendation.[63] If a blocked duct occurs, warm compresses should be applied and the area massaged to encourage opening of the blockage.

When nursing, the infant's chin and nose should be angled toward the blocked duct to help drain the area. Application of *cabbage leaves* or *potato slices* to the breasts is also commonly suggested to relieve blocked ducts and engorgement, though the limited research performed has not validated this traditional advice.[64]

When engorgement and blocked ducts progress into an infectious mastitis of the breast tissue, conservative management will often relieve the infection within 24 hours. Ibuprofen is the preferred treatment for pain relief and fever control and also helps decrease inflammation in the breast. Frequent emptying of the breast is paramount to prevent further milk stasis, evacuate the bacteria, and prevent abscess development. Massage and warm compresses also aid in milk drainage. Unfortunately, as many as 1 in 10 women are incorrectly advised to stop breastfeeding due to mastitis, increasing the risk of further complications and unnecessarily resulting in the discontinuation of breastfeeding.[61] Nursing does not put the infant at risk for infection, as typically both mother and infant are colonized with the same bacteria. Reeducation of medical professionals in the proper management of mastitis is an important part of breastfeeding promotion. Occasionally, a nursing infant may refuse the breast during a bout of mastitis, due to a change in the taste of the milk in the setting of infection. Pumping to empty the breast should be performed in this setting or to augment milk expression.

If conservative treatment of mastitis fails to improve symptoms after 24 hours, antibiotic treatment is indicated. The most common bacteria present is *Staphylococcus aureus* and, thus, the recommended antibiotic regimen should be directed at this organism, most commonly cephalexin or dicloxacillin. If standard antibiotic treatments fail to improve symptoms, the breast milk should be cultured and sensitivities obtained in order to rule out a methicillin-resistant organism (MRSA) and antibiotics adjusted accordingly. Resistant mastitis should also prompt examination and an ultrasound to rule out an underlying breast abscess.

Thrush

Candida mastitis, or thrush, is generally considered to be the etiology of a common collection of symptoms that includes significant nipple pain, deep, shooting pain within the breast, and pink, inflamed nipples. It is typically only diagnosed in the setting of persistent breast and nipple pain which occurs in the absence of any other clinical features of bacterial mastitis, engorgement, or blocked ducts. The infant in the breastfeeding dyad may or may not display signs of oral candidiasis, but commonly does not. Medical treatments usually involve treatment of the infant with oral nystatin, fluconazole, or gentian violet and treatment of the mother with oral fluconazole and topical nystatin application to the nipples. There is actually, however, limited quality evidence in support of these common treatment regimens, despite multiple case reports and anecdotal stories detailing improvement of this type of breast pain with antifungals.[65–69] There is, likewise, a lack of evidence in support of common prevention strategies including maternal intake of probiotics, dietary restriction of sugar and dairy, and frequent changing of bras and breast pads. Furthermore, more recent research calls into question whether the correct organism is even being treated in response to these symptoms, with some studies failing to show clinically significant levels of *candida* in the milk of mothers identified as having symptoms consistent with commonly diagnosed *candida* mastitis. Alternatively, most mothers with this collection of symptoms demonstrated strep or staph growth within their breast milk, suggesting these symptoms may represent a subacute mastitis, rather than a fungal infection.[70] Furthermore, the presence of bacteria has been shown to augment yeast overgrowth, indicating that treating yeast in this circumstance may be addressing only one symptom of a subclinical bacterial mastitis, rather than the root cause of the problem. This view is supported by the frequently cyclical nature of thrush. Yet, follow-up research has not, to date, been published expanding upon whether antibiotics may be an alternative therapy to alleviate pain in these patients without evidence of acute, infectious mastitis. With this limited evidence-based guidance, it would seem a combined approach, addressing the possibility of both bacterial and yeast overgrowth, may be reasonable in patients presenting with this pattern of pain.

PHYSICAL RECOVERY

I will tell you some of the many dirty secrets no one else tells you about becoming a mother. You are going to be wetting your pants every time you cough or sneeze, you will still look 6 months pregnant when you go home from the hospital, so bring maternity pants, and the weight is not just going to fall off. With all this, no sleep, and everything that goes on "down there," sex seems like a distant memory. I didn't even want my husband to look at me for almost a year and, even for some time after that, I felt like I had become asexual or something. It didn't matter to me if we never had sex again.

—A. P., new mother

Perineal Healing

Perineal tears or episiotomies affect approximately 85% of women who deliver vaginally.[71] Perineal trauma is associated with moderate to severe discomfort when sitting, going to the bathroom, or walking and can take up to several weeks to heal. If proper healing does not occur, perineal tears can lead to prolonged perineal discomfort, painful intercourse, or incontinence. The wound may also break down and need to be surgically repaired. Thankfully, the majority of tears heal quickly and well. Remedies that have been shown to relieve pain and/or promote healing include:

- Oral tylenol and ibuprofen
- Localized cooling with ice packs, gel packs, or cool sitz baths[72,73]
- Lidocaine sprays or gels[74,75]
- Aloe vera and calendula ointment[76]
- Lavender oil[77]

Witch hazel is also commonly used, though specific studies examining its efficacy have not been performed. New mothers should also change pads frequently, bathe or shower daily, and practice good hand hygiene to minimize the risk of perineal wound infection or breakdown. If there is concern that a perineal wound is not healing normally or breaking down, women should be evaluated by their obstetrician or midwife without delay.

Pelvic Floor Strengthening and Sexual Function

Pelvic floor disorders are also common following pregnancy and delivery. The symptoms and severity of pelvic floor dysfunction vary widely but include a general sense of vaginal "openness" or "gaping," urinary incontinence, flatulence incontinence, fecal incontinence, and pelvic organ prolapse. The reported incidence of these conditions also varies widely and, while the evidence suggests pregnancy in general increases the risk of pelvic floor disorders, vaginal delivery, particularly operative vaginal delivery, prolonged pushing, large babies, and maternal obesity are specific risk factors.[78–81] There is also an association between pelvic floor weakness and sexual dysfunction.[82,83] Sexual dysfunction is common in the postpartum period and can include symptoms such as dyspareunia, or painful intercourse, and hypoactive desire and/or arousal.

Treatments that may aid in pelvic floor strengthening, reducing symptoms of pelvic floor dysfunction, and improved postpartum sexual function include *pelvic floor muscle training (PFMT)*, more commonly known as *Kegel exercises, biofeedback, electrical stimulation*, and *vaginal cones or balls.* PFMT has been most widely studied of these individual treatments and has been shown to reduce symptoms of pelvic dysfunction, as well as improve sexual function.[83–86] These exercises may be initiated in the immediate postpartum period, without significant discomfort, and may be performed individually or with the aid of a medical professional, generally a pelvic floor physical therapist.[87] The other treatments for pelvic floor dysfunction are nearly always administered in the setting of professional pelvic floor physical therapy sessions, typically in combination with PFMT, and the limited research available suggests this combination of therapies and professional treatment may be more beneficial than individual PFMT alone.[88,89]

Women should be questioned about signs of pelvic floor dysfunction as a standard part of their postpartum care. While all postpartum women may benefit from PFMT, symptomatic women, as well as women with significant perineal trauma, should strongly be encouraged to begin these exercises and pelvic floor physical therapy may be considered as well. Any concerns about resumption of intercourse should be addressed and breastfeeding women should be encouraged to use a lubricant, as breastfeeding decreases natural vaginal lubrication. In follow-up exams, women should be questioned about their sexual health and treatments recommended if there is a concern. Often providers will perform an "annual" at postpartum exam; however, it may be better to defer an "annual" for 3 to 6 months after delivery, so that any lingering postpartum concerns may be better addressed.

HOW TO PERFORM PFMT OR KEGELS

1. Locate the pelvic floor muscles either by stopping your urine stream midway through voiding or placing a finger in the vagina and using your pelvic muscles to squeeze your finger.
2. Start each exercise session with several short, quick contractions of the pelvic floor muscles to both localize the muscles and practice your contraction.
3. Then perform 3 sets of 10 slow contraction-release sequences.
4. Daily pelvic floor exercise is the goal.
5. Intermittently, up to three times weekly, combine with pelvic tilt: lay flat on the floor, with knees bent, and feet planted firmly on the floor and slowly lift your bottom off the floor, contracting your pelvic muscles with the lift and relaxing as you return to the floor.

Core Strengthening and Weight Loss

The desire to "lose the baby weight" is also strong among most new mothers. However, pregnancy is known to be associated with excessive weight gain, long-term weight retention, and obesity.[90] This can increase the risk of health complications later in life, as well as in subsequent pregnancies. While there is no one right way to help women lose weight, as evidenced by the multibillion dollar weight-loss industry, studies have demonstrated that active postpartum weight loss programs do help mothers lose significantly more postpartum weight than the simple "eat right and exercise" advice typically provided at postpartum visits.[91,92] Both diet modification alone and combined diet and exercise programs have demonstrated efficacy. However, as with health and wellness promotion in the antepartum period, providers are often time restricted and have difficulty putting these programs in place.

One simple solution that could be easily provided by obstetricians or midwives in their waiting rooms after-hours or developed by new mothers themselves in their community is *new mother health and wellness groups*. These groups, which meet monthly or bimonthly, offer dietician-led nutritional guidance, in a less cost-prohibitive group setting, weigh-ins, and group motivation. Wellness groups also serve as a source of friends and exercise partners and group dynamics encourage better long-term adherence to healthy lifestyle modifications.

However, for mothers working individually, the guidance for postpartum weight loss is not substantially different than outside of childbearing, even when mothers are breastfeeding. Women should reduce excess carbohydrates and processed foods in the diet, increase their intake of protein and fresh fruits and vegetables, and maximize their water intake. Exercise goals should consist of three-times weekly exercise, combining both cardiovascular and weight-resistant activity. Weight checks should be performed weekly.

Core Strength and Rectus Muscle Diastasis

Core strength is often of particular concern to new mothers. Rectus muscle diastasis refers to the separation of the two bellies of the rectus abdominus muscle and is found in as many as 60% of new mothers at the 6-weeks postpartum and persists past 1 year after delivery in as many as one in three women.[93] It is generally diagnosed by palpating along the midline of the abdomen while a woman lies flat and contracts her abdominal muscles. Rectus muscle diastasis is identified when a significant indentation is felt, generally a separation of more than 2 cm, wide enough to fit more than two fingers. While there are no documented negative associations with the condition, it is believed to contribute to poor pelvic floor function and a weakened core and is cosmetically unpleasing for most women, causing abdominal distention known as the "mummy tummy."

There is a substantial amount of articles and online discussion concerning the condition and possible remedies; however, the research regarding those treatments is limited. Most advice centers on avoiding any aggressive abdominal exercise, such as sit-ups, crunches, or other exercises that push the belly out, putting further strain on the muscles and pulling them apart. Instead, women are encouraged to perform exercises that pull the abdomen inward, such as pelvic tilts, heel slides, and single-leg stretches. Reviews of the literature have been inconclusive as to whether this advice is actually valid; however, it also is unlikely to hurt and some exercise focusing on rebuilding core strength is certainly better than no exercise.[94,95] Additionally, the condition may be prevented by exercise in the antenatal period and avoidance of repetitive lifting of more than 20 lb.

EMOTIONAL HEALTH AND WELL-BEING

I was really struggling three months into life with my daughter. I don't remember who said it to me, but someone reminded me of that moment in the airplane where they tell you to put the oxygen mask on yourself before you assist anyone else. That really resonated with me. I had been living for my daughter, but I was slowly dying inside and before long I wasn't going to have anything left to give. I began taking better care of myself and got some help and, in turn, I began taking better care of my child.

—B. P., new mother

Aside from the challenges of breastfeeding and physical recovery after pregnancy and childbirth, mothers also face an enormous life transition as they either become mothers for the first time or introduce a new child into their family and navigate that disruption to their established family structure. Caring for a newborn is often stressful and exhausting. There is little time for any self-care or even sleep after the relentless cycle of feeding, burping, changing, and putting down has been completed. New mothers also face a complete change in their identity and may find their new role isolating or, even at times, unfulfilling or understimulating. Partner dynamics shift has new parents negotiate their change from friends and lovers to co-parents and back again, hopefully somehow finding a way to be all three simultaneously.

It is no wonder that rates of postpartum depression and anxiety are as high as they are, when these stresses are compounded by the hormonal adjustments that occur in the postpartum period. Care providers, communities, and families must work together to better support new mothers and families in order to begin to reduce these disorders. The importance of *partner support* cannot be overemphasized. Parenting should be approached as a team, both to distribute the workload and prevent new mothers from being overwhelmed, but also to share in the emotional responsibility of parenting, which can be as burdensome as providing for the physical needs of new infants. Decisions should be made collaboratively and partners should avoid simply deferring to the mother. *Family support* in the first days and weeks should also be encouraged and sought out by new parents, if not prohibited by geographical restrictions or strained relationships. However, family members should be more than just baby visitors. They can and should help with food preparation, household chores, or childcare either for the new baby or other children, even if only for an hour or two so the new parents may sleep, shower, or go for a walk.

Postpartum doulas are another valuable resource that can be accessed by new parents. Postpartum doulas provide assistance in the home with infant care, breastfeeding, meal preparation, household tasks, partner support, as well as valuable social and emotional support for the new mother.[96] While research has not yet been performed evaluating doulas efficacy in providing this type of support and preventing postpartum mood disorders, it is anticipated that this level of care would be incredibly valuable for new mothers based on the evidence supporting other types of in-home care. Much of the world outside the United States considers nurse or midwife *home visits* to be an integral part of postpartum care. Studies have shown significant improvements in nutrition and healthy behaviors, breastfeeding, rates of postpartum mood disorders, and infant care among mothers who receive in-home postpartum visits by a trained professional when compared to women who receive standard postpartum care.[97,98] Home visits and postpartum doulas, unfortunately, are not reimbursed within the current global-fee payment structure of most American insurance companies, nor are they offered through government public health resources. However, given the benefits home visits offer, it would make sense for providers and hospitals to negotiate reimbursements for this service or engage private nursing groups that could individually obtain reimbursement.

Peer support groups are another source of positive social and emotional support. Groups may either be peer led or facilitated by a medical or mental health professional and may help eliminate maternal feelings of isolation through the acknowledgment of shared experiences. Support groups can also be a source of valuable advice and friendship with other women in similar life circumstances. Furthermore, meetings may also help minimize feelings of guilt, as members realize and celebrate the universal perfect imperfection of new motherhood. Meetings are also simply an excuse to get out of the house and gain some new exposure and interaction outside of infant care.

Professional counseling may also be helpful and necessary for mothers and their partners. If an expecting mother has a history of mental health struggles prior to or during pregnancy, she should have an appointment arranged with her mental health provider for the postpartum period. However, the postpartum period can be so challenging, this may be something all mothers should consider. Couples counseling may also help parents who are having difficulty co-parenting or simply relating to each other and redefining their relationship post-baby. Certainly, if any signs of postpartum depression or anxiety are present, professional help should be sought without delay.

SIGNS OF POSTPARTUM DEPRESSION AND ANXIETY[99]

- Feeling that you should not have become a mother or had another child
- Intense feelings of guilt or ineptitude
- Lack of bonding with your baby
- Extreme irritation, anger, and impatience
- Feelings of numbness and emptiness
- Feelings of hopelessness
- Frequent crying
- Loss of appetite

- Trouble sleeping or staying asleep
- Feeling that you want to run away, disappear, or hurt yourself or your baby
- Racing thoughts or the need to be doing something at all times
- Feelings of constant worry and fear
- Occasional or frequent disturbing thoughts
- Feeling the need to constantly check things or the baby

Apart from utilizing these resources, mothers should also be encouraged to schedule some personal time for themselves during early motherhood. They should utilize partners, family, and child care providers in order to have time to exercise, spend time with friends and family, or simply spend some quiet time alone. Meditation may also help mothers reduce stress and anxiety. Taking this time is especially important when new mothers resume work, as understandably mothers report a hesitancy to spend any additional time away from their child after spending the workday away. However, this tendency to de-prioritize self-care emotionally drains mothers, reduces healthy behaviors, and should be discouraged by health care providers and families alike.

Supporting the social and emotional needs of mothers is obviously complicated and the results of interventions are difficult to quantify. However, the emotional health of mothers directly impacts both their physical health and their children's well-being. Directing resources and energy toward promoting maternal wellness is not only good for mothers, but makes sense from a public health standpoint as well.

Postpartum care is too important to simply be an afterthought. The goal of all stages of maternal–child care, antepartum, intrapartum, and postpartum, should be to maximize both the physical and emotional health of women and their babies and build strong family foundations. This can only be done through a broad, holistic approach along all points of the pregnancy and parenting journey, with providers, hospitals, birth workers, and communities working collaboratively to provide women-centered care. It will be necessary for everyone working within this team to be open to new ideas and solutions in order to really provide what new mothers and families want and need. A change of pace is also necessary. Whether in the office, delivery room, or postpartum, it is only when we slow down that we can really be present to a new mother and it is only in truly being present with new mothers that we can really see them, see their needs, understand their motivations, and help them achieve their mothering goals in a happy and healthy way.

REFERENCES

1. Entsieh AA, Hallström IK. First-time parents' prenatal needs for early parenthood preparation—a systematic review and meta-synthesis of qualitative literature. *Midwifery.* 2016;39(Aug):1-11. doi:10.1016/j.midw.2016.04.006.
2. World Health Organization. *The Optimal Duration of Exclusive Breastfeeding: Report of an Expert Consultation.* Geneva, Switzerland: World Health Organization; 2001. Available at http://www.who.int/nutrition/publications/infantfeeding/WHO_NHD_01.09/en/index.html. Accessed Aug 2017
3. Kramer MS, Kakuma R. Optimal duration of exclusive breastfeeding. *Cochrane Database Syst Rev.* 2012;(8):1-139.
4. Lumbiganon P, Martis R, Laopaiboon M, et al. Antenatal breastfeeding education for increasing breastfeeding duration. *Cochrane Database Syst Rev.* 2016;(12). doi:10.1002/14651858.CD006425.pub4.
5. Artieta-Pinedo I, Paz-Pascual C, Grandes G, et al. Antenatal education and breastfeeding in a cohort of primiparas. *J Adv Nurs.* 2013;69(7):1607-1617. doi:10.1111/jan.12022.
6. Haroon S, Das JK, Salam RA, Imdad A, Bhutta ZA. Breastfeeding promotion interventions and breastfeeding practices: a systematic review. *BMC Public Health.* 2013;13(suppl 3):S20. doi:10.1186/1471-2458-13-S3-S20.
7. The Baby-Friendly Hospital Initiative. Available at https://www.babyfriendlyusa.org/about-us. Accessed Aug 2017.
8. Naylor AJ. Baby-Friendly Hospital Initiative. Protecting, promoting, and supporting breastfeeding in the twenty-first century. *Pediatr Clin North Am.* 2001;48(2):475-483.
9. Kramer MS, Chalmers B, Hodnett ED, et al. Promotion of Breastfeeding Intervention Trial (PROBIT): a randomized trial in the Republic of Belarus. *JAMA.* 2001;285(4):413-420.
10. Ten Steps and International Code. Available at https://www.babyfriendlyusa.org/about-us/10-steps-and-international-code. Accessed Aug 2017.
11. Braun MLG, Giugliani ERJ, Soares MEM, et al. Evaluation of the impact of the Baby-Friendly Hospital Initiative on rates of breastfeeding. *Am J Public Health.* 2008;93(8):1277-1279.
12. Venancio SI, Saldiva SR, Escuder MM, Giugliani ER. The Baby-Friendly Hospital Initiative shows positive effects on breastfeeding indicators in Brazil. *J Epidemiol Community Health.* 2012;66(10):914-918.
13. Merten S, Dratva J, Ackermann-Liebrich U. Do Baby-Friendly hospitals influence breastfeeding duration on a national level? *Pediatrics.* 2005;116(5):e702-e708.
14. Hawkins SS, Stern AD, Baum CF, Gillman MW. Evaluating the impact of the Baby-Friendly Hospital Initiative on breastfeeding rates: a multi-state analysis. *Public Health Nutr.* 2015;18(2):189-197.
15. Howe-Heyman A, Lutenbacher M. The Baby-Friendly Hospital Initiative as an intervention to improve breastfeeding rates: a review of the literature. *J Midwifery Womens Health.* 2016;61(1):77-102.
16. Chien LY, Tai CJ, Chu KH, et al. The number of Baby Friendly hospital practices experienced by mothers is positively associated with breastfeeding: a questionnaire survey. *Int J Nurs Stud.* 2007;44(7):1138-1146.

17. Patel S, Patel S. The effectiveness of lactation consultants and lactation counselors on breastfeeding outcomes. *J Hum Lact.* 2016;32(3):530-541.

18. Liu L, Zhu J, Yang J, et al. The effect of a perinatal breastfeeding support program on breastfeeding outcomes in primiparous mothers. *West J Nurs Res.* 2017;39(7): 906-923.

19. Wouk K, Chetwynd E, Vitaglione T, Sullivan C. Improving access to medical lactation support and counseling: building the case for Medicaid reimbursement. *Matern Child Health J.* 2017;21(4):836-844. doi:10.1007/s10995-016-2175-x.

20. McFadden A, Gavine A, Renfrew MJ, et al. Support for healthy breastfeeding mothers with healthy term babies. *Cochrane Database Syst Rev.* 2017;(2):1-292. doi:10.1002/14651858.CD001141.pub5.

21. Ogbo FA, Eastwood J, Page A, et al. Prevalence and determinants of cessation of exclusive breastfeeding in the early postnatal period in Sydney, Australia. *Int Breastfeed J.* 2016;12(16). doi:10.1186/s13006-017-0110-4.

22. Mannion CA, Hobbs AJ, McDonald SW, Tough SC. Maternal perceptions of partner support during breastfeeding. *Int Breastfeed J.* 2013;8(1):4. doi:10.1186/1746-4358-8-4.

23. Maycock BR, Scott JA, Hauck YL, et al. A study to prolong breastfeeding duration: design and rationale of the Parent Infant Feeding Initiative (PIFI) randomised controlled trial. *BMC Pregnancy Childbirth.* 2015;15:159. doi:10.1186/s12884-015-0601-5.

24. Tohotoa J, Maycock B, Hauck YL, et al. Dads make a difference: an exploratory study of paternal support for breastfeeding in Perth, Western Australia. *Int Breastfeed J.* 2009;4:15. doi:10.1186/1746-4358-4-15.

25. Gatti L. Maternal perceptions of insufficient milk supply in breastfeeding. *J Nurs Scholarsh.* 2008;40(4):355-363. doi:10.1111/j.1547-5069.2008.00234.x.

26. Sheehan D, Krueger P, Watt S, et al. The Ontario Mother and Infant Survey: breastfeeding outcomes. *J Hum Lact.* 2001;17(3):211-219.

27. Galipeau R, Dumas L, Lepage M. Perception of not having enough milk and actual milk production of first-time breastfeeding mothers: is there a difference? *Breastfeed Med.* 2017;12:210-217. doi:10.1089/bfm.2016.0183.

28. Savenije OEM, Brand PLP. Accuracy and precision of test weighing to assess milk intake in newborn infants. *Arch Dis Child Fetal Neonatal Ed.* 2006;91(5):F330-F332. doi:10.1136/adc.2005.091876.

29. Colin WB, Scott JA. Breastfeeding: reasons for starting, reasons for stopping and problems along the way. *Breastfeed Rev.* 2002;10(2):13-19.

30. Lewallen LP, Dick MJ, Flowers J, et al. Breastfeeding support and early cessation. *J Obstet Gynecol Neonatal Nurs.* 2006;35(2):166-172.

31. McCarter-Spaulding DE, Kearney MH. Parenting self-efficacy and perception of insufficient breast milk. *J Obstet Gynecol Neonatal Nurs.* 2001;30(5):515-522.

32. Brownell E, Howard CR, Lawrence RA, Dozier AM. Does delayed onset lactogenesis II predict the cessation of any or exclusive breastfeeding? *J Pediatr.* 2012;161(4):608-614. doi:10.1016/j.jpeds.2012.03.035.

33. Marshall AM, Nommsen-Rivers LA, Hernandez LL, et al. Serotonin transport and metabolism in the mammary gland modulates secretory activation and involution. *J Clin Endocrinol Metab.* 2010;95(2):837-846. doi:10.1210/jc.2009-1575.

34. Dewey KG, Nommsen-Rivers LA, Heinig MJ, Cohen RJ. Risk factors for suboptimal infant breastfeeding behavior, delayed onset of lactation, and excess neonatal weight loss. *Pediatrics.* 2003;112(3 pt 1):607-619.

35. Hurst NM. Recognizing and treating delayed or failed lactogenesis II. *J Midwifery Womens Health.* 2007;52(6):588-594.
36. Stuebe AM, Grewen K, Pedersen CA, et al. Failed lactation and perinatal depression: common problems with shared neuroendocrine mechanisms? *J Womens Health.* 2012;21(3):264-272. doi:10.1089/jwh.2011.3083.
37. Watkins S, Meltzer-Brody S. Early breastfeeding experiences and postpartum depression. *Obstet Gynecol.* 2011;118(2 pt 1):214-221. doi:10.1097/AOG. 0b013e3182260a2d.
38. Borra C, Iacovou M, Sevilla A. New evidence on breastfeeding and postpartum depression: the importance of understanding women's intentions. *Matern Child Health J.* 2015;19(4):897-907.
39. Lemay DG, Ballard OA, Hughes MA, et al. RNA sequencing of the human milk fat layer transcriptome reveals distinct gene expression profiles at three stages of lactation. *PLoS ONE.* 2013;8(7):e67531. doi:10.1371/journal.pone.0067531.
40. Glueck CJ, Wang P. Metformin before and during pregnancy and lactation in polycystic ovary syndrome. *Expert Opin Drug Saf.* 2007;6(2):191-198.
41. Daly SE, Kent JC, Owens RA, Hartmann PE. Frequency and degree of milk removal and the short-term control of human milk synthesis. *Exp Physiol.* 1996;81(5): 861-875.
42. Jones E, Dimmock P, Spencer SA. A randomised controlled trial to compare methods of milk expression after preterm delivery. *Arch Dis Child Fetal Neonatal.* 2001;85(2):F91-F95.
43. Ndikom CM, Fawole B, Ilesanmi RE. Extra fluids for breastfeeding mothers for increasing milk production. *Cochrane Database Syst Rev.* 2014;(6):CD008758. doi:10.1002/14651858.CD008758.pub2.
44. Whichelow MJ. Letter: calorie requirements for successful breastfeeding. *Arch Dis Child.* 1975;50(8):669.
45. Abe SK, Balogun OO, Ota E, Takahashi K, Mori R. Supplementation with multiple micronutrients for breastfeeding women for improving outcomes for the mother and baby. *Cochrane Database Syst Rev.* 2016; (18):CD010647. doi:10.1002/14651858. CD010647.pub2.
46. Zuppa AA, Sindico P, Orchi C, et al. Safety and efficacy of galactogogues: substances that induce, maintain and increase breast milk production. *J Pharm Pharm Sci.* 2010;13(2):162-174.
47. Academy of Breastfeeding Medicine Protocol Committee. ABM Clinical Protocol#9: use of galactogogues in initiating or augmenting the rate of maternal milk secretion (First Revision January 2011). *Breastfeed Med.* 2011;6(1):41-49. doi:10.1089/ bfm.2011.9998.
48. Forinash AB, Yancey AM, Barnes KN, Myles TD. The use of galactogogues in the breastfeeding mother. *Ann Pharmacother.* 2012;46(10):1392-1404. doi:10.1345/ aph.1R167.
49. Mortel M, Mehta SD. Systematic review of the efficacy of herbal galactogogues. *J Hum Lact.* 2013;29(2):154-162. doi:10.1177/0890334413477243.
50. Alade RL. Sucking technique and its effect on success of breastfeeding. *Birth.* 1992;19(4):185-189.
51. Kent JC, Ashton E, Hardwick CM, et al. Nipple pain in breastfeeding mothers: incidence, causes and treatments. *Int J Environ Res Public Health.* 2015;12(10):12247-12263. doi:10.3390/ijerph121012247.

ANTEPARTUM & POSTPARTUM CARE

52. Chow S, Chow R, Popovic M, et al. The use of nipple shields: a review. *Front Public Health*. 2015;3:236. doi:10.3389/fpubh.2015.00236.

53. Kupietzky A, Botzer El. Ankyloglossia in the infant and young child: clinical suggestions for diagnosis and management. *Pediatr Dent*. 2004;27:40-46.

54. Ghaheri BA, Cole M, Fausel SC, Chuop M, Mace JC. Breastfeeding improvement following tongue-tie and lip-tie release: a prospective cohort study. *Laryngoscope*. 2017;127(5):1217-1223.

55. Emond A, Ingram J, Johnson D, et al. Randomised controlled trial of early frenotomy in breastfed infants with mild-moderate tongue-tie. *Arch Dis Child Fetal Neonatal Ed*. 2014;99(3):F189-F195.

56. Francis DO, Krishnaswami S, McPheeters M. Treatment of ankyloglossia and breastfeeding outcomes: a systematic review. *Pediatrics*. 2015;135(6):e1467-e1474. doi:10.1542/peds.2015-0658.

57. Buryk M, Bloom D, Shope T. Efficacy of neonatal release of ankyloglossia: a randomized trial. *Pediatrics*. 2011;128(2):280-288.

58. Spencer JP. Management of mastitis in breastfeeding women. *Am Fam Physician*. 2008;78(6):727-731.

59. Anderson JE, Held N, Wright K. Raynaud's phenomenon of the nipple: a treatable cause of painful breastfeeding. *Pediatrics*. 2004;113(4):e360-e364. doi:10.1542/peds.113.4.e360.

60. Dennis CL, Jackson K, Watson J. Interventions for treating painful nipples among breastfeeding women. *Cochrane Database Syst Rev*. 2014;(12):1-72. doi:10.1002/14651858.CD007366.pub2.

61. Scott JA, Robertson M, Fitzpatrick J, et al. Occurrence of lactational mastitis and medical management: a prospective cohort study in Glasgow. *Int Breastfeed J*. 2008;3:21. doi:10.1186/1746-4358-3-21.

62. Crepinsek MA, Crowe L, Michener K, Smart NA. Interventions for preventing mastitis after childbirth. *Cochrane Database Syst Rev*. 2012;(10):1-42. doi:10.1002/14651858.CD007239.pub3.

63. Lecithin use while breastfeeding. Available at https://www.drugs.com/breastfeeding/lecithin.html. Accessed Aug 2017.

64. Roberts KL, Reiter M, Schuster D. Effects of cabbage leaf extract on breast engorgement. *J Hum Lact*. 1998;14(3):231-236.

65. Brent NB. Thrush in the breastfeeding dyad: results of a survey on diagnosis and treatment. *Clin Pediatr*. 2001;40(9):503-506.

66. Chetwynd EM, Ives TJ, Payne PM, Edens-Bartholomew N. Fluconazole for postpartum candidal mastitis and infant thrush. *J Hum Lact*. 2002;18(2):168-171.

67. Shepherd J. Thrush and breastfeeding. *Pract Midwife*. 2002;5(11):24-27.

68. Stamatakos M, Kontzoglou K, Sargedi C, et al. Mammary candidiasis. A breast infection difficult to handle. *Chirurgia*. 2008;103(5):583-586.

69. Kaplan YC, Koren G, Ito S, Bozzo P. Fluconazole use during breastfeeding. *Can Fam Physician*. 2015;61(10):875-876.

70. Jiménez E, Arroyo R, Cárdenas N, et al. Mammary candidiasis: a medical condition without scientific evidence? Smidt H, ed. *PLoS ONE*. 2017;12(7):e0181071. doi:10.1371/journal.pone.0181071.

71. Smith LA, Price N, Simonite V, Burns EE. Incidence of and risk factors for perineal trauma: a prospective observational study. *BMC Pregnancy Childbirth*. 2013;13:59. doi:10.1186/1471-2393-13-59.

72. East CE, Begg L, Henshall NE, et al. Local cooling for relieving pain from perineal trauma sustained during childbirth. *Cochrane Database Syst Rev.* 2012;(5):1-154.
73. Ramler D, Roberts J. A comparison of cold and warm sitz baths for relief of postpartum perineal pain. *J Obstet Gynecol Neonatal Nurs.* 1986;15(6):471-474.
74. Corkill A, Lavender T, Walkinshaw SA, Alfirevic Z. Reducing postnatal pain from perineal tears by using lignocaine gel: a double-blind randomized trial. *Birth.* 2001;28(1):22-27.
75. Delaram M, Dadkhah N-K, Jafarzadeh L. Comparison of indomethacin suppository and lidocaine cream on post-episiotomy pain: a randomized trial. *Iran J Nurs Midwifery Res.* 2015;20(4):450-453. doi:10.4103/1735-9066.160995.
76. Eghdampour F, Jahdie F, Kheyrkhah M, et al. The impact of aloe vera and calendula on perineal healing after episiotomy in primiparous women: a randomized clinical trial. *J Caring Sci.* 2012;2(4):279-286. doi:10.5681/jcs.2013.033.
77. Sheikhan F, Jahdi F, Khoei EM, et al. Episiotomy pain relief: use of lavender oil essence in primiparous Iranian women. *Complement Ther Clin Pract.* 2012;18(1):66-70. doi:10.1016/j.ctcp.2011.02.003.
78. Ng K, Cheung RY, Lee LL, et al. An observational follow-up study on pelvic floor disorders to 3-5 years after delivery. *Int Urogynecol J.* 2017;28(9):1393-1399.
79. Dietz HP, Schierlitz L. Pelvic floor trauma in childbirth—myth or reality? *Aust N Z J Obstet Gynaecol.* 2005;45(1):3-11.
80. Baytur YB, Serter S, Tarhan S, et al. Pelvic floor function and anatomy after childbirth. *J Reprod Med.* 2007;52(7):604-610.
81. Fitzpatrick M, O'Herlihy C. The effects of labour and delivery on the pelvic floor. *Best Pract Res Clin Obstet Gynaecol.* 2001;15(1):63-79.
82. Ozdemir FC, Pehlivan E, Melekoglu R. Pelvic floor muscle strength of women consulting at the gynecology outpatient clinics and its correlation with sexual dysfunction: a cross-sectional study. *Pak J Med Sci.* 2017;33(4):854-859. doi:10.12669/pjms.334.12250.
83. Lowenstein L, Gruenwald I, Gartman I, Vardi Y. Can stronger pelvic muscle floor improve sexual function? *Int Urogynecol J.* 2010;21(5):553-556. doi:10.1007/s00192-009-1077-5.
84. Gagnon LH, Boucher J, Robert M. Impact of pelvic floor muscle training in the postpartum period. *Int Urogynecol J.* 2016;27(2):255-260. doi:10.1007/s00192-015-2822-6.
85. Boyle R, Hay-Smith EJ, Cody JD, Mørkved S. Pelvic floor muscle training for prevention and treatment of urinary and faecal incontinence in antenatal and postnatal women. *Cochrane Database Syst Rev.* 2012;(10):1-115. doi:10.1002/14651858.CD007471.pub2.
86. Ferreira CH, Dwyer PL, Davidson M, et al. Does pelvic floor muscle training improve female sexual function? A systematic review. *Int Urogynecol J.* 2015;26(12):1735-1750. doi:10.1007/s00192-015-2749-y.
87. Neels H, De Wachter S, Wyndaele JJ, et al. Does pelvic floor muscle contraction early after delivery cause perineal pain in postpartum women? *Eur J Obstet Gynecol Reprod Biol.* 2017;208:1-5. doi:10.1016/j.ejogrb.2016.11.009.
88. Rivalta M, Sighinolfi MC, De Stefani S, et al. Biofeedback, electrical stimulation, pelvic floor muscle exercises, and vaginal cones: a combined rehabilitative approach for sexual dysfunction associated with urinary incontinence. *J Sex Med.* 2009;6(6):1674-1677. doi:10.1111/j.1743-6109.2009.01238.x.

ANTEPARTUM & POSTPARTUM CARE

89. Sun Z, Zhu L, Lang J, et al. Postpartum pelvic floor rehabilitation on prevention of female pelvic floor dysfunction: a multicenter prospective randomized controlled study. *Zhonghua Fu Chan Ke Za Zhi.* 2015;50(6):420-427. Chinese.

90. Lipsky LM, Strawderman MS, Olson CM. Maternal weight change between 1 and 2 years postpartum: the importance of 1 year weight retention. *Obesity.* 2012;20(7):1496-1502. doi:10.1038/oby.2012.41.

91. Wilkinson SA, van der Pligt P, Gibbons KS, McIntyre HD. Trial for reducing weight retention in new mums: a randomised controlled trial evaluating a low intensity, postpartum weight management programme. *J Hum Nutr Diet.* 2015;28(1):15-28. doi:10.1111/jhn.12193.

92. Huseinovic E, Bertz F, Leu Agelii M, et al. Effectiveness of a weight loss intervention in postpartum women: results from a randomized controlled trial in primary health care. *Am J Clin Nutr.* 2016;104(2):362-370. doi:10.3945/ajcn.116.135673.

93. Sperstad JB, Tennfjord MK, Hilde G. Diastasis recti abdominis during pregnancy and 12months after childbirth: prevalence, risk factors and report of lumbopelvic pain. *Br J Sports Med.* 2016;50(17):1092-1096. doi:10.1136/bjsports-2016-096065.

94. Mommers EHH, Ponten JEH, Al Omar AK, et al. The general surgeon's perspective of rectus diastasis. A systematic review of treatment options. *Surg Endosc.* 2017;31(12):4934-4949. [Epub June 8, 2017]. doi:10.1007/s00464-017-5607-9.

95. Benjamin DR, van de Water AT, Peiris CL. Effects of exercise on diastasis of the rectus abdominis muscle in the antenatal and postnatal periods: a systematic review. *Physiotherapy.* 2014;100(1):1-8. doi:10.1016/j.physio.2013.08.005.

96. Campbell-Voytal K, McComish JF, Visger JM, et al. Postpartum doulas: motivations and perceptions of practice. *Midwifery.* 2011;27(6):e214-e221. doi:10.1016/j.midw.2010.09.006.

97. Milani HS, Amiri P, Mohseny M, et al. Postpartum home care and its effects on mothers' health: a clinical trial. *J Res Med Sci.* 2017;22:96. doi:10.4103/jrms.JRMS_319_17.

98. Mirmolaei ST, Valizadeh MA, Mahmoodi M, Tavakol Z. Comparison of effects of home visits and routine postpartum care on the healthy behaviors of Iranian low-risk mothers. *Int J Prev Med.* 2014;5(1):61-68.

99. The symptoms of postpartum depression and anxiety (in plain mama English). Available at http://www.postpartumprogress.com/the-symptoms-of-postpartum-depression-anxiety-in-plain-mama-english. Accessed Aug 2017.

Note: Page numbers followed by *f* and *t* refer to figures and tables, respectively.